Obstetric Myths
Versus
Research Realities

Obstetric Myths Versus Research Realities

A Guide to the Medical Literature

Henci Goer

Foreword by Don Creevy, M.D.

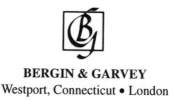

BERGIN & GARVEY
Westport, Connecticut • London

The author of this book is neither a physician nor a midwife. The information contained in this book is not a substitute for professional medical advice. While the advice and information in this book are believed to be true and accurate at the date of going to press, neither the author nor the publisher can accept any legal responsibility for any errors or omissions that may be made. The publisher makes no warranty, express or implied, with respect to the material contained herein. Readers should consult their physician or midwife before acting on any of the information contained in this volume.

Library of Congress Cataloging-in-Publication Data

Goer, Henci.
    Obstetric myths versus research realities : a guide to
the medical literature / Henci Goer ; foreword by Don Creevy, M.D.
        p. cm.
    Includes bibliographical references and index.
    ISBN 0–89789–242–9 (alk. paper).—ISBN 0–89789–427–8 (pbk.: alk. paper)
    1. Obstetrics—Popular works.   2. Natural childbirth.   I. Title.
RG525.G5137   1995
618.2—dc20   94–17337

British Library Cataloguing in Publication Data is available.

Library of Congress Catalog Card Number: 94–17337
ISBN: 0–89789–242–9
        0–89789–427–8 (pbk.)

First published in 1995

Bergin & Garvey, 88 Post Road West, Westport, CT 06881
An imprint of Greenwood Publishing Group, Inc.

Printed in the United States of America

The paper used in this book complies with the
Permanent Paper Standard issued by the National
Information Standards Organization (Z39.48–1984).

10 9 8 7 6 5 4

Copyright Acknowledgment

The author and publisher gratefully acknowledge permission for use of the following material:

Excerpts from "Anesthesia and You . . . Planning Your Childbirth," © 1992, of the American Society of Anesthesiologists. A copy of the full text can be obtained from ASA, 520 N. Northwest Highway, Park Ridge, Illinois 60068–2573.

*To my husband, Don, and my children, Evan, Elana, and Sarah,
for their understanding and patience while I have been "with book"*

Facts can be disproved, and theories based on them will yield in time to rational arguments and proof that they don't work. But myth has its own furious, inherent reason-to-be because it is tied to desire. Prove it false a hundred times, and it will still endure because it is true as an expression of feeling. . . . It is illogical—or at least, pre-logical; but from this very fact it gains a certain strength: logic may disprove it, but it will not kill it.

Elizabeth Janeway, *Man's World, Woman's Place*, 1971

Contents

Part III: The Case for an Alternative System

Foreword

Don Creevy, M.D.

Is obstetrics an art or a science?

As pre-medical students, we study physical and biological science, and we learn about the scientific method.

In the first two years of medical school, we study the "basic sciences" of medicine, including biostatistics. The purpose of the biostatistics course is to teach us to discriminate fact from fiction. We are taught to read scientific articles with a healthy skepticism based on a knowledge of basic scientific and statistical methods.

We are told that no new method or technique should be adopted or change made in current practice, unless research has shown that such methods, techniques, or changes have value and do no harm. We are taught that studies should, where methodology and ethical considerations permit, be randomized, controlled, and double blind. This means that patients are randomly assigned to experimental and control groups, and neither investigators nor subjects know a given subject's group until after completion of the study. We are taught that research should be published in peer-reviewed journals, meaning each article submitted must be approved by one or more experts in the field before being accepted for publication.

In the third and fourth years of medical school, we study the "clinical sciences." Now we are taught to apply the basic principles of medicine that we learned in the first two years to evaluation and treatment of living human beings. We are taught by physicians who have had more experience than we: interns, residents, and faculty physicians. We begin to model ourselves after these more advanced physicians, for better or for worse, trusting that their training and experience have made them wise.

In the postgraduate years of internship and residency, we continue our clinical studies with a narrower focus than in medical school. In the final preparation before beginning our professional career, we concentrate in a medical specialty, such as obstetrics and gynecology.

As our education progresses, we are exposed increasingly to the "art of medicine," as more of our teachers are clinicians and fewer are basic scientists. Somewhere between the beginning of the third year of medical school and the completion of residency, many of us seem to lose our ability to discriminate fact from belief as we are exposed more and more to practical techniques that "seem" to work and less and less to scientific theory and proof that our theories and practices are scientifically valid.

I believe this book provides good evidence for this phenomenon. Obstetricians, initially trained in the scientific method, adopt clinical practices, many of which have no scientific basis whatever. These practices are passed down from doctor to doctor as being scientifically valid, yet there is little or no proof of their validity in the peer-reviewed obstetric literature.

Oddly, many obstetricians criticize midwives, calling their practices unscientific. In fact, as this book shows, these "poor relations" of obstetricians may be practicing in a manner *more* scientifically valid that that of their scientifically trained physician colleagues! How can this be?

The answers to this and to many related questions lie within this book. The reader will learn of the research evidence against such practices as artificial rupture of the fetal membranes, routine episiotomy, epidural anesthesia, and liberal use of the cesarean operation. This should prove to be of great value to birth educators, obstetrical nurses, nurse practitioners, midwives, and physicians as well as expectant couples. Because they provide ready access to the research data, the abstracts that form the bulk of most chapters will be especially useful when differences of opinion arise about the validity of obstetric customs and techniques.

As for the question posed at the beginning of this preface, obstetrics should be both art and science. The science lies in what we know to be true, the art in how that information is used for greatest benefit to mothers and babies. However, as this book makes clear, at least as typically practiced today, obstetrics cannot legitimately claim to be either.

Dr. Creevy is a board-certified obstetrician-gynecologist in private practice in Portola Valley, California. He holds a clinical assistant professorship at Stanford University School of Medicine. He served as medical director of The Birth Place, *a freestanding birth center, during its 14-year existence.*

Acknowledgments

I thank the members of my writers' group, Alexis Rubin and Cindy Tolliver, for their innumerable helpful comments. So many people have inspired or helped me that if I try to list them all, I am afraid I will inadvertently omit someone. However, I must single out Penny Simkin, who is my model, my mentor, and my friend. I honor too the researchers who discarded their prejudices and followed where the evidence led, even though this commonly resulted in attack and ridicule by their colleagues. Without them, this book could hardly exist. Finally, I always said that if I ever wrote a book, I would acknowledge P.K., who, while intending no such benefit, reminded me that one of the things I could do was write.

1

Introduction

As a childbirth educator and a doula (someone who does labor support), I have read or heard obstetric myths—old doctors' tales, if you like—many times. Here are some examples, along with the disinformation they convey:

- "My doctor says trying to turn the baby from breech to head down would be like driving on the wrong side of the road at 90 miles per hour."
  Myth: External cephalic version is unacceptably risky.
- "They said if I didn't want the electronic fetal monitor, I would have to sign a paper saying they could not be held responsible if anything went wrong with my baby."
  Myth: Electronic fetal monitoring prevents fetal death and brain damage.

And, of course, the perennial favorite,

- "When I asked about episiotomy, he said, 'Which would you rather have: a nice, clean cut or a jagged tear?'"
  Myth: Episiotomies prevent perineal injury.

Anyone working to improve the childbearing experience and help women avoid unnecessary intervention can fill in the blank on a long, frustrating list that begins, "But the doctor said . . . ," where the doctor was wrong. And while the evidence in the medical literature is solidly, often unequivocally, against whatever "the doctor said," without access to that evidence the pregnant woman is quite reasonably going to believe her doctor, who she presumes is the expert.

This book is my attempt to make the medical literature on a variety of obstetric issues accessible to people who do not have the time, expertise, access, or proximity to a medical library to research it on their own. This includes those who teach pregnant women, those who care for them, those who plan maternity care, and the women themselves. My goal is a compact reference, scholarly yet understandable to people without medical training, and organized so that readers can readily find the information they want. Secondarily, I want to explain the huge gap that yawns between common obstetrical practice, which claims to be research based, and what that research actually says. This paradox puzzled me greatly, as I think it must trouble all those trying to reform maternity care.

Accordingly, an introductory chapter gives basic information about the different types of medical studies, how to evaluate them, and some basic statistical concepts. (Don't worry, you don't need to know a lot about statistics. A little knowledge will take you a long way.) Mostly you need to know some commonsense questions to ask and what to look for while reading through an article. Because a major stumbling block in reading the medical literature is the specialized vocabulary, I provide a glossary at the end of the book and define terms in the text as well.

The Glossary and Chapter 2, on evaluating studies, will provide enough background to read the abstracts (summaries) I have written of medical papers or to tackle the studies directly. (Many medical school libraries are open to the general public. Many hospitals also maintain libraries.) One of the better-kept secrets of medicine is that it is not an arcane body of knowledge comprehensible only to doctors.

The main body of the book is divided into three parts. Part I is entitled "The Cesarean Epidemic" because our outrageous cesarean rate—nearly one out of four women gives birth by major surgery—is the hottest of the birth issues. It begins with a general overview followed by a closer look at the four most common indications for cesarean section in order of frequency. Part II, "Pregnancy and Labor Management," takes pregnancy and labor chronologically, dealing with some myths of mainstream medical practice. (I have by no means covered them all.) Part III, "The Case for an Alternative System," argues for midwives, their noninterventive approach, and out-of-hospital birth.

Each chapter follows a pattern:

1. A stated myth followed by a quotation from the literature stating the reality.

2. An essay that analyzes mainstream belief, pointing out its fallacies.

3. A list of significant points gleaned from the studies and keyed to my abstracts.

4. The outline by which the abstracts will be grouped.

5. The numbered abstracts themselves.

I have had to be selective but have included enough to make my case. Surprisingly few issues were controversial. In most cases the evidence was overwhelmingly on one side. I have also liberally sprinkled my abstracts with quotations because I think it is important to have what the researchers say in their own words without filtering through me.

Each abstract begins with its citation structured in this way:

Author's last name and initials, next author or et al. if there are more than three. Title of the article, with only the first word capitalized. *Journal Title Abbreviated* year;volume(issue):page numbers.

For example:

4. **Thorp JM and Bowes WA. Episiotomy: can its routine use be defended?** *Am J Obstet Gynecol* 1989;160(5):1027-1030.

Sometimes I have inserted my own comments or definitions, which appear in brackets, in the body of the abstract itself. Occasionally I have added explanatory notes to an outline heading.

I have confined myself to articles published from 1980 on with few exceptions, . For example, some of the randomized controlled trials of electronic fetal monitoring took place in the 1970s. Articles grouped under each subheading are listed in ascending chronological order of publication to enable you to follow how subsequent studies built on previous findings or filled in holes. Sometimes I make exceptions if the studies are connected, as when a group of researchers studied a population and then later presented follow-up data on the same population.

I have tried to make this book responsive to many different needs. Some people will stop with the overview essay and significant points. Others may use the numbers keyed to those points to look up the abstracts that contain evidence for that particular statement. Yet others will use the broader groupings of my outline similarly. Still others may use the abstracts to decide if they want to see the whole article.

Naturally, additional studies will have been published since I completed this book. Nonetheless, once there is a body of well-done studies that reach the same conclusion, future studies rarely invalidate that conclusion.

The closing chapter synthesizes the work of medical anthropologists and others to explain why Western obstetrics operates (in both senses of the word) contrary to its own research findings and what forces shape its beliefs and practices. This chapter amplifies a running theme in the essays that begin each chapter in the main body of the book. It also explains why normally assertive women have docilely accepted a system that manifestly serves them poorly.

Because I have biases (although I hope I am not prejudiced), I think you should know more specifically what those biases are. I believe we have a maternity care system whose unconscious principles and resultant conscious practices fail those who should be its primary beneficiaries.

I am not antitechnology, but I am opposed to the routine use of intervention. I have attended labors in which the judicious use of technology probably saved the baby and even in a case or two, possibly the mother, but the key word is judicious. I believe the injudicious use of technology is doing considerable physical and psychological harm to mothers and babies.

I am not antiobstetrician, and I personally know and know by reputation some very fine obstetricians. Here is what I think defines good care. Good doctors and midwives:

- Believe childbearing to be a fundamentally healthy and normal part of a woman's psychosexual life.
- Treat women holistically, taking into consideration their thoughts, feelings, concerns, and priorities.
- Respect the right of women to make informed decisions for themselves and their babies.
- Respect labor as an experience with its own lessons and rewards.
- Offer supportive rather than interventive care.
- Evaluate individually and do not treat by rule.
- Start small when intervention becomes necessary.
- Keep abreast of the medical literature.

I believe most doctors want to do well by their patients, although I have seen, experienced, and read about enough instances of arrogance, indifference, ignorance, and even cruelty to have no illusions. This book itself contains numerous examples of all of the above. Still, the main problem is differing definitions of "doing well." Korte and Scaer (*A Good Birth, A Safe Birth*) explain:

If all childbirth is seen to be dangerous, the overriding concern of the obstetrician becomes, naturally, "a safe birth." . . . [From the obstetrician's viewpoint] there are six key elements; a "safe birth"

- Is actively managed
- Is predictable
- Is controlled by the obstetrician
- Takes place in the hospital
- Is attended by an obstetrician
- Is solely measured by a live baby and a live mother

I understand where this viewpoint comes from. One way of gaining an illusion of control over an essentially unpredictable process is to set up rigid rules. The doctor feels less helpless if he or she is orchestrating events especially if he or she also believes that less aggressiveness will lead to a dead or damaged baby, a malpractice suit, or the disapprobation of peers (more about this later). However, Korte and Scaer point out that a "good experience" and a "healthy baby" are not either-or propositions. This is the point of my book too. I see the doctor's role as lifeguard at the beach, watching out for sharks and intervening should one appear, but believing in women's innate competency as swimmers.

You may be wondering about my credentials to write this book since I am not a doctor—either M.D. or Ph.D. I respond with a story. Penny Simkin, well-known educator, writer, speaker, and editor, was called on the carpet by an anesthesiologist, irate that she had written a handout listing the potential trade-offs of epidural anesthesia when she was not a doctor (although he did not dispute her accuracy). "What are your credentials?" he demanded. "I can read," was her reply. So can I. For that matter, you can too.

I would like to hear from you if you find any errors so that they can be corrected in future editions. I have been as careful as I could, but no doubt some have crept in despite my efforts. I hope you find my book useful. I'd be interested to know if you did.

REFERENCE

Korte D and Scaer R. *A good birth, a safe birth.* 3d rev. ed. Boston: Harvard Common Press, 1992.

2

The Nature of Evidence: How to Read the Medical Literature

Myth: *By picking and choosing studies, you can make the research show anything.*

Reality: *"Clinicians who can critically read the medical literature, and understand and accept the uncertainty that exists, are better able to draw meaningful conclusions."*

MK Riegelman 1981

Medical research certainly has its flaws. It suffers from all the problems that beset obstetric practice, particularly the tendency to seek to reinforce beliefs rather than to discover truth. It has, however, a redeeming feature: it is the only means of seeking knowledge that acknowledges this bias and, in the better-done studies at least, takes it into account. Moreover, much, if not most, of the medical research done all over the world is reported in English. This means we have access to work done by people working from different sets of cultural assumptions. In this sense medical research is like democracy: it is far from ideal, but it beats the alternatives, which, in this case, are practices based on authoritarian pronouncements, habit, horror stories shared at the scrubroom sink, and unreasoning fear of malpractice suits.

Research is our only hope of obtaining objective information, but we must learn to discern the good from the bad to make use of it. This, fortunately, is not all that difficult. This chapter will help by describing the different types of studies, offering a few basics on how statistics are used to evaluate data, and pointing out some common pitfalls to which studies are prone. This knowledge should enhance your understanding of the abstracts I have written or allow you to dive into the medical literature on something better than a sink-or-swim basis.

TYPES OF ARTICLES

Case Reports

Case reports usually document a single instance or several instances of an unusual event, such as the reports of deaths due to a rare and rapidly progressing infection of the episiotomy incision. Case reports are useful for pointing the way toward further research, alerting care providers to potential reactions or symptoms, or sounding a general alarm.

Observational Studies

These usually present data culled from records, questionnaires, and the like. For example, cesarean section for all breech babies was believed to improve outcomes by eliminating the hazards of vaginal birth. However, when a hospital compared two different time periods, the cesarean rate for breech went from 22% to 94%, but the incidence of adverse outcome did not change (Green et al. 1982).

Retrospective or Case Control Studies

As the name implies, retrospective studies look backward. Researchers collect a population with a particular outcome or problem, and then, using records or interviews, they look into the past for characteristics or events not shared by a comparison population free of that outcome or problem. For example, when unusual numbers of babies with limb deformities were reported, researchers studied them and discovered that their mothers had all taken thalidomide in early pregnancy.

Retrospective studies are usually quicker and cheaper to do than prospective studies or clinical trials, but definitive conclusions cannot be drawn. Records and recall are notoriously unreliable, and the nature of retrospective studies makes it difficult to establish causality. For example, epidural anesthesia associates with an increased forceps rate. Is this because women with big or malpositioned babies are more likely to have more painful labors and want an epidural, or did the epidural cause problems with the baby's descent or rotation? Retrospective studies cannot answer such questions, but they are useful for suggesting fruitful territory for prospective studies or clinical trials.

Prospective Studies

Prospective studies assemble a population with certain common characteristics and follow it forward to see if its members are more likely to have some particular outcome compared with a similar population not sharing the target characteristics. For example, one prospective study found that a subgroup of women who planned epidural anesthesia had the same incidence of forceps and fetal malposition as the overall group, which mostly had the epidural for "medical reasons" (Hoult, MacLennan, and Carrie 1977).

Prospective studies have the advantage that medical technique, data gathering, and statistics are uniform because they are controlled by the researchers doing the study. And since prospective studies move forward in time, it is easier to establish (or discredit) a cause-and-effect relationship.

Clinical Trials

In clinical trials researchers take two or more similar groups, submit them to different treatments (or no treatment, i.e., "controls"), and compare outcomes. The most convincing type of clinical trial is the double-blind, randomized controlled trial because it minimizes the chance of bias. *Randomization* means that the population was randomly allocated to the various groups, which ensures that these groups are truly similar. *Double-blinding* means that neither the subjects nor those administering treatment know which group had (or did not have) what. This eliminates the placebo effect on the subject's side and observer bias (seeing what you want to see) on the researcher's side. For example, a double-blind, randomized controlled trial concluded that taking folic acid (a B vitamin) supplements around the time of conception reduced the incidence of neural tube defects in the babies of women who had a prior affected fetus. Women were randomly assigned to groups, all took identical-looking capsules, and no one knew until the study was over who had taken folic acid (MRC Vitamin Research Group 1991). Although a blinded randomized controlled trial produces the strongest evidence, blinding or even randomizing trial participants is not always possible.

Review/Clinical Practice Paper

These are articles in which investigators collect and analyze the research on a particular topic and write about their findings to summarize the state of knowledge, make an argument for a particular viewpoint, or advise practitioners on clinical practice.

Meta-Analysis

A new type of study, meta-analyses use sophisticated statistical analyses to pool data from multiple small studies. The difficulty here is accounting for the dissimilarities among studies so that they can be considered collectively. The advantage is that with larger populations, firmer conclusions can be drawn.

STATISTICS

Significance Testing

All studies begin with a hypothesis, test it, and analyze the data to see how likely it is that the results were due to chance. Statistical analysis deals in probabilities, not certainties. Unlike mathematical proofs, you cannot prove an experimental hypothesis to be true; you can only show how unlikely it is to be false (called proving the null hypothesis). In other words, if you suspect a pair of dice are loaded, the null hypothesis would be, "The dice are not loaded." If repeatedly rolling the dice showed that "7" turned up more often than would be expected by chance, you would have disproved the null hypothesis or shown it to have failed, which would mean the dice were, indeed, loaded. If rolling the dice showed no excess of a particular number, you would conclude the dice were not loaded. However, there is always a statistically quantifiable probability, however remote, that results were due to chance.

The most common way of expressing that probability is the *p-value* as in "*p* < 0.01*," which says the odds are less than 1 out of 100 that the difference in outcome was due to chance. The lower the *p*-value, the more certain you can be of this. By convention, a *p*-value of 0.05 (5 out of 100, or 1 in 20) or less is considered *significant*, meaning that the observed difference is considered a real difference and not due to chance. This value seemed a reasonable cut-off for making that distinction, although occasionally a study requires a more rigorous standard. Note, however, that while the possibility that chance caused the difference can be vanishingly small, it can never be zero. This inherent problem can cause a *Type I error*, meaning a significant difference may be found that is, in fact, due to chance.

Another type of significance testing is applied to *odds ratios* and *risk ratios*, which compare two rates of occurrence by dividing one into the other. Usually you will see a number followed by a range as in "RR [relative risk] = 0.6, CL [confidence limit or sometimes CI, confidence interval] 0.4-1.3." This means the calculated value is 0.6, but the actual value has a 95% probability of falling somewhere between 0.4 and 1.3, another instance where we can quantify only the uncertainty. If the range includes 1.00, as it does here, then the result is not significant because a value of 1.00 means that one of the possible ratios is 1:1 (1/1), meaning no difference between the two rates.

Power

In newer studies the *power* of the study may be given. Power indicates the ability of the study to detect a significant difference between the experiment and control groups given a particular population. Power calculations quantify the possibility that a true difference will be missed (*Type II error*). Type II errors usually occur because the population tested was too small to detect a difference, although, as with Type I errors, chance may play a role. So, for example, you may read that for 125 subjects, the power was 80% for detecting a 25% difference, which means a population of this size had an 80% probability of detecting a true difference of 25% in the primary outcome measured.

Returning to our suspect dice, this means that if we rolled the dice 125 times, we would have an 80% probability (four chances out of five) of detecting that they were loaded if the odds of "7" turning up were at least 25% greater than expected by chance. The power calculation also lets us know that if we rolled the dice only 10 times, we would not be likely to observe a true difference of 25%.

Evaluating a Test

When evaluating a test, the question of diagnostic accuracy is answered by measuring the *sensitivity*, or what percentage of the population tested will be accurately identified as being diseased, and the *specificity*, or what percentage of the population will be correctly diagnosed as disease free. From these can be calculated the *false-negative rate*, or the percentage of people diagnosed as healthy who, in fact, have the disease, and the *false-positive rate*, or the percentage of healthy people incorrectly identified as being diseased (Figure 2.1).

Because these measurements are percentages, they are not affected by the *prevalence* of the disease, meaning how common the disease is in the population under study. While sensitivity and specificity are useful for research comparisons precisely because the values are constant regardless of prevalence, practitioners can be easily misled by high sensitivity and specificity values.

Positive and *negative predictive* values are more useful for practitioners because they take the likelihood of disease into account (Figure 2.1). Bernard Ewigman (1992) illustrates the importance of prevalence in determining whether every pregnant woman should have an ultrasound scan to rule out intrauterine growth retardation (IUGR). In a very high-risk group of 1000 women who smoke two packs of cigarettes a day, have a previous undersized baby, and at 34 weeks gestation have had no increase in uterine fundal height for four weeks, 700 (70%) will have true IUGR and 300 (30%) will be normal. A superb ultrasonographer will correctly diagnose IUGR 90% of the time (*sensitivity*), which means he or she will incorrectly diagnose IUGR 10% of the time (*false-positive* rate).

$$700 \text{ (true IUGR)} \times 0.90 = 630 \text{ (true IUGR)}$$
$$300 \text{ (normal)} \times 0.10 = 30 \text{ (false positive)}$$
$$630 + 30 = 660 \text{ (total number diagnosed as IUGR)}$$

$$\text{positive predictive value} = \text{true IUGR/IUGR diagnosed}$$
$$= 630/660$$
$$= 0.95$$

Therefore, a care provider can say with 95% confidence that a woman with these characteristics who has been diagnosed as having IUGR actually has it.

Now perform the same calculations on a low-risk population of 1000 women of whom 40 (4%) have IUGR and 960 (96%) are normal.

$$40 \text{ (true IUGR)} \times 0.90 = 36 \text{ (true IUGR)}$$
$$960 \text{ (normal)} \times 0.10 = 96 \text{ (false positive)}$$
$$36 + 96 = 132 \text{ (total number diagnosed as IUGR)}$$

$$\text{positive predictive value} = 36/132$$
$$= 0.27$$

This time only 27% of women diagnosed with IUGR have an undersized fetus, and the other 73% will be subjected to chronic anxiety (not good during pregnancy), further testing, and possibly premature termination of the pregnancy—all for a normal baby.

Figure 2.1

		Gold Standard ("the truth")		
		subjects have the condition	subjects do not have the condition	
Test Result (conclusion drawn from results of the test)	Positive (subjects appear to have condition)	TRUE POSITIVES (a)	FALSE POSITIVES (b)	a + b
	Negative (subjects appear not to have condition)	(c) FALSE NEGATIVES	(d) TRUE NEGATIVES	c + d
		a + c	b + d	a + b + c + d

Stable Properties

$a/(a + c)$ = sensitivity
$d/(b + d)$ = specificity
$b/(b + d)$ = false-positive rate
$c/(a + c)$ = false-negative rate

Frequency-Dependent Properties

$(a + c)/(a + b + c + d)$ = prevalence
$a/(a + b)$ = positive predictive value
$d/(c + d)$ = negative predictive value

Source: Grant 1984, Riegelman 1981

PITFALLS

As you read through a study, consider this series of questions:

Is there a clearly stated hypothesis? A fuzzy hypothesis makes it difficult, if not impossible, to determine whether the study did what it intended. Statistical evaluation depends on proving or disproving the null hypothesis, so if there is no hypothesis or the hypothesis was formulated after data collection ("data churning"), any statistical analysis will be worthless.

Example: Some years back the American College of Obstetrics and Gynecology (ACOG) hypothesized that home birth was dangerous, citing as proof that death certificates showed significantly higher death rates for babies born at home compared with babies born in the hospital. What did ACOG mean by "home birth"? ACOG intended to condemn planned home births with a trained attendant. A better-formulated hypothesis would have made clear that death certificates will not produce evidence to the point. Death certificates do not distinguish these births from unplanned home births (often preterm) or planned home births with an untrained or no attendant. In fact, planned home birth with a trained attendant has never been shown to be riskier than hospital birth.

How was the population selected? Is it an appropriate population to prove or disprove the hypothesis? If the researchers are not looking at the right group of people, their conclusions will be invalid.

Example: Many of the early studies of the risks of gestational diabetes, now cited as proving those risks, selected a population for blood sugar testing on the basis of such problems as hypertension or previous stillbirth and then compared outcomes with the general population. Selecting a population at greater risk than the general population before testing for the target characteristic defeated the purpose of the study.

Was the study size sufficient? When power is not given, be wary. The smaller the study (or subgroup) is, the more likely the outcome is to be due to chance. Never fall prey to impressive percentages. An apocryphal story tells of the researchers who announced a new treatment for a disease of chickens by saying, "33.3% were cured, 33.3% died—and the other one got away" (Cohn 1989).

Example: Anesthesiologists have reassured laboring women that epidurals are safe, saying they have never seen a life-threatening problem. But because life-threatening problems are rare, this means only that the doctor's "population sample" does not have sufficient power to show the risk.

If the study was randomized, could the randomization method be easily subverted? Did the researchers establish that the groups were similar? The most common method to confirm that randomization succeeded is to compare the groups with respect to characteristics that might affect outcome.

Example: The only randomized controlled trial to show that electronic fetal monitoring (EFM) reduced perinatal mortality used a coin toss to make the allocation (Vintzileos et al. 1993). Moreover, differences among groups were highly unlikely to be due to chance.

Could lack of blinding affect the results?

Example: In the sole study showing that treating gestational diabetes reduced operative delivery rates, the doctors assigning the women to the treatment or control groups were responsible for labor management (Coustan and Imarah 1984). Knowing which women had had insulin therapy and believing (which they did) that insulin treatment made for smaller babies could well affect the decision to use forceps or perform a cesarean.

Have researchers made assumptions? Researchers may approach a problem conditioned by their beliefs. Bias acts like blinders. Those without bias (or at least with a different bias) will see both the problem and the potential solutions differently.

Example: A clinical practice article (O'Leary and Leonetti 1990) offering a systematic approach to the causes and cures of shoulder dystocia (the baby's head has been born, but the shoulders are stuck), exemplifies a classic obstetric belief: mother and child must be rescued from the inept natural process by the doctor; therefore all problems are her fault, all solutions the doctor's. The article presumes the universal delivery position to be with the mother on her back with feet in stirrups, which prevents consideration of this position as a cause of shoulder dystocia or alternative birth positions as both prevention and cure. All predispositions to shoulder dystocia blame mother or baby (e.g., obesity, short stature, glucose intolerance, oversized baby). None implicate medical management (e.g., epidural anesthesia, poor positioning for delivery, or use of forceps). The "cure" depends solely on maneuvers performed by medical staff on a passive woman as in, "The McRoberts maneuver . . . consists of removing the patient's legs from the stirrups and sharply flexing them against the abdomen."

Have the researchers accounted for the human factor? Records are often in error, memory of past events inaccurate (recall bias), and people (both medical personnel and research subjects) may not do what they were asked to do (noncompliance). People tell researchers what they think they want to hear and feel better if they think they are supposed to (placebo effect). The people lost to follow-up are likely to be people who were dissatisfied or had problems. Did the study account for these possibilities?

Example: Some studies of the effect of diet on gestational diabetes measured blood glucose during doctor visits. In one study, women admitted eating differently on test days so as to get a good value (Goldberg et al. 1986).

Did the authors account for possible confounding variables? Confounding variables are extraneous factors that can affect outcomes.

Example: A study of caffeine consumption and fetal growth adjusted for the fact that heavy coffee drinkers are more likely to be cigarette smokers, alcohol users, and less educated (Fenster et al. 1991).

Did the authors manipulate the data? Thomas Huxley said, "The great tragedy of science is the slaying of a beautiful hypothesis by an ugly fact." Some people, consciously or unconsciously, cannot bear to let a pet theory die and will skew the data or their interpretation so as to get the answer they seek. Researchers may also be tempted to fiddle with the data because both medical journals and grant underwriters prefer studies that "got results." Be especially skeptical of studies in which the trial's funder stands to gain financially based on the results.

Examples: Rudick et al. (1983) argued that epidural anesthesia did not increase instrumental delivery rates because the year before epidural anesthesia was introduced at their hospital, the instrumental delivery rate was 9%, and the year after introduction, it was 11%—except that only 37% of women had epidurals. *Among women who had epidurals* the rate jumped to 25%, almost a threefold increase.

The study mentioned above that found that EFM greatly reduced perinatal mortality had its funding and equipment supplied by a monitor manufacturing company.

Did the researcher prove causality? Just because two things happen during the same time frame does not mean one caused the other.

Example: A British researcher showed slides to a medical audience correlating the decline in perinatal mortality with other factors. The audience nodded approvingly as he showed perinatal mortality dropping with the decrease in home births, the rise in cesarean sections, and the rise in electronic fetal monitoring. They were puzzled when the next slide showed correlation with the decreasing number of children per family, the increased number of households with T.V. sets, and the election of the Thatcher government. They roared with appreciative laughter when the final slide showed equal correlation with the rise in British unemployment, the rise in violent crime in the U.S., and the declining stork population in Holland (Enkin, Hunter, and Snell 1984).

Are the results clinically relevant? Studies may show "significant" results that aren't of use or importance.

Example: Oleske et al. (1991) found a highly significant difference ($p < 0.001$) between primary (first) cesarean rates at teaching hospitals (14.4%) versus nonteaching hospitals (15.6%). The difference in percentages means 1 fewer woman per 100 had a primary cesarean at a teaching hospital, a trivial difference, however "significant."

Do the researcher's conclusions match results? Bias can affect both what researchers see and their weighing of risks versus benefits. This is one compelling reason to read the whole paper, not just the abstract.

Examples: A study of epidurals and profound fetal bradycardia (slowing of the fetal heart rate) concluded that while epidurals caused episodes of bradycardia, they were safe because all the babies turned out fine (Stavrou, Hofmeyr, and Boezaart 1990). Yet among the data was the statement that two women had emergency cesareans for fetal bradycardia directly attributable to their epidurals.

Two other studies of epidurals concluded that delaying pushing did not increase spontaneous birth rates (Gleeson and Griffith 1991; Manyonda, Shaw, and Drife 1990). Gleeson and Griffith claimed that pushing was delayed until either the head was visible on the perineum or three hours had elapsed. However, the average delay was only 52 minutes and 64% of the "delayed pushing" group had a forceps delivery, suggesting that the head was not on the perineum before pushing began. Manyonda, Shaw, and Drife "recommended" a two-hour delay before pushing, but 72% of the women began pushing less than one hour after full dilation. Neither study actually tested what it said it did.

Are the results applicable to populations differing from the one studied? Valid conclusions for the group studied might not hold true for a population that is, for example, healthier or has a different racial mix or enjoys higher socioeconomic status or was treated differently.

Example: Extrapolating from the the knowledge that premature rupture of membranes in preterm infants leads to a high mortality rate from infection, doctors instituted the "24-hour rule": if prematurity is not an issue, once membranes rupture, deliver the baby within 24 hours. The 24-hour rule meant inducing labor within a few hours if labor did not begin spontaneously, which led to a high cesarean rate because if the body is not ready to labor, oxytocin will not force it.

What is true for preterm fetuses, however, is not true for term fetuses. Preterm fetuses are especially vulnerable to infection and, in many cases, a preexisting infection caused the rupture, not vice versa. In addition, care providers were *causing* infections by performing cervical checks. This procedure inoculated the cervix with vaginal bacteria carried up on the examination glove, and with membranes gone, no barrier prevented entry to the uterus. Several studies comparing policies of "no vaginal examinations, watch and wait" with early induction for rupture of membranes at term have shown that waiting for spontaneous labor results in equally low infection rates and substantial reductions in cesarean rate.

What do other studies have to say? Findings are much more convincing if there is a cluster of well-done studies with the same results.

Example: One African study of external cephalic version (turning a breech head down from the outside) found an unacceptably high perinatal mortality rate and recommended against the procedure (Kasule, Chimbera, and Brown 1985). No other study, including some extensive ones, has had any perinatal deaths or even serious morbidity attributable to the version.

REFERENCES

Cohn V. *News and numbers*. Ames, Iowa: Iowa State University Press, 1989.

Coustan DR and Imarah JI. Prophylactic insulin treatment of gestational diabetes reduces the incidence of macrosomia, operative delivery, and birth trauma. *Am J Obstet Gynecol* 1984;150:836-842.

Enkin MW, Hunter DJ, and Snell L. Episiotomy: effects of a research protocol on clinical practice. *Birth* 1984;11(3):145-146.

Ewigman B. Ultrasound screening and perinatal outcome: The NIH study on routine antenatal diagnostic imaging with ultrasound (RADIUS). Paper presented at Innovations in Perinatal Care: Assessing Benefits and Risks, tenth conference presented by *Birth*, Boston, Oct 31-Nov 1 1992.

Fenster L et al. Caffeine consumption during pregnancy and fetal growth. *Am J Public Health* 1991;81:458-461.

Gleeson NC and Griffith AP. The management of the second stage of labour in primiparae with epidural analgesia. *Br J Clin Pract* 1991;45(2):90-91.

Goldberg JD et al. Gestational diabetes: impact of home glucose monitoring on neonatal birth weight. *Am J Obstet Gynecol* 1986;154:546-550.

Grant A. Principles for clinical evaluation of methods of perinatal monitoring. *J Perinat Med* 1984;12:227-231.

Green JE et al. Has an increased cesarean section rate for term breech delivery reduced the incidence of birth asphyxia, trauma, and death? *Am J Obstet Gynecol* 1982;142:643-648.

Hoult IF, MacLennan AH, and Carrie LES. Lumbar epidural analgesia in labour: relation to fetal malposition and instrumental delivery. *Br Med J* 1977;1:14-16.

Kasule J, Chimbira THK, and Brown I. Controlled trial of external cephalic version. *Br J Obstet Gynaecol* 1985;92:14-18.

Manyonda IT, Shaw DE, and Drife JO. The effect of delayed pushing in the second stage of labor with continuous lumbar epidural analgesia. *Acta Obstet Gynecol Scand* 1990;69:291-295.

MRC Vitamin Study Research Group. Prevention of neural tube defects: results of the Medical Research Council vitamin study. *Lancet* 1991;338:131-137.

O'Leary JA and Leonetti HB. Shoulder dystocia: prevention and treatment. *Am J Obstet Gynecol* 1990;162:5-9.

Oleske DM et al. The cesarean birth rate: influence of hospital teaching status. *Health Serv Res* 1991;26(3):325-337.

Riegelman RK. *Studying a study and testing a test*. Boston: Little, Brown, 1981.

Rudick V et al. Epidural analgesia during labor in 1,200 monitored patients. *Isr J Med Sci* 1983;19:20-24.

Stavrou C, Hofmeyr GJ, and Boezaart AP. Prolonged fetal bradycardia during epidural analgesia. *S Afr Med J* 1990;77:66-68.

Vintzileos AM et al. A randomized trial of intrapartum electronic fetal heart rate monitoring versus intermittent auscultation. *Obstet Gynecol* 1993;81(6):899-907.

Part I

THE CESAREAN EPIDEMIC

In memory of Joshua Greening,
born May 31, 1992; died June 3, 1992

3

The Cesarean Rate

Myth: *I only do cesareans when they are necessary.*

Reality: *"[I]t does seem clear to us that today's rates are in large measure a result of socioeconomic and not medical factors."*

Hurst and Summey 1984

The percentage of women in the United States who give birth by major abdominal surgery soared from 5.5% in 1970 to 24%—nearly one woman in four—in 1986, and it has not budged since. "The Cutting Edge," a page from a national report on hospital cesarean rates using 1989-90 data, listed 104 U.S. hospitals with rates of 37% or more (VanTuinen and Wolfe 1992). An analysis of 1984-86 data from New York state noted that out of 2126 obstetricians, only 187 had a cesarean rate under 10%. Seven doctors had cesarean rates between 40% and 50% (Zdeb and Logrillo 1989). Cesarean section is *the* most common operation performed in the U.S. (VanTuinen and Wolfe 1992).

How has this come about? Mortimer Rosen, Columbia University chairman of obstetrics and gynecology, wrote that doctors have bought a set of myths about cesarean section: "that cesareans are as safe as vaginal birth, that they are necessary in a wide range of cases, and that they guarantee a good outcome" (Rosen and Thomas 1989).

Examples of these beliefs abound. In a San Jose newspaper (1985) article, the president of the county society of obstetrician-gynecologists says, "When we do a cesarean section, we're sure we're going to get a good result." In the same article, the chief of obstetrics at a local hospital remarks, "Maybe the hospitals with low cesarean section rates are not doing some they should do," and "[T]he purpose of having a baby is having a baby—not going through labor." On the other coast, a Boston obstetrician observes, "When women look to vaginal delivery as the goal of their pregnancy—and there are those out there who tell them they should . . . you have a lot of dead and damaged babies along the way" (Knox and Karagianis 1984).

What these doctors share is a fervent belief that the natural processes of pregnancy and birth are inherently problematic and that technology is the solution. Believing that technology is a panacea blinds doctors to seeing that their interventions cause cesareans, for, as we shall see in later chapters, antenatal testing, labor induction, electronic fetal monitoring (EFM), and epidural anesthesia all increase cesarean rates without improving outcomes. Furthermore, it creates an ever-widening pool of indications for cesarean or for procedures that make cesarean more likely: suspected macrosomia (large baby), preterm delivery, twins, breech presentation, and positive fetal surveillance test (a result on any of a number of tests of fetal well-being that suggests there may be a problem). This belief creates a self-reinforcing vicious cycle: as more and more women "require" cesarean section, the assumption that the natural process is dangerous and that c-section is the cure is reinforced. This cycle has culminated in serious proposals that all women have prophylactic cesareans to avoid exposing themselves and their babies to the "dangers" of vaginal birth (Pascoe 1990; Feldman and Freiman 1985).

In fairness, some doctors deplore this mass surgical assault. Commenting on colleagues who perform c-sections on half their patients, Dr. Richard Porreco (1991a, 1991b), whose Denver hospital clinic staff have maintained cesarean rates around 6% for the last decade with excellent infant outcomes, said sarcastically, "It's hard to 'section everyone even if you want to, but I'm impressed at how well some doctors are doing when they try!" Eugene Pearce, a Kansas doctor, witheringly commented that the idea these days seems to be, "If it doesn't fall out, cut it out" (Socol et al. 1993, abstracted below). But all too many doctors refuse to confront the problem: "With so few data on how the cesarean-section rate is affected by the factors that appear to drive it, a 'correct' rate can hardly be identified" (Golde 1989); "Until there are reasonable data about long-term maternal and fetal morbidity [injuries, disease, or medical complications] as it relates to cesarean rates, we will continue to make decisions about cesareans on an individual basis rather than trying to 'achieve' any particular rate" (Gribble and Meier 1992).

"Reasonable data" about the risks of cesarean section abound. Cesarean-related surgical complications threatening the mother's life or well-being include infection, hemorrhage, embolism, anesthesia problems, and injuries to other organs. Complication rates are estimated to be five to ten times that of vaginal birth (National Institutes of Health 1981).

Wide regional and temporal variations and the fact that complications may lead to surgery make it difficult to determine the death rate directly attributable to cesarean section. Rosen and Thomas, however, state that the cesarean maternal death rate is 40.9 per 100,000, four times higher than the vaginal birth mortality rate. Elective repeat cesareans, a good proxy for cesarean-caused deaths, have twice the maternal death rate. A study using data as recent as 1986, which excluded indirect deaths, women with acute medical problems, and women who had emergency prepartum cesareans, concluded that cesarean section carried 5.1 times the mortality risk of vaginal birth (31/100,000 versus 6/100,000) (Lilford et al. 1990). These numbers may seem small, until they are put into perspective: the death rate in automobile accidents for women ages 15 through 34 is 20 per 100,000 (Petitti 1985). What is more, the c-section numbers are almost certainly low. Data culled from vital statistics undercount cesarean death rates by 40% to 50% (Rochat et al. 1988; Rubin et al. 1981).

A cesarean section casts a shadow over the rest of a woman's reproductive life (Chazotte and Cohen 1990; Hall et al. 1989, Rosen and Thomas 1989; Hemminki 1987). Scar tissue or adhesions may cause long-term pain, bowel obstruction, infertility, or miscarriage and may make repeat surgery more difficult. The uterine scar may rupture during a subsequent pregnancy or labor and its presence may cause placenta accreta (the placenta grows into the wall of the uterus) or placenta previa (the placenta implants low, covering the cervix). As a result, the perinatal mortality rate is higher in subsequent children compared with women with a prior vaginal birth, and statistically the babies are born sooner, smaller, and sicker.

In addition, a woman who has a cesarean starts motherhood behind a physiological and psychological eight-ball. She faces recovery from major surgery while trying to care for a newborn, and she must either cope with or suppress the host of negative feelings that swirl around both any experience of major surgery and the issues of needing an operation to have a baby.

As we have seen, cesareans are neither safe nor easy. Rosen's other myths—that they are frequently necessary and improve infant outcomes—will be refuted in the abstracted papers of this chapter and the other chapters in Part I.

Although obstetricians also offer defensive medicine as an excuse for the astronomical U.S. cesarean rate, malpractice did not become an issue until the late 1970s—*after* the cesarean rate had already tripled. Canada, where malpractice has never been an issue, has shown a parallel rise (Notzon 1990, abstracted below). No one, by the way, has shown that this pervasive belief is more than another myth. Most malpractice lawsuits between 1976 and 1979 were associated with cesarean surgery rather than failure to perform surgery because the more invasive and risky the intervention was, the more likelihood there was of something going wrong (O'Reilly et al. 1986). In any case, deliberately performing unnecessary surgery in the belief it avoids lawsuits is indefensible. That many obstetricians seem oblivious to this profound violation of ethical principles is shocking.

Finally, the most common reason women have cesareans is that they have had one before. Obstetricians used to say that labor after a cesarean was too dangerous, but now that an avalanche of data has shown that to be false, the excuse for elective repeats has become patient preference. Safety and patient choice will be taken up in detail in Chapter 4, but suffice it to say of the latter that where obstetricians are truly committed to vaginal birth after cesarean (VBAC), the elective repeat cesarean rate is nil (Porreco 1991b; and Iglesias, Burn, and Saunders 1991; Sanchez-Ramos et al. 1990; and Myers and Gleicher 1988, last three abstracted below).

The reality is that doctors have had no motivation to change their practices, and they and hospitals have had strong disincentives for changing. One disincentive is convenience: "Most physicians have not jumped into [VBAC] right away because of the requirements that they have to stop everything they're doing to sit with a woman in labor" (*San Jose Mercury News* 1985). (See also "The Convenience Factor"in Chapter 5.) Another is money. When Myers and Gleicher (1988, abstracted below) reduced the cesarean rate from 17.5% to 11.5% over two years, the hospital lost $1 million in revenue—not, according to the article, that they minded, of course (Koska 1989).

With new national health care policies on the horizon, there may be motivation to change. A window of opportunity is opening that will likely have a far greater impact on lowering the cesarean rate than self-recognition among obstetricians that the cesarean rate is too high, a recognition that has had pitifully little effect so far. Even so, because the underlying belief system is unaffected, the changes may not be benign. A recent article concluded that elective induction does not increase maternal or fetal risk, overlooking that the cesarean rate among induced nulliparous women (those who have not given birth previously) was 34% (probably because it was 22% among nulliparous women beginning labor spontaneously). An obstetrician commented, "I believe that the trend in obstetrics will continue toward managed labor because traditional care for the normal woman in labor is no longer cost-effective. It is no longer feasible for individual physicians who have invested 12 years in training at a cost of hundreds of thousands of dollars to dedicate extended periods to observing one normal woman in labor" (Macer, Macer, and Chan 1992).

What is a reasonable cesarean rate? A World Health Organization conference report (1985) stated, "Countries with some of the lowest perinatal mortality rates in the world have cesarean section rates of less than 10%. There is no justification for any region to have a rate higher than 10-15%." Edward Quilligan (1985), editor of the *American Journal of Obstetrics and Gynecology*, argued that cesarean section rates should range between 7.8% and 17.5%, depending on the mix of low- to high-risk patients—although a Bronx maternity unit run by midwives and Chicago and Jacksonville, Florida, teaching hospitals serving indigent, high-risk populations achieved 10% to 12% cesarean rates (Haire and Elsberry 1991; Sanchez-Ramos et al. 1990 and Myers and Gleicher 1988, the last two abstracted below). Lomas et al. (1989) surveyed the medical literature and concluded, "From the national data available, little improvement in outcome appears to occur when [cesarean] rates rise above about seven percent."

Generously assuming that half the current 24% cesarean rate is reasonable, approximately 500,000 unnecessary cesareans are performed in the U.S. every year. Using Lilford et al.'s mortality figures (6/100,000 versus 31/100,000), this means 125 women die needlessly every year, not to mention the thousands more with cesarean-related morbidity. In 1991 the difference in cost between the average vaginal birth and cesarean section was $3100 (U.S. Department of Health and Human Services 1993). Halving the cesarean rate would not only reduce the human cost but would save more than $1.5 billion annually.

In recent years both total and primary cesarean rates rates have plateaued (see Figure 3.1). If this inclines anyone to optimism, consider these facts: (1) using data through 1987, Stafford (1990) predicted that even extrapolating a 50% VBAC rate, the cesarean rate would rise to 34% by the year 2000; (2) a 1993 U.S. national health objective is to reduce the cesarean rate to 15% by the year 2000 (U.S. Department of Health and Human Services 1993), the same rate that was viewed with such alarm in 1980 that a national consensus conference was convened; and (3) even if we are turning the corner, the overall cesarean rate will not fall to reasonable levels for years. A lot of women and babies will suffer before then, and some of them will die.

SUMMARY OF SIGNIFICANT POINTS

- Cesarean rates depend on factors having nothing to do with medical indication. These factors are: individual philosophy and training, convenience, the patient's socioeconomic status, peer pressure, fear of litigation, and possibly financial gain. (Abstracts 7-17, 25, 28)

- In many cases of cesarean section, the true culprit was obstetric management practices, not medical indication. (Abstracts 6, 13-15, 18-25, 28)

- Perinatal mortality and morbidity rates bear no relationship to cesarean rates. (Abstracts 1-7, 10, 14-19)

- Far from doing better, babies born by cesarean fare worse. (Abstracts 7-8)

- Cesarean section substantially increases maternal risk. (Abstracts 1, 8)

- High cesarean rates affect all of us by enormously increasing unnecessary health care expenditures. (Abstracts 15, 29)

- Evidence and education do not change practices. (Abstracts 26-29)

ORGANIZATION OF ABSTRACTS

C-sections Are Not Responsible for Improved Perinatal Outcomes

Figure 3.1: Cesarean Section Rates

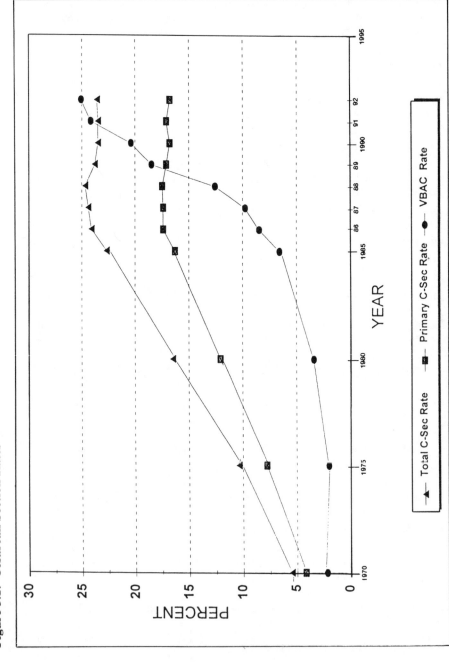

Nonmedical Factors Influencing Cesarean Rates

The Women Having C-sections Are the Women Least Likely to Need Them

Studies Reducing the Cesarean Rate

Evidence and Education Do Not Affect Practice

C-SECTIONS ARE NOT RESPONSIBLE FOR IMPROVED PERINATAL OUTCOMES

1. Minkoff H and Schwarz RH. The rising cesarean section rate: Can it safely be reversed? *Obstet Gynecol* **1980;56(2):135-143.**
Despite common belief that the decline in perinatal mortality is due to the rise in cesarean rates, a causal relationship has not been demonstrated. Between 1961 and 1968 at Downstate Medical Center-Kings County Hospital in Brooklyn, perinatal mortality fell by one-third while cesarean section rates remained constant (5-6.5%). Between 1972 and 1977, the cesarean rate rose from 12% to 17%, while perinatal mortality remained constant. Moreover, perinatal mortality declined by one-third over the 16-year period among women having repeat cesareans. Since the cesarean rate was 100%, it cannot be responsible for this improvement.

The 1977 maternal mortality rate was 10.8 per 10,000 cesarean sections versus 1.7 per 10,000 vaginal births, and the incidence of postpartum morbidity has consistently been at least ten times greater. "Unfortunately, . . . a 'when in doubt, section' sentiment has occasionally replaced hard thought when deciding on the mode of delivery. . . . [I]t remains for obstetricians to be willing to consider each case carefully and not rush to operate in problematic situations. The risk to mothers with cesarean section is still far beyond that from vaginal deliveries."

2. O'Driscoll K and Foley M. Correlation of decrease in perinatal mortality and increase in cesarean section rates. *Obstet Gynecol* **1983;61(1):1-5.**
Between 1965 and 1980, 108,987 births occurred at the National Maternity Hospital in Ireland. The cesarean section rate remained constant (4.1-4.8%) during those years, while perinatal mortality declined from 42.1 to 16.8 per 1000 for infants weighing over 500 g. "Perinatal mortality improved along parallel lines [with the U.S.], although the incidence of cesarean section remained substantially unchanged. These contemporary events constitute strong evidence that cesarean birth rates and perinatal mortality rates are not necessarily closely linked."

3. Pearson JW. Cesarean section and perinatal mortality. *Am J Obstet Gynecol* **1984;148(2):155-159.**
At an Indianapolis hospital serving low-income women, the cesarean rate between 1973 and 1982 fluctuated between 5.8% and 8.2%, while the perinatal mortality rate for infants weighing more than 500 g was halved (35/1000 to approximately 18/1000). The prematurity rate remained stable at 9% to 10%. "The inexorable growing cesarean section rate in the United States is the result of one of the least controlled clinical experiments that has occurred in medicine. . . . [We] remain unconvinced that cesarean section and perinatal mortality rates necessarily need have a reciprocal relationship."

4. Notzon FC. International differences in the use of obstetric interventions. *JAMA* **1990;263(24):3286-3291.**

Data were obtained from Australia, Bavaria (Germany), Brazil, Canada, Czechoslovakia, Denmark, England and Wales, Greece, Hungary, Italy, Japan, the Netherlands, New Zealand, Norway, Portugal, Puerto Rico, Scotland, Spain, Sweden, Switzerland, and the U.S. Using 1985 or the most recent year, the lowest cesarean rate per 100 hospital births was 7% (Czechoslovakia and Japan); the rest of the countries ranged from 10% to 16%, and the top four were Canada (19%), the U.S. (23%), Puerto Rico (29%), and Brazil (32%). The Dutch cesarean rate was 10%, but when "the large proportion" of home births were included, it dropped to 6.6%. The 1985 perinatal mortality ranged from 7.3 per 1000 (Sweden) to 21.0 per 1000 (Puerto Rico) and bore no relation to cesarean rates. The Netherlands, with the lowest cesarean rate, was 9.9 per 1000 and the U.S., with the third highest rate, was 10.8 per 1000. Brazil's rate was not available. "A nation may achieve a low level of early infant mortality while maintaining a low rate of cesarean delivery."

5. Rockenschaub A. Technology-free obstetrics at the Semmelweis Clinic. *Lancet* **1990;335:977-998.**

Data from 1966 to 1985 are presented on 42,500 births at a Viennese clinic that avoided technological intervention and compared with data from Vienna as a whole from 1974 to 1985. The clinic cesarean rate remained at 1% to 2%, while Vienna's rate rose from 6.3% to 10.3%. Neonatal mortality and stillbirth rates at the clinic declined in exact parallel with Vienna's (neonatal mortality: clinic 16.2 to 7.2/1000, Vienna 17.1 to 8.1/1000; stillbirth: clinic 9.7 to 6.5/1000, Vienna 8.9 to 5.4/1000).

6. Sepkowitz S. Birth weight-specific fetal deaths and neonatal mortality and the rising cesarean rate. *J Okla State Med Assoc* **1992;85(5):236-41.**

Between 1968 and 1987, the total cesarean rate at an Oklahoma community hospital rose from 4.7% to 25.7%. Between 1973 and 1987 the primary cesarean rate went from 4.9% to 12.2%. The distribution of indications for primary cesarean was relatively stable except for "fetal distress," which jumped from 5.3% to 16.4%, concurrent with acquiring electronic fetal monitors. While crude neonatal mortality rates declined as cesarean rates went up, when corrected for congenital anomalies, the neonatal mortality for infants weighing over 2499 g was a constant 1 per 1000. Among stillbirths, the decline was due to a reduction in antepartum, not intrapartum, deaths. "This analysis . . . indicates that a five-fold rise in the annual cesarean rate has contributed little, if anything, to reductions in fetal and neonatal mortality during this time."

NONMEDICAL FACTORS INFLUENCING CESAREAN RATES

7. Goyert GL et al. The physician factor in cesarean birth rates. *N Engl J Med* **1989 Mar;320(11):706-709.**

This study examined whether individual management practices correlated to differences in neonatal outcomes by analyzing cesarean rate versus outcome for all patients (*N* = 1533) of 11 obstetricians during 1986-87 at a Detroit hospital serving affluent "very-low-risk private patients." The total cesarean rate averaged 26.9%, and individual rates ranged from 19.1% to 42.3%. The primary cesarean rate averaged 17.2% and ranged from 9.6% to 31.8%. Only nulliparity ($p < 0.0001$) had a stronger influence on the probability of cesarean than the doctor ($p < 0.001$). Low one-minute Apgars correlated positively with cesarean section ($p < 0.001$). Results could not be attributed to differences among the doctors' patient populations. "[W]e were unable to demonstrate objective evidence that higher cesarean-section rates reduced neonatal morbidity."

8. Demott RK and Sandmire HF. The Green Bay cesarean section study. I. The physician factor as a determinant of cesarean birth rates. *Am J Obstet Gynecol* **1990;162(6):1593-1602.**

All singleton cesarean deliveries performed by 11 obstetricians at 2 Wisconsin hospitals from 1986 through 1988 ($N = 1030$) were compared with the next singleton vaginal birth by the same doctor. Cesarean rates ranged from 5.6% to 19.7%, with a mean rate of 14.0%. [The national average was 24%.]

No differences could be found among the doctors' patient populations. All women had continuous EFM, and none had epidurals. No significant differences between doctors were found for adverse infant outcomes. After low-birth-weight infants were eliminated, transient tachypnea [abnormally rapid breathing] (wet lung) occurred 4.5 times more often after a cesarean. Among cesarean deliveries, endometritis [uterine infection] occurred in 1.8% of cases and hemorrhage requiring transfusion in 1.9%. Eighty-four percent had no complications. Among vaginal births, only one woman had endometritis, 1.6% required transfusion, and 96% had no complications.

"Our data clearly demonstrate no difference in the condition of newborn infants from cesarean and vaginal births. . . . Therefore the physicians with low cesarean rates do not place infants at greater risk by the avoidance of many cesarean sections."

In the discussion that followed, Sandmire said, "[T]he burden of proof somehow has fallen on advocates of fewer operative deliveries, when in fact those who contend higher cesarean rates improve outcome are the ones who should have to present justifying data." S. Bottoms commented, "I think it is important to stop fooling ourselves and saying 'Oh, well there might be some difference between these patients if you studied everything on God's earth' and we start to deal with the issue because everybody who's had any experience in the delivery room knows that some people are going to go to the knife a whole lot faster."

9. Tussing AD and Wojtowycz MA. The cesarean decision in New York State, 1986. Economic and noneconomic aspects. *Med Care* **1992;30(6):529-540.**

The authors analyzed 1986 data on all deliveries ($N = 68,847$) by all New York obstetricians (excluding New York City) to determine the factors influencing cesarean rate (27.8%). Source of payment did not affect cesarean rates, except that self-pay women were less likely to undergo cesarean. Maximizing income was not a factor, except more cesareans were done where the difference in fee between vaginal and cesarean birth was greatest. Convenience (time management in a busy practice) positively affected cesarean rates, as did peer influence (both county and individual hospital rates significantly affected whether a birth would be a cesarean). No association was found with fear of malpractice suit, but since comparisons were made between areas, its influence on the group as a whole could not be judged. Teaching institutions and hospitals with neonatal intensive care units had lower cesarean rates. Board-certified obstetricians and foreign medical school graduates were more likely to perform cesareans. More recent graduates were not more likely to perform cesareans.

10. Localio AR et al. Relationship between malpractice claims and cesarean delivery. *JAMA* **1993;269(3):366-373.** (Like Abstract 9, these are also New York data.)

This study looked at the relationship between cesarean rates and risk of malpractice at 31 hospitals in New York State during 1984. Hospital cesarean rates varied from 10.7% to 33.8% [!]. Rates of individual doctors with 50 or more births ranged from 0 to 61% [!]. Of the 31 hospitals, 10 had doctors with cesarean rates of 40% or more and 24 had physicians with rates of 30% or more. Physician malpractice premiums varied almost threefold across regions. After controlling for hospital characteristics, doctor characteristics, and patient clinical and socioeconomic factors, the odds ratio (OR) for cesarean in high-premium versus low-premium areas was 3.00, $p < 0.0001$, and the OR for physician-perceived risk of suit (as measured by a survey of doctors) was 1.96, $p < 0.0001$. The risk of cesarean was slightly increased where there were more claims against a hospital's obstetric staff (OR 1.15, $p < 0.027$), but it was not related to the individual doctor's claims history. "Although ORs are not large for any of the claims measures, the populations at risk are large. . . . Pregnancy is not a rare condition, cesarean section is a common procedure, and high malpractice exposure is wide-spread."

11. Haas JS, Udvarhelyi S, and Epstein AM. The effect of health coverage for uninsured pregnant women on maternal health and the use of cesarean section. *JAMA* **1993 270(1);61-64.**

In 1985 in Massachusetts, state-funded health coverage was instituted for low-income, uninsured pregnant women. This study evaluated its effect on maternal health outcomes and cesarean section. The analysis focused on incidence of severe hypertension, placental abruption, and prolonged length of hospital stay because these outcomes are coded on hospital discharge abstracts and potentially can be prevented. (A previous study reported that the program had no effect on newborn health status.)

In 1984 adverse outcome rates for uninsured women were 5.5% versus 5.1% for privately insured women, and cesarean rates were 17.2% versus 23.0%. In 1987 cesarean rates were 22.4% versus 25.9%. The gap in cesarean rates closed by 2.3% (CI 0.4-4.2%), but the gap in rates of adverse outcome widened (6.0% versus 4.9%, NS). Similarly, adverse outcome rates in 1984 for study women versus women with Medicaid were 5.5% versus 6.5% and cesarean rates were 17.2% versus 19.4% In 1987 adverse outcome rates were 6.0% versus 6.4% (NS), although the cesarean rate had surpassed the rate for Medicaid women (22.4% versus 20.8%). Since the state program did not pay more for cesareans, doctors had no financial incentive, nor did women switch from public to community hospitals, which have higher cesarean rates. Perhaps doctors were more willing to perform cesareans on insured patients because they perceived them as being of higher social class, or perhaps doctors worried more about malpractice. "Our work demonstrates that the rate of cesarean section is responsive to a change in payor status."

THE WOMEN HAVING C-SECTIONS ARE THE WOMEN LEAST LIKELY TO NEED THEM

12. Hurst M and Summey PS. Childbirth and social class: the case of cesarean delivery. *Soc Sci Med* **1984;18(8):621-631.**

Postulating a variation of the "inverse care law"—the availability of good medical care tends to vary inversely with the need for it in the population served—the authors used cesarean rates to examine whether "the amount of medical care women receive in labour and delivery varies inversely with their actual medical need for that care." Analyzing data from other studies showed that poor women, the population at greatest medical risk, were least likely to undergo cesarean. For example, the average cesarean rate in 1980 at New York City municipal hospitals was 15.0%, at proprietary hospitals it was 22.5%, and at voluntary hospitals, which serve both clinic and private patients, the clinic rate was 16.4% while the private rate was 22.5%. The effects of profit incentive, fear of lawsuits, convenience, identification with the patient (the women most like the doctor in social class and culture got what the doctor believed to be the "best" treatment), style ("the 31 busiest New York private obstetricians practicing at one hospital had cesarean delivery rates for 1980 ranging from 13 to 52%") were discussed.

13. Haynes de Regt R et al. Relation of private or clinic care to the cesarean birth rate. *N Engl J Med* 1986;315(10):619-624.

To look for differences in cesarean rate between clinic and private patients, births at four Brooklyn hospitals between 1977 and 1982 were compared ($N = 65,647$). Clinic patients were significantly more likely ($p < 0.001$) to be nonwhite, have medical problems, be teenagers, and have babies weighing under 2000 g. However, private patients underwent significantly ($p < 0.001$) more cesareans (odds ratio [OR] 1.32), more primary cesareans (OR 1.25), and more repeat cesareans (OR 1.34). Private patients with diagnoses of dystocia [difficult labor] (OR 2.23), fetal distress (OR 1.96), or malpresentation (OR 3.01) were more likely to undergo cesarean than clinic patients with the same diagnosis ($p < 0.001$). Low-risk private patients, whether primiparous (OR 1.18) or multiparous (OR 1.59), were more likely to have cesareans compared with low-risk clinic patients ($p < 0.001$). Controlling for birth weight, private patients were more likely to have babies with low Apgar scores or birth injuries (OR 1.28, $p = 0.001$). While babies of private patients were less likely to die, the difference occurred primarily among infants weighing less than 2000 g, and less than 3% of cesareans were done in this weight group. "Although they cared for patients with significantly fewer medical complications and higher-birth-weight infants, private physicians performed significantly more cesarean deliveries without significantly improving perinatal outcome."

14. Gould JB, Davey B, and Stafford RS. Socioeconomic differences in rates of cesarean section. *N Engl J Med* 1989;321(4):233-239.

Birth certificate data for singleton infants born in Los Angeles County during 1982-83 were analyzed ($N = 245,854$) using census tract data as a proxy for socioeconomic status. The overall cesarean rate was 17.8%, with a rate of 13.2% for median income below $11,000 and 22.9% (75% more) where median income exceeded $30,000. Age and parity had independent effects ($p < 0.05$) on the primary cesarean rate, but taking this into account, increasing income maintained its independent association. Birth weight had an effect, but increasing income associated with increasing cesarean rate in all birth weight categories. Within each race or ethnic group, cesarean rates increased with increasing income. The reported incidence of complications, the rates of cesarean in the presence of complications, and the cesarean rate in the absence of reported complications all increased with increasing income. "[W]e found a consistent and statistically significant relation between socioeconomic status and the use of cesarean section . . . independent of maternal age, parity, birth weight, and race or ethnic group. . . . We speculate that differences in both the health care setting and clinical decision making contribute to the observed socioeconomic differences in the use of cesarean section."

15. Stafford RS. Cesarean section use and source of payment: an analysis of California hospital discharge abstracts. *Am J Public Health* **1990;80(3):313-315.**

This report investigates the relationship between hospital payment source and cesarean section for all births ($N = 461,066$) at nonmilitary California hospitals during 1986. The overall cesarean rate was 24.4%. The rate for women with private insurance was 29.1%, health maintenance organizations (HMOs) 26.8%, Medi-Cal [California's insurance program for those with low income] 22.9%, Kaiser Permanente (a hospital-based HMO) 19.7%, self-pay 19.3%, and indigent services 15.6%.

Examining the four main indications for cesarean, repeat cesarean rates were ordered similarly to overall rates and ranged from 91.9% for private insurance to 75.2% for indigent services. The VBAC rate for indigent services (24.8%) was three times that of private insurance (8.1%). Fetal distress showed a similar ordering and ranged from 33% for HMOs to 21.6% for indigent women. Cesarean rate patterns with breech presentation were distinctive, with Kaiser highest (88.3%) and indigent women lowest (78.5%). Cesarean rates in the presence of dystocia for private insurance, HMOs, and Medi-Cal were all 64% to 66%; self-pay was 61.4%; and indigent services and Kaiser were significantly lower [no p value given], at 56.9% and 58.8% respectively.

These results suggest that reimbursement plays a role. Of note is that HMOs other than Kaiser resemble private insurance. Only Kaiser operates its own hospitals, which makes cost containment a factor. Given the 1986 cost differential between cesarean and vaginal birth ($5000 versus $2720), adopting Kaiser's cesarean section patterns could save $51 million annually by avoiding 22,500 cesarean sections. "This may be an underestimate of cost savings, however, because Kaiser's rate is nearly twice that suggested as an optimal cesarean section rate."

16. Oleske DM et al. The cesarean birth rate: influence of hospital teaching status. *Health Serv Res* **1991;26(3):325-337.**

Using 1986 data from all births ($N = 130,249$) at 198 Illinois hospitals and adjusting for higher-risk populations at teaching hospitals, women were less likely to have a primary cesarean section (OR 0.76, $p < 0.001$) at a teaching hospital. Unadjusted primary cesarean rates were: teaching hospital 14.4% versus nonteaching 15.6% ($p < 0.001$). Unadjusted total rates were 20.4% versus 23.1% ($p < 0.001$).

17. McKenzie L and Stephenson PA. Variation in cesarean section rates among hospitals in Washington State. *Am J Public Health* **1993;83(8):1109-1112.**

This study compared hospital-specific cesarean rates in 1987 for all hospitals in Washington state with 12 or more births. Proprietary hospitals had significantly higher rates than church, district, military, private nonprofit, or public hospitals. The other types had mean and median rates between 17.5% and 22.4%, and rates ranged from 0.9% to 32.5%. Proprietary hospitals had both a mean and median cesarean rate of 36.0%, and rates ranged from 29.2% to 42.8%, although they did not serve higher-risk populations and their populations were similar to other hospital types. No significantly different rates were found for teaching versus nonteaching, urban versus nonurban, or among hospitals with Level I, II, or III neonatal care. The 42.8% cesarean rate was at a hospital with no residency program and a Level I nursery. As other studies have found, low-income women were more likely to have complications ($p < 0.05$) but less likely to have cesareans.

STUDIES REDUCING THE CESAREAN RATE

18. Gilstrap LC, Hauth JC, and Toussaint S. Cesarean section: changing incidence and indications. *Obstet Gynecol* 1984;63(2):205-208.

At a Texas medical center, total cesarean rates rose from 8.2% in 1970 to a peak of 19.5% in 1976, then declined to an average of 15.2% between 1978 and 1981 ($p < 0.02$). Primary cesarean rates rose from 5.6% to a peak of 15% in 1976 then declined to an average of 9.6% between 1978 and 1981. The decline was attributed to establishing criteria and policies to ensure adequate trial of labor, ensure fetal distress was persistent and ominous, and allow selected breeches a trial of labor. Despite the reduction in cesarean rate, perinatal mortality for 1978-81 declined to an average of 14.6 per 1000 compared with 16.1 per 1000 in 1976-77.

19. Porreco RP. High cesarean section rate: a new perspective. *Obstet Gynecol* 1985;65(3):307-311.

Outcomes were compared during 1982-83 between clinic and private patients at a Denver hospital. The clinic protocol was:

1. Trial of labor after one previous cesarean with low transverse scar and no new indication.
2. Possible trial of labor with two or more previous cesareans.
3. Fetal scalp sampling to confirm fetal distress.
4. Prostaglandin E_2 gel to ripen cervix before induction of labor.
5. External version for breech presentation.
6. Selected vaginal delivery with breech.
7. Viral cultures for women with herpes.
8. An "appreciation of" the latent phase of labor, the usefulness of ambulation in labor, and the "judicious" use of Pitocin when diagnosing failure to progress.

The clinic service total cesarean rate was 5.7% versus the private rate of 17.6%. The primary rate was 4.3% versus 11.0%. Perinatal outcomes were identical. "It is the author's conclusion that excellent perinatal results can be obtained in the modern practice of obstetrics with cesarean section rates well below 10% in unselected patients." [As of 1991, annual cesarean rates continued to range from 6% to 8% (personal communication).]

20. Peter J, Amir W, and Eitan P. Reversing the upward trend in the cesarean section rate. *Eur J Obstet Gynecol Reprod Biol* 1987;25:105-113.

Between 1965 and 1982 the cesarean section rate at an Israeli tertiary care hospital rose from 3.5% to 12.2%, plateaued, then dropped to 9.7% in 1985. The primary cesarean rate rose from 2% to 7% in 1980, plateaued, then dropped to 5% in 1985.

Rates were affected by several factors: Only one-third of women with a prior cesarean had a vaginal birth between 1970 and 1980; in 1985 the number had risen to one-half. Reductions in the primary rate further reduced the number of repeat cesareans. Although the cesarean rate for dystocia rose from 0.5% in 1970 to 1.5% in 1985, it was not a major contributor to increased cesarean rates. The relative proportion of cesareans for dystocia was stable at 11% to 16%. EFM was introduced in 1970. Cesarean rates for fetal distress increased sixfold from 0.18% to 1.2% by 1980, declined to 0.7% in 1981, plateaued through 1984, and fell to 0.4% in 1985. This suggests that with improved interpretation and fetal scalp blood sampling, EFM need not elevate the cesarean rate. Cesarean for breech rose from 0.2%, peaked at 2.8% in 1980, dropped to 2.1% in 1981-84, and fell to 1% in 1985. Performing more external cephalic versions and (as of 1983) allowing multiparous women to give birth vaginally reduced the cesarean rate for breech. Excluding malformed fetuses, the intrapartum mortality rate fell from 19 per 1000 in 1965 to 6 per 1000 in 1980, where it has remained.

21. Myers SA and Gleicher N. A successful program to lower cesarean-section rates. *N Engl J Med* 1988;319(23):1511-1516.

This Level III Chicago teaching hospital serving mostly inner-city poor women reduced its cesarean rate by instituting new policies on the clinic service. The cooperation of private doctors was voluntary. Policies were:

1. Second opinion for all nonemergency cesareans,
2. Trial of labor for all women with previous cesarean(s) (which led to 86% trial-of-labor rate),
3. Diagnosis of dystocia only after two hours of no progress with adequate contractions (41% had oxytocin),
4. Diagnosis of fetal distress to be corroborated with fetal scalp blood sample,
5. Vaginal delivery of breech fetuses except for true neck hyperextension [the baby's head is tipped back instead of curled forward, which may cause neurologic injury during the birth] or estimated weight greater than 4300 g and
6. Peer review process.

Total cesarean rates fell from 17.5% in 1985 to 11.5% in 1987 ($p < 0.05$), and primary rates fell from 12% to 7.5% ($p < 0.05$). Neonatal mortality and Apgar scores were unaffected.

22. Sanchez-Ramos L et al. Reducing cesarean sections at a teaching hospital. *Am J Obstet Gynecol* 1990;163(3):1081-1088.

A Florida teaching hospital serving indigent women reduced total cesarean rates from 27.5% in 1986 to 10.5% in 1989 and primary cesarean rates from 19.5% to 7.2% ($p < 0.0001$) by the following means:

• All women were candidates for trial of labor except for previous classic incision, more than two cesareans, prior uterine surgery, or unknown scar.

• Elective cesarean was not an option.

- When contractions were adequate (spontaneous or augmented), a diagnosis of dystocia required arrest of dilation for 2 hours or arrest of descent for 1 hour in primiparas or 30 minutes in multiparas.

- When contractions were weak, the diagnosis required arrest of dilation for four hours on oxytocin.

- Cervical ripening with prostaglandin gel would precede induction of labor with unripe cervix.

- Fetal distress must be confirmed with fetal scalp blood sampling or acoustic stimulation.

- Breeches would undergo external cephalic version, and vaginal birth was possible in selected cases.

The cesarean rate further decreased to 8.6% over the first six months of 1990.

Perinatal mortality decreased from 31.8 to 14.9 per 1000 and neonatal mortality from 16.4 to 6.4 per 1000 ($p < 0.0001$) during the same period. [The changes in protocol were instituted by a faculty perinatologist hired in 1986 who doubtless also improved the care of high-risk pregnancies and babies.]

23. Iglesias S, Burn R, and Saunders LD. Reducing the cesarean section rate in a rural community hospital. *Can Med Assoc J* 1991;145(11):1459-1464.

In this rural Canadian hospital staffed by family physicians and serving mostly low-risk women, the total cesarean rate fell from 23% in 1985 to 13% in 1989 ($p = 0.001$) and the primary rate from 23% to 11% ($p = 0.069$) when staff adopted a modified version of the Canadian National Consensus on Aspects of Cesarean Birth criteria. [These numbers are still high for a low-risk population.] The major change in primary rate was due to a drop in dystocia-related cesareans. The new diagnostic definition required dilation to 4 cm or more and the use of oxytocin to establish adequate contractions. Among VBAC eligible women, the cesarean rate dropped from 93% to 36%. The proportion of women agreeing to labor after a cesarean rose from 7% to 79% [which shows that acceptance of trial of labor is doctor, not mother, driven]. The VBAC rate was 81%, with little variation over the years. One neonatal death occurred from a prolapsed umbilical cord.

24. Treacy BJ, Mathews NB, and Rayburn WF. The escalating cesarean section rate: a 25 year experience at the University of Nebraska Medical Center. *Neb Med J* 1991;76(8):271-273.

After instituting peer review and enforcing new guidelines, the total cesarean rate dropped from 21.9% in 1989 to 16.9% [still too high] in 1990. The proportion of repeat cesareans did not change (37.8% versus 42.2%) because "many such cases had either other accompanying conditions...or patient reluctance toward an attempted vaginal delivery despite our encouragement." [Since "anticipated large fetus" is on the list of contraindications for VBAC, although many women subsequently give birth to big babies after previous cesareans and other studies have overcome "patient reluctance," one wonders how committed these doctors were.] The guidelines were those of Myers and Gleicher [see Abstract 21].

25. Socol ML, et al. Reducing cesarean births at a primarily private university hospital. *Am J Obstet Gynecol* **1993;168(6 Pt 1):1748-1758.**

This Illinois private tertiary care hospital "encouraged" VBAC, "recommended" active management of labor (a randomized controlled trial had been done there), and circulated individual annual cesarean rates because, while effective, a "centralized approach to intrapartum decision making . . . is unlikely to be well received by the obstetric community at large." While Illinois rates remained stable, the total, primary, and repeat cesarean rates at the hospital fell from 27.3% to 16.9%, 18.2% to 10.6%, and 9.1% to 6.4%, respectively (*p* < 0.0001 for all rates) between 1986 and 1991. Cesarean rates declined for both private (OR 0.54, CI 0.48-0.61) and clinic patients (OR 0.49, CI 0.40-0.62). However, private patients were more likely to have a cesarean in both 1986 (30.3% versus 20.8%) and 1991 (19.1% versus 11.5%). This held true for all birth weight groups. Not only did trials of labor after cesarean increase (27.2% versus 58.3%, *p* < 0.0001), but more resulted in VBACs (67.4% versus 80.0%, *p* < 0.01). Despite the overall drop, total and primary cesarean rates for doctors attending 100 private patients or more per year ranged from 5.2% to 42.3% and 3.0% to 26.1%, respectively, in 1988 and from 6.5-41.1% and 4.6-21.1%, respectively in 1991. The perinatal mortality rate declined from 19.5 to 10.3 per 1000 (*p* < 0.001) between 1986 and 1991.

H. Sandmire, discussant: "[C]an a . . . facility with a private patient cesarean rate . . . almost twice the clinic rate . . . be regarded as successful in reaching their goal, which was the 'curtailment of unnecessary cesarean sections'? To achieve success the authors need to find ways to raise the quality of labor management . . . to the level currently provided to their clinic patients."

EVIDENCE AND EDUCATION DO NOT AFFECT PRACTICE

26. Porreco RP. Meeting the challenge of the rising cesarean birth rate. *Obstet Gynecol* **1990;75(1):133-136.**

By making educational presentations on management of previous cesarean, fetal distress, dystocia, breech, twins, and herpes to physicians, nurses, and interested public groups between 1982 and 1986, the author hoped to reduce the Denver cesarean rate. Thirty formal presentations were given to physicians, with at least one formal presentation at each Denver hospital. For nurses, 22 presentations were given as part of the continuing-education programs nurses need to renew their licenses. Fifteen presentations were made to area childbirth educators and various support groups. Nevertheless, the Denver cesarean rate in these same years increased from 17.3% to 19.3%. At the author's hospital, the private service cesarean rate increased from 15.4% to 17.6%, while the clinic service rate held steady at 6%. [Staff presentations at Porreco's hospital were not included in the study statistics because "they occurred on a frequent and ongoing basis."]

27. Lomas J et al. Do practice guidelines guide practice? The effect of a consensus statement on the practice of physicians. *N Engl J Med* **1989;321(19):1306-1311.**

Data on cesarean rates for Ontario hospitals were collected pre- and postpublication of nationally endorsed cesarean section guidelines published in 1986. Obstetricians were surveyed on their knowledge of and response to the guidelines. While most obstetricians knew of them (87-94%) and most agreed with them (82.5-85%), and one-third reported a change in practice and a reduction in cesarean rates as a result of them, knowledge of the content of the recommendations was poor (67% correct responses), and cesarean rates were essentially unchanged two years after release of the guidelines. "[T]he dissemination of research evidence in the form of practice guidelines issued by a national body is unlikely to have much effect on inappropriate practices that are sustained by powerful nonscientific forces."

28. Soliman SR and Burrows RF. Cesarean section: analysis of the experience before and after the National Consensus Conference on Aspects of Cesarean Birth. *Can Med Assoc J* **1993;148(8):1315-1320.** (Like Abstract 27, these are also Ontario data.)

In order to judge the effect of the Canadian Consensus Conference recommendations published in 1986, outcomes were compared for births between 1982 ($N = 4121$) and 1990 ($N = 4431$) for two Ontario hospitals: a tertiary care referral center and a teaching hospital with a Level II nursery. Trial of labor after cesarean was offered 93% more often (33.1% in 1982 versus 63.8% in 1990, $p = 0.0002$), which reduced the repeat cesarean rate by 15%. However, "previous cesarean" as an indication for cesarean fell by 19.9%, and the rate of vaginal births increased by only 2.6%. The discrepancy is explained by an increase in the "other" category of indications for cesarean. "It appeared that physicians were encouraging VBAC at first but then were opting out of that choice . . . thus, the cesarean sections were not being classified as repeat." The primary cesarean rate was unchanged (15.7% versus 14.8%). Despite conference recommendations, incidence and treatment of dystocia remained unchanged, as did the rate of cesarean for breech. Fetal distress was the indication in 12.1% of cesarean deliveries in 1990. However, most infants with this diagnosis had Apgar scores above 7 at one and five minutes. Fetal distress was rarely confirmed with fetal scalp-blood pH measurement. The major predictors of cesarean in 1990 were prior cesarean section (OR 20.0, $p < 0.0001$) and induction (OR 7.1, $p < 0.0001$). For multiparous women with no prior cesarean (OR 12.5, $p < 0.0001$) and nulliparous women (OR 4.5, $p < 0001$), it was induction. "[T]he strongest correctable predictor of cesarean section is labour induction."

29. Dillon WP et al. Obstetric care and cesarean birth rates: a program to monitor quality of care. *Obstet Gynecol* **1992;80(5):731-737.**

In 1987 a joint task force was formed in New York State by the Department of Health, American College of Obstetrics and Gynecology, and NAACOG [now called the Association of Women's Health, Obstetric and Neonatal Nurses (AWHONN)] to lower cesarean rates by enhancing in-hospital reviews, improving quality of care, and standardizing terminology. A format for in-hospital reviews was developed, and voluntary external reviews with follow-up contacts were conducted at 24 hospitals during 1989 and 1990. The hospitals selected for review were diverse in terms of geographic location, size, and cesarean rate. In 1986 individual hospital rates varied from 11.2% to 40.2% [!]. From 1987 to 1990 the statewide cesarean rate fell from "over 25%" to 23.6%. Compared with nonreviewed hospitals, the cesarean rate for reviewed hospitals was higher in 1987 ([about] 28% versus 25%), and declined faster than non-reviewed hospitals (to [about] 25% versus 24%) in 1990 [I am making estimates from a graph]. With 300,000 births annually in New York State, every percentage point decline in cesarean rates saves about $9 million. "Conclusion: A successful quality assurance program can be jointly developed by a state regulatory agency and a medical specialty society." [This minimal improvement can hardly be described as success. Note, too, the lack of control group. Other states may have had equal or superior declines without instituting a formalized program.]

REFERENCES

Chazotte C and Cohen WR. Catastrophic complications of previous cesarean section. *Am J Obstet Gynecol* 1990;163(3):738-742. (abstracted in Chapter 4)

Feldman GB and Freiman JA. Prophylactic cesarean at term? *N Engl J Med* 1985;312(19):1264-1267.

Golde SH. A program to lower cesarean-section rates. *N Engl J Med* 1989;320(25):1692-1693.

Gribble RK and Meier PR. Effect of epidural anesthesia on the primary cesarean rate. *Obstet Gynecol* 1992;79(1):155-156.

Haire DB and Elsberry CC. Maternity care and outcomes in a high-risk service: the North Central Bronx Hospital experience. *Birth* 1991;18(1):33-37. (abstracted in Chapter 15)

Hall MH et al. Mode of delivery and future fertility. *Br J Obstet Gynaecol* 1989;96:1297-1303.

Hemminki E. Pregnancy and birth after cesarean section: a survey based on the Swedish birth register. *Birth* 1987;14(1):12-17.

Knox RA and Karagianis. Birth by cesarean section. *Boston Globe Magazine,* Oct 21, 1984.

Koska MT. Reducing cesareans—a $1 million trade-off. *Hospitals* 1989;63(5):26.

Lilford RJ et al. The relative risks of caesarean section (intrapartum and elective) and vaginal delivery: a detailed analysis to exclude the effects of medical disorders and other acute pre-existing physiological disturbances. *Br J Obstet Gynaecol* 1990;97:883-892.

Lomas J et al. Caesarean section. In *A guide to effective care in pregnancy and childbirth.* Enkin M, Keirse MJNC, and Chalmers I, eds. Oxford: Oxford University Press, 1989.

Macer JA, Macer CL, and Chan LS. Elective induction versus spontaneous labor: a retrospective study of complications and outcome. *Am J Obstet Gynecol* 1992;166(6 Pt 1):1690-1697. (abstracted in Chapter 5)

National Institutes of Health. *Cesarean childbirth* NIH Publication 82-2067. Washington, D.C. : U.S. Department of Health and Human Services, 1981.

"News." *Birth* 1994;21(2):114.

O'Reilly W et al. Childbirth and the malpractice insurance industry. In *The American way of birth,* Eakins PS, ed. Philadelphia: Temple University Press, 1986.

Pascoe JM. The cesarean section rate [letter]. *JAMA* 1990;26(8):971.

Petitti DB. Maternal mortality and morbidity in cesarean section. *Clin Obstet Gynecol* 1985;28(4):763-769.

Porreco R. Decreasing unnecessary cesareans. Presented at 1991 convention of the International Childbirth Education Association, Denver, Aug 16-18, 1991a.

——. Telephone interview with author, Feb 1991b.

Quilligan EJ. Cesarean section: modern perspectives. In *Management of high-risk pregnancy.* 2d ed. Queenan, JT, ed. Oradell NJ: Medical Economics Books, 1985.

Rochat RW et al. Maternal mortality in the United States: report from the maternal mortality collaborative. *Obstet Gynecol* 1988;72(1):91-97.

Rosen M and Thomas L. *The cesarean myth.* New York: Penguin Books, 1989.

Rubin G et al. The risk of childbearing re-evaluated. *Am J Public Health* 1981;71(7):712-716.

San Jose Mercury News. The losing battle to reduce cesareans. Feb 17, 1985.

Stafford RS. Recent trends in cesarean section use in California. *West J Med* 1990;153(5):511-514.

Taffel SM, Placek PJ, and Kosary CL. U.S. cesarean section rates 1990: an update. *Birth* 1992;19(1):21-22.

U.S. Department of Health and Human Services. Rates of cesarean delivery—United States, 1991. *MMWR* 1993;42(15):285-300.

VanTuinen I and Wolfe M. *Unnecessary cesarean sections: halting a national epidemic.* Washington, D.C.: Public Citizen Health Research Group, 1992.

World Health Organization. Appropriate technology for birth. *Lancet* 1985;2(8452):436-437.

Zdeb MS and Logrillo VM. Cesarean childbirth in New York State: trends and directions. *Birth* 1989;16(4):203-207.

4

Vaginal Birth After Cesarean

> Myth: *"Once a cesarean, always a cesarean."*
>
> EB Craigin
>
> Reality: *"The concept of routine repeat cesarean birth should be replaced by a specific indication for a subsequent abdominal delivery."*
>
> ACOG 1988

Craigin's famous dictum, penned in 1916, has condemned millions of women to run the gantlet of repeated cesarean delivery. Today the most common reason for having a repeat cesarean section is solely that the woman has had one before. When women do not schedule a repeat cesarean, their chance of having a vaginal birth after cesarean (VBAC) is about 70%. In the U.S., in 1992, 25.1% of women with a prior cesarean had a vaginal birth after cesarean (VBAC) ("News" 1994). If this represents 70% of those who tried labor, then only 36% of U.S. women tried labor after a prior cesarean, which says we have a long way to go before labor after cesarean becomes the norm. How did an untested, unsupported statement made so long ago gain such credence that we have yet to exorcise it?

When anyone talks about labor after a cesarean, the overarching fear is of uterine rupture. This fear may have been reasonable years ago when doctors made vertical ("classical") uterine incisions. Because they are made through the uterine muscle, these incisions occasionally rupture during pregnancy, generally with catastrophic results. The force of labor contractions presumably adds additional stress. However, the lower uterine segment transverse incision, in standard use by the 1970s (Martin, Morrison, and Wiser 1988, abstracted below), is made through an area that is mostly connective tissue. As study after study has shown, it rarely gives way, and when it does, the separation is usually like opening a zipper: neat, bloodless, and benign. By the mid-1980s, enough evidence had accumulated on this point that fear of rupture was no longer valid as a reason for elective repeat cesarean. Despite this the VBAC rate remained in the single digits (Taffel et al. 1991).

Symptomatic ruptures do occur, of course, and doctors have used the hospital's inability to perform a timely emergency cesarean as another reason to refuse VBAC. The cumulative number of ruptures in the articles I abstracted was 46 ruptures in 15,154 trials of labor, or 0.30%. According to Enkin (1989), the probability of any laboring woman's needing an emergency cesarean for other unpredictable conditions, such as fetal distress, umbilical cord prolapse, or hemorrhage, is 2.7%, roughly 10 times the rate of rupture during labor. The American College of Obstetricians and Gynecologists' (ACOG) guidelines for VBAC stipulate the ability to perform cesarean section within 30 minutes, "as is standard for any obstetric patient in labor" (ACOG 1988). Based on these guidelines, the National Association of Childbearing Centers (NACC) supports VBAC with a documented low transverse uterine incision at freestanding birth centers, provided they can meet the ACOG 30-minutes-to-cesarean rule (NACC 1992). Hospitals have no excuse. If a hospital does not think it can meet the ACOG guidelines, then it is saying it cannot handle labor, period.

Another roadblock to VBAC is the common practice of putting severe limitations on who should be permitted trial of labor (TOL). Aided by an unquestioned (and unfounded) belief in the safety of planned cesarean section, doctors feel justified in refusing TOL to anyone they think unlikely to give birth vaginally or who they believe has an increased risk of scar separation. This reasoning does not hold up either. In particular, more than half the women who had a cesarean for cephalopelvic disproportion (CPD) (the baby is too large to pass through the mother's pelvis) or failure to progress (FTP) will give birth vaginally if allowed to labor—many to a bigger baby—as will those whose fetus is adjudged macrosomic (predicted birth weight 4000 g or 8 lb 13 oz or more). No association has been found between rupture and uterine distention, previous infection, and so forth.

Protocols, too, often work to exclude candidates or reduce the odds of vaginal birth. Some forbid using oxytocin to induce or augment VBAC labor, but oxytocin bears little or no association with rupture. (I may disagree that oxytocin is indicated—see Chapters 9 and 10—but that is cold comfort to a woman who had a repeat cesarean because her doctor thought it was and would not use it.) Time limitations on length of labor, elective induction, hospital admission in early labor, and so forth all increase the odds of repeat cesarean without conferring benefits. On the theory that it would mask the pain of rupture, epidural anesthesia has also been refused, undoubtedly frightening away many women whose prior labor was long and difficult. Pain, however, does not reliably signal rupture, so epidurals are not contraindicated.

Bruce Flamm, whose lifework has been VBAC research, believes women with a prior transverse cesarean(s) should be treated normally, with one exception: because fetal distress is the most reliable symptom of rupture and onset of distress may be sudden, he thinks continuous electronic fetal monitoring (EFM) is beneficial (Flamm 1990), but even this has been disputed (Flamm, MacDonald, Shearer, and Mahan 1992). MacDonald, Shearer, and Mahan observe that EFM has never been shown to be superior to auscultation (listening to fetal heart tones periodically) at detecting fetal distress, and without evidence to the contrary, we cannot assume EFM would prove superior here. MacDonald warns, "Before . . . giving the opinion or impression that monitoring is essential every time VBAC is attempted, let us have some solid data. . . . Otherwise, . . . the legal profession will use such opinion as if it were factual." Shearer adds that women laboring with a scar are no more likely to have emergency problems than other laboring women. She reminds us that "lack of sufficient nursing staff" is often cited as a reason for EFM. "Less careful or frequent attention from hospital staff . . . could . . . lead to delay in response to fetal distress caused by any reason, and potentially a poorer outcome." Shearer's concern is more than theoretical. One study reported a 20-minute delay in diagnosing one rupture despite EFM and intrauterine pressure catheter (IUPC), and in another, a 40-minute delay in performing a cesarean after diagnosis of fetal distress resulted in the death of the baby (Arulkumaran, Chua, and Ratnam 1992; Stoval et al. 1987, both abstracted below). Mahan states that unnecessary monitoring increases costs and could decrease the odds of VBAC because EFM confines women to bed.

Another reason proffered for low VBAC rates is patient preference. An ACOG survey (1990) reported that 92% of the 2200 obstetricians responding said they "encouraged VBAC," but 42% of women refused. This statistic poses a philosophical problem:

Women are not normally allowed to choose cesarean if they have not had one before. Why does a prior cesarean make a difference? One could argue that a woman should be allowed to choose a primary cesarean on the basis that people have the right to elective surgery. Indeed, a few doctors have argued that very point (Feldman and Freiman 1985; Kirk et al. 1990), but the ability to choose a cesarean is not really about freedom of choice. As Beth Shearer, a noted cesarean educator and VBAC advocate, says, the ability to choose a cesarean is about the only choice women are allowed to make. The same doctors who say, "Shouldn't she be allowed to choose?" would not let her choose vaginal birth if they thought a cesarean advisable (Shearer 1989). One study of how 100 women with a prior cesarean decided on birth route for the next baby described negotiation strategies "to gain decision making power," which in all cases meant the power to choose a cesarean, *never* vaginal birth (McClain 1987). The doctors who believed in "once a cesarean, always a cesarean" refused to negotiate. Does a woman really have freedom of choice if all she can say is "no" to vaginal birth and "yes" to a cesarean?

Digging deeper, let us look at why women choose cesareans. McClain found that medical risks and benefits played no part. Women wanted the convenience of scheduling the delivery or control over the unpredictability of labor, poor reasons to expose themselves to the risks and pain of major surgery. A similar study of 160 women found that 25% of those electing cesareans listed "danger to the mother," an inaccuracy because VBAC is safer for the mother; 40% listed "fear of labor pain," although epidural anesthesia should be available and pain following a cesarean is considerable, continuous, and lasts for days; 27% listed "convenience of timing the birth"; and 38% put "knew what to expect." To repeat, none of these is a good reason to have major surgery (Kirk et al. 1990).   Joseph, Stedman, and Robichaux (1991) noted that despite "encouragement" to try labor, women listed fear and convenience as reasons for choosing repeat cesarean.   Kline and Arias (1993) comment on the "puzzling fact" that so few women at their hospital opt for VBAC. They then unwittingly reveal that the source of that refusal lies in their own biases. They write that women are "reluctant to suffer . . . the pain and inconveniences of labor" when they can have the "convenience and safety of a scheduled operative delivery."

The reasons women elect repeat cesarean bring up another problem with the ACOG survey: if women are making decisions based on misinformation and misconceptions, what constitutes encouragement? If it means giving women the information to make an informed choice, then these women's doctors have been derelict. But even accurate information may not go far enough. The reasons why women turn down VBAC suggest that knowing they are good candidates is not enough. The doctor must also address the woman's desire for control and predictability and her fears about labor, and few doctors see that as their department. Without coming to terms with these, as a midwife would help her do (Laufer et al. 1987), she has no real alternative to another cesarean section.

Many obstetricians don't even get as far as advising patients of what is medi- cally best. They opt for "neutrality." Neutrality, however, is a sham; not to be for VBAC is to be against it. Kirk et al. (1990) found that when women believed their doctor to be neutral, only 10% of women chose labor, and 41% chose a c-section.

The premise of all three studies of decision making is that the woman has complete autonomy and the obstetrician only limited influence. That mani- festly is not true. Both Kirk et al. and Joseph, Stedman, and Robichaux found that *no* woman chose labor contrary to her doctor's advice. Sadly (and ironi- cally because their chances of VBAC would have been better than 50-50), in the latter study 24 women who wanted to labor were later dissuaded because their doctors said the baby was too big. Another study found that of 220 women undergoing repeat cesarean, only 11% had a discussion of VBAC noted in their chart, whereas of 117 women whose charts noted a VBAC discussion, 79% agreed to try it (Norman, Kostovcik, and Lanning 1993).

That women *believe* they have made a free choice and are satisfied does not signify true autonomy. The supreme exercise of power occurs when people's preferences are so manipulated that they act against their own interests but they themselves are content (Shapiro et al. 1983).

Other doctors, despite the overwhelming evidence, actively discourage VBAC or damn it with such faint praise that it amounts to the same thing. Lomas et al. (1991) document the difficulties of persuading obstetricians to promote VBAC. They found that having a respected and influential doctor on site actively lobbying colleagues on behalf of VBAC yielded the best results. Nevertheless, over half of eligible women at such sites were still undergoing elective repeat cesarean at the end of their two-year study—not much different from the two-thirds of women having elective repeat cesareans at control hospitals. Three-fourths of the women were offered labor (versus half of control women), but only 38% accepted (versus 28% of control women).

Why do obstetricians resist VBAC? Kirk et al. list "respect for patient autonomy, a reluctance to change long-held positions, a wish to avoid a failed vaginal birth after cesarean section [that concern about avoiding failed vaginal birth does not seem to keep doctors from performing the first cesarean] . . ., or *fear of litigation*" (italics mine). Some doctors may honestly think they are honoring patients' rights, but most, subconsciously or consciously, are simply shirking their duty to advocate for the best medical option. The twist here is that, under the guise of patient autonomy, the victim is made responsible.

With increasing pressures (mostly on economic grounds) to make VBAC the standard of care, a backlash is developing. Some doctors are looking for reasons to rethink encouraging VBAC. Two alarming reports on uterine rupture appeared in an issue of *Obstetrics and Gynecology* (Jones et al. 1991; Scott 1991). Jones et al. noted eight cases in the Denver area that led to one perinatal death, two cases of neonatal asphyxia, one case of maternal bladder tears, and one hysterectomy. Richard Porreco (1990) points out that this "epidemic" calculates out to an incidence of 0.5%, well within normal expectations, but "perinatal morbidity (indeed mortality), with rare exceptions *should not occur* in properly attended patients." Scott reports on 14 ruptures over nine years in Salt Lake City, 12 of which occurred from 1987 to 1991. They resulted in four perinatal deaths, two cases of brain damage, two hysterectomies, and one instance of serious postoperative complications. Porreco's comment applies equally well to Scott.

Both reports ignored morbidity from elective cesarean. Surgical complications and hysterectomies are ever-present risks of elective cesarean, increasingly so with multiple scars. Furthermore, no study in the VBAC literature has recorded a maternal death attributable to VBAC, but several have occurred as a result of cesarean section.

Scott and Jones et al. imply that repeat cesarean is safer for the baby, but babies are more likely to have breathing difficulties after a cesarean than after vaginal birth (Flamm 1990). Additionally, each succeeding cesarean makes subsequent pregnancies more hazardous for both mother and baby. The incidence of the life-threatening complications placenta accreta (the placenta grows into the muscular wall of the uterus) and placenta previa (the placenta implants low so as to partially or completely cover the cervix) goes up markedly with the number of scars (Chazotte and Cohen 1990; Clark, Koonings, and Phelan 1985, both abstracted below).

Any labor carries a certain amount of risk, VBAC or not, and resubjecting the mother to major surgery unnecessarily is not the way to solve that problem. Says Lawrence Roberts (1991, abstracted below), "Obstetricians should remember that to allow a patient to labour is not a treatment, it is a virtually unavoidable consequence of pregnancy."

Note: VBAC terminology uses loaded language. Studies speak of "successful VBAC," implying that repeat cesarean is a failure. "Attempted VBAC" also implies that labor is not the norm and vaginal birth is doubtful, as does "trial of labor." I have tried to avoid this terminology with the exception of TOL, which I have used because of its brevity. I feel this is justified because the medical model, with its "guilty until proven innocent" attitude, regards all labors as a TOL.

SUMMARY OF SIGNIFICANT POINTS

- Lower uterine segment transverse scars rarely reopen and rarely cause problems when they do. Proper monitoring minimizes morbidity from rupture. Labor does not increase the risk of dehiscence. (Abstracts 3-10, 12-13, 15, 19-24, 26-34, 38, 42-47, 50)

- Vertical fundal scar increases the risk of rupture, with many ruptures occurring in pregnancy. The risks of low vertical scar are unknown and probably depend on the degree of extension into the fundus. T- or J-shaped scars are also believed dangerous. (Abstracts 3, 5-6, 9-10, 12, 16, 24, 47-48)

- Preterm cesareans are usually low vertical or sometimes classical incisions because the lower uterine segment is not developed. Since many VBAC protocols exclude vertical incision, having a vertical incision often restricts women to repeat cesareans. (The hazards of repeat cesarean and multiple scars for mother and subsequent children should be considered when weighing risks versus benefits of preterm cesarean.) (Abstracts 10, 13-16, 18, 22-28, 30, 32-33, 36-37)

- The incidence of placenta previa and accreta increases markedly with the number of uterine scars. These complications kill mothers and babies, and placenta accreta often requires hysterectomy. (Abstracts 1-2, 5-6, 16, 19, 21, 30, 44-47)

- Serious complications are more common with cesarean section than vaginal birth. (Abstracts 2, 4, 9-13, 15-16, 19, 21, 24-25, 38, 45-47, 49)

- Women can labor safely after more than 1 cesarean. The overall VBAC rate (calculated from Abstracts 42-47) was 69%. Over half of women will have a VBAC even after two prior cesareans for labor dystocia. (Abstracts 8-12, 28, 39, 41-47)

- Because today over 90% of scars are lower segment transverse, TOL with unknown scar type should be permitted. (Abstracts 10, 12, 48-49)

- Broad versus limited selection of VBAC candidates does not correlate with VBAC rates. (Abstracts 14-39, 45-47)

- The odds of VBAC when the prior cesarean was for CPD (cephalopelvic disproportion), FTP (failure to progress), or labor dystocia, so-called recurrent indications, or where macrosomia (birth weight 4000 g or more) is anticipated are good enough that TOL is still the best choice (Figure 4.1). (Abstracts 8-19, 21-25, 28, 30, 32-33, 37, 39, 45-47, 50-52)

- Women with one prior scheduled cesarean are equally likely to have a VBAC (79%). (Abstract 29)

- X-ray pelvimetry does not reliably predict vaginal birth. (Abstracts 8, 14, 18, 33, 53-54)

- Twin pregnancies and vaginal breeches have safely been VBACs, but few data exist. (Abstracts 8, 10-12)

- VBAC rates in some studies are artificially low because women were allowed to elect a cesarean in labor or because women were not given adequate time in labor. (Abstracts 8-9, 15, 17-19, 24, 26, 36, 38, 47, 56)

- VBAC rates most often fall into the 70% to 79% range (Figure 4.1). (Abstracts 2, 4, 8-10, 12-40, 49)

- Women with no prior vaginal birth child have labor lengths more like primiparous women than multiparous women. (Abstracts 55-56)

Figure 4.1: VBAC Rates Reported in the Abstracted Studies

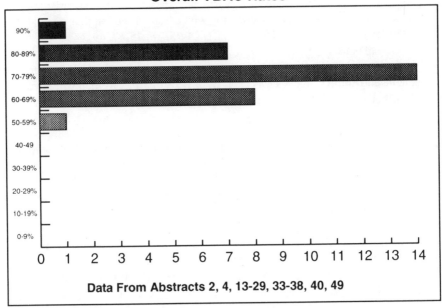

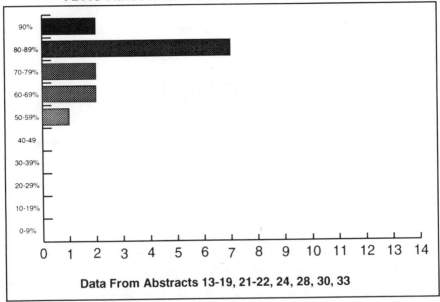

NOTE: VBAC rates have been corrected by excluding women who elected cesarean section in labor

VBAC Rates With Prior Cesarean For Fetal Distress

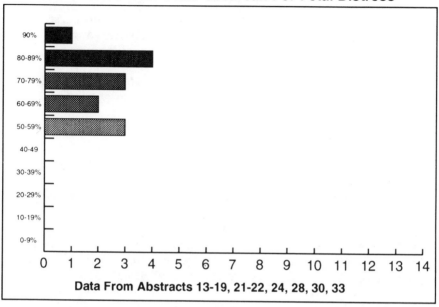

Data From Abstracts 13-19, 21-22, 24, 28, 30, 33

VBAC Rates With Prior Cesarean For FTP/CPD/Dystocia

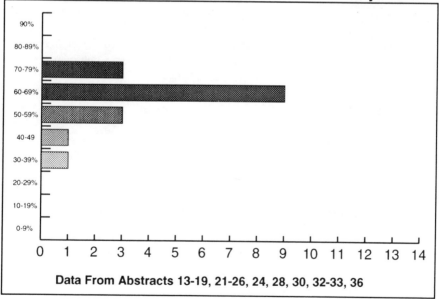

Data From Abstracts 13-19, 21-26, 24, 28, 30, 32-33, 36

- Pain at the scar site does not reliably indicate rupture. Cesareans performed for this reason often find intact scars. (Abstracts 5, 19, 22, 25)

- Changes in contraction strength do not reliably indicate rupture, so routine intrauterine pressure catheters (IUPC) have little value. (Abstracts 27-28, 45, 63)

- Epidurals should be permitted in TOLs. Their effect on the VBAC rate varies. (Abstracts 3, 8-12, 15, 17, 20-21, 23, 27, 29-30, 33-34, 45)

- When judiciously used, oxytocin is generally found to be safe, but whether it is used and how often it is used bear no correlation with VBAC rates. (Abstracts 3, 5, 8-16, 18-30, 32-35, 37-38, 42-46, 49-51, 57-62)

- Induced labors generally have lower VBAC rates than spontaneous or augmented labors. (Abstracts 29, 35, 38, 57-62)

- Most inductions are for premature rupture of membranes or postdates (questionable indications; see Chapters 9 and 10). Routine induction for postdates confers no benefits. (Abstracts 52, 59, 61-62)

- Women admitted in active labor had higher VBAC rates than women admitted in early labor. (Abstract 19)

- Manual exploration of the scar results in both false positives and false negatives. False positives lead to unnecessary surgery. Symptomless dehiscences probably need no repair anyway. The exploration (which is painful) may introduce infection and could potentially convert a dehiscence into a rupture. (Abstracts 3, 6-7, 10, 12, 22, 28, 64)

- Women do not refuse TOL when care providers truly encourage them. (Abstracts 13, 22, 25, 36)

- TOLs can be safely managed by midwives using their typically less interventive protocols. (Abstracts 36-37)

ORGANIZATION OF ABSTRACTS

Note: Because so many VBAC studies have been done, I have presented them in table form (Tables 4.2 through 4.9).

The Risks of Repeat Cesarean

The Risks of Uterine Rupture

Review Paper
Studies

VBAC Articles

Review Papers
VBAC Studies Conducted by Obstetricians
VBAC Studies Conducted by Midwives

Exclusions

Arguments for Liberal Inclusions When Selecting for TOL
Labor with a Multiple Scar (Review)
Studies of Labor with Multiple Scar
Studies of Labor with Unknown Scar
Studies of Labor with Macrosomic Baby
Study of Labor with Postterm Pregnancy
Studies of the Predictability of Pelvimetry

Labor Protocol Issues

Note: I have no separate section on the safety of epidurals, but VBAC reports consistently confirmed that epidural anesthesia is not contraindicated.

Labor Takes Longer
Labor with Oxytocin
Intrauterine Pressure Catheter Is Unnecessary
Manual Exploration of Scar Is Unnecessary

THE RISKS OF REPEAT CESAREAN

1. Clark SL, Koonings PP, and Phelan JP. Placenta previa/accreta and prior cesarean section. *Obstet Gynecol* **1985;66(1):89-92.**

The records of all women giving birth at a single hospital between 1977 and 1983 were examined ($N = 97,799$); 4882 (5%) had one cesarean or more. The risk of placenta previa was 0.26% in an unscarred uterus, 0.65% with one cesarean scar, 1.8% with two, 3.0% with three, and 10% with 4 or more, a 38-fold increase. The risk of placenta accreta in conjunction with placenta previa rose from 5% in an unscarred uterus to 24% with one scar, 47% with two, 40% with three, and 67% with four or more cesarean scars. When women had both conditions, 58% required hysterectomy with an unscarred uterus whereas, 82% required hysterectomy with a scar(s).

Normally, placentas implanting low are carried away from the cervix by differential growth as the uterine muscle grows. Scar tissue in the lower segment could impair this process, thus causing placenta previa. The more scars there are, the greater the effect. As for placenta accreta, the decidual layer is thin in the lower uterine segment, and scar tissue may thin it further, thus increasing the likelihood of placental tissue invading the muscular layer. "All obstetricians should be aware of the strong association between placenta previa in a scarred uterus and placenta accreta. The fact that the risk of this life-threatening condition continues to rise with multiple prior uterine incisions gives further support to attempted vaginal delivery after a cesarean section."

2. Chazotte C and Cohen WR. Catastrophic complications of previous cesarean section. *Am J Obstet Gynecol* 1990;163(3):738-742.

This analysis looked at data on 711 women from 1986 to 1989 who had a prior cesarean (VBAC rate was 312 of 414, or 74%). Seventeen women (2.4%)—one woman in 42—had one or more catastrophic complications (defined as maternal or fetal death, hemorrhage requiring five units of blood or more, hysterectomy or artery ligation, or uterine rupture).

Two women died: one from hemorrhage with placenta previa and percreta during her third elective repeat cesarean and the other from pulmonary embolus following cesarean hysterectomy after rupture of vertical incision was found at elective repeat cesarean. Three fetal deaths occurred, all preterm: (1) death from rupture of unknown scar type (prior cesarean for preterm delivery); (2) induction done after fetal death and during c-section for failed induction (two prior c-sections) rupture and abruptio placenta were found; and (3) death from bleeding from placenta previa (one prior cesarean). All three mothers had hysterectomies. Hemorrhage occurred in 11 women, necessitating hysterectomy in 8. In three it was due to rupture and in the others to placenta previa, often in association with placenta accreta. Nine women had uterine ruptures, five occurring during labor. "[T]he observed frequency and nature of complications . . . emphasizes the importance of performing cesarean section only when the benefits . . . outweigh potential risks."

THE RISKS OF UTERINE RUPTURE

Review Paper

3. Clark SL. Rupture of the scarred uterus. *Obstet Gynecol Clin North Am* 1988;15(4):737-744.

The incidence of scar separation after a low transverse incision ranges from 1% to 2%. The rate appears to be the same whether or not the woman has labored, suggesting that labor does not increase the incidence. Most separations are benign. When they are not, proper monitoring for fetal distress and prompt intervention should avoid perinatal morbidity. With classic incisions, the risk of rupture is much greater, with many ruptures occurring preterm. The perinatal mortality rate and maternal complication rates are high. The risk with low vertical incision is unknown.

Judicious use of oxytocin is safe. Epidural anesthesia should not be withheld because "pain is neither a sensitive nor a specific symptom of rupture." Women with multiple scars can have TOLs. Only a few hundred women have been studied (versus thousands with one scar), but dehiscence rates did not increase.

When asymptomatic scar dehiscences ("windows") are found, repair is best even in women desiring sterilization because of the morbidity associated with cesarean hysterectomy. When a window is discovered after vaginal birth, many authorities advocate no action. Subsequent vaginal birth has been reported, but cesarean section may be more prudent.

Studies

4. Finley BE and Gibbs CE. Emergent cesarean delivery in patients undergoing a trial of labor with a transverse lower-segment scar. *Am J Obstet Gynecol* **1986;155(5):936-939.**

Between 1978 and 1982, 1156 women labored after a cesarean, and 745 (62%) had a VBAC. Three women had cesareans for suspected rupture as evidenced by fetal distress or death, vaginal bleeding, or maternal shock. Rupture was found in only one case (0.09%): a woman was being expectantly managed for ruptured membranes. Fetal heart tones were lost, surgery revealed complete rupture, and the baby was stillborn. The rupture was repaired. Among 411 repeat cesareans, 4 dehiscences were incidental findings at surgery. Three were repaired; one was "difficult to repair," and hemorrhage led to hysterectomy. Another woman in this group had a hysterectomy for hemorrhage caused by uterine atony. The cesarean rate for fetal distress was similar to that in women with no scar. Over the five-year period of this review, three out of the four ruptures that occurred during pregnancy occurred in women scheduled for repeat cesarean.

5. Meehan FP and Magani IM. True rupture of the caesarean section scar (a 15 year review, 1972-1987). *Eur J Obstet Gynecol Reprod Biol* **1989;30(2):129-135.**

A 15-year review (1972-1987) at this hospital revealed 2434 women with a prior cesarean, of whom 1084 (44.5%) had planned cesareans and 1350 had TOL (VBAC rate 81%). In the TOL group, six women had ruptures (0.44%). Oxytocin did not associate significantly with rupture. Of the six women, four had parities five or more children. [Grand multiparity predisposes to rupture even in an unscarred uterus.] Three women had vaginal births, one of them with forceps. The forceps delivery was a stillbirth. [Details given suggest death was prior to labor.] Two women had hysterectomies. The other three women had emergency cesareans: of this group, two babies died; one woman had a hysterectomy; and the other two needed no repair. [With one of the deaths there was fetal distress but no bleeding and no need to repair scar, suggesting rupture was not responsible.] Pain was not reported in any of the cases, and only two of the six women had an epidural. Four women had ruptures prior to labor, one of a classical scar. That baby was stillborn. The other three had placenta accreta or percreta. The other three babies survived, but two of their mothers died [!]. All four women had hysterectomies.

6. Nielson TF, Ljungblad U, and Hagberg H. Rupture and dehiscence of cesarean section scar during pregnancy and delivery. *Am J Obstet Gynecol* **1989;160(3):569-573.**

Records were examined for 2044 women who had prior cesarean sections between 1978 and 1987, of whom 1008 had a TOL. Six ruptures occurred in the TOL group (0.6%), one found after vaginal birth. None of the six had oxytocin, nor did rupture associate with prior postpartum infection. One baby had a 10-minute Apgar of 6, but recovered, and one woman had endometritis. Two women with a T incision (not candidates for TOL) ruptured during pregnancy: one mother ruptured at 33 weeks, had a hysterectomy, and her baby spent 29 days in intensive care but recovered. The other mother ruptured at 38 weeks; the baby was fine, and the rupture repaired. "[T]he potential benefit of scar examination [after VBAC] is obscure, and many asymptomatic scars have been untreated, with no apparent adverse consequences."

7. Farmer RM et al. Uterine rupture during trial of labor after previous cesarean section. *Am J Obstet Gynecol* **1991;165(4 Pt 1):996-1001.**

All charts of women at a Los Angeles hospital who had uterine scar separations during TOL from 1983 to 1989 ($N = 137$) were examined. During that period 7598 women had a TOL. The uterine rupture rate was 0.8%; 47.5% of women who had ruptures had a known transverse scar, 41.0% had unknown scar type, 8.2% had a classic scar, and 3.3% had a vertical scar. [Therefore the rate for known transverse scar was 0.8% × .475 = 0.38%. Assuming all women with unknown scar had transverse scars, the rate would be 0.71%.] Of the 61 women who had ruptures, seven had vaginal births, 14 required hysterectomies, one fetus died, and one mother died of a postpartum hemorrhage after a vaginal birth. Manual exploration had revealed no scar separation, but 2½ hours later, the mother had a cardiac arrest. Laparotomy revealed a 10-centimeter left lateral rupture that disrupted the left uterine artery. [It would not seem that it was the scar that ruptured, or if it was, it does not appear that the mother had a transverse scar.]

VBAC ARTICLES

Review Papers

8. Davies JA and Spencer JA. Trial of scar. *Br J Hosp Med* **1988;40(5):379-381.**

A survey of studies between 1924 and 1980 reveals a perinatal mortality rate due to rupture during labor of 0.93 per 1000 births, almost all due to rupture of a vertical scar. Summarizing 11 reports published between 1983 and 1987, the TOL rate ($N = 10,448$) after one c-section was 47% (range 16-82%), and the VBAC rate was 82% (range 60-94%). In the study with the lowest VBAC rate [Ngu and Quinn, Abstract 18), many women were allowed a maximum of five hours in labor. Summarizing five studies of TOL after more than one cesarean ($N = 220$), the VBAC rate was 69% (range 57-81%). Summarizing six reports breaking down VBAC rate by prior cesarean indication yielded the following information: CPD/FTP: 774 TOLs, VBAC rate 66%; fetal distress: 317 TOLs, VBAC rate 75%; breech: 467 TOLs, VBAC rate 84%; other: TOLs 584, VBAC rate 73%. Other factors that improved the odds of VBAC were previous vaginal birth, short time in labor before prior cesarean, birth weight in this pregnancy less than 4000 g, and admission to hospital for TOL at 3 cm dilation or more [probably because inductions are less likely to end in VBAC but possibly also because maternal or physician anxiety over the length of labor led to premature abandonment of TOL in women admitted at an earlier stage].

The incidence of dehiscence during TOL ranged from 0.4% to 3.2%. For non-TOL women it ranged from 0% to 3.9%. The rate of rupture was not affected by febrile morbidity after prior cesarean, the number of previous cesareans, the number of subsequent VBACs, the degree of uterine distention [big baby or twins], or the use of oxytocin. Perinatal complications did not increase with TOL. A few breeches ($N = 96$) have been VBACs without increased morbidity.

The conclusions are:

- Scar rupture is rare even with classical scar.
- X ray pelvimetry [measuring pelvic dimensions] appears to do little to help select TOL candidates.

- Neither epidural anesthesia nor oxytocin is contraindicated.
- Labor should be monitored carefully.

9. Haq CL. Vaginal birth after cesarean delivery. *Am Fam Physician* 1988;37(6):167-171.

The risk of fetal distress from scar rupture is less than the risk of distress from cord prolapse, and the risk of hemorrhage from rupture is less than that from placenta previa or abruptio placenta. Therefore, any hospital offering obstetric care should be able to offer VBAC. The risk of rupture is 4% with a classical incision and 0.5% for low transverse scar. A review of VBACs from 1950 to 1980 found 12 of 14 fetal deaths involved classical scars. No maternal death due to rupture during TOL has been recorded since 1970. Fever, endometritis, and excessive blood loss with repeat cesarean (18%) exceed that of planned cesarean (10%) but are comparable to primary cesarean (20-30%).

VBAC means less febrile morbidity and blood loss and fewer cases of iatrogenic prematurity. The maternal mortality rate is 27 times lower compared with cesarean. Hospital stays are shorter, and VBACs cost less than half that of cesarean section.

VBAC rates now approach an average of 80%. Highest VBAC rates are among those with prior vaginal birth (94%) or prior breech (91%). Even with prior CPD, up to 77% have a VBAC. Women with more than one prior cesarean show no increased risk of rupture. Macrosomia and postterm pregnancy do not associate with increased risk nor does prior endometritis. Oxytocin does not increase risk of rupture when carefully monitored, and epidural anesthesia is not contraindicated.

The most common reason for repeat cesarean is CPD/FTP followed by "patient request." Women chose planned cesarean because the prior cesarean rescued them from a difficult labor or they feared the uncertainty of VBAC. Some did not have the option in their community.

10. Martin JN, Morrison JC, and Wiser WL. Vaginal birth after cesarean section: the demise of routine repeat abdominal delivery. *Obstet Gynecol Clin North Am* 1988;15(4):719-736.

Arguments against VBAC are rebutted:

Uterine rupture: Of all perinatal rupture-related deaths, 96% were of classical scars. Rupture of the unscarred uterus occurs more often and does more harm than rupture of the scarred uterus. The emergency cesarean rate during TOL is the same as for women laboring with no scar.

Maternal safety: No maternal death associated with VBAC has been reported for decades, and more than 11,500 women [as of this study] have undergone VBAC. The repeat cesarean mortality rate is 1 per 500-1000, and the vaginal birth mortality rate is 1 per 2000-4000.

Fetal safety: One study found greater risk associated with elective repeat cesarean. It found that eliminating iatrogenic prematurity would equalize the risks, but only if amniocentesis-associated risks for determining fetal maturity were not factored in.

Lawsuits: The standard of care is such that VBAC with adverse outcome would be considered negligent only if the doctor departed from generally accepted guidelines. Lawsuits have arisen from complications following elective repeat cesarean.

The deterrents to VBAC were these:

Disincentives for the doctor: "Convenience of scheduling and . . . time management

. . . are often-stated powerful deterrents[!]." Cesareans are more profitable, although insurance companies are moving to equalize payments.

Patient refusal: Women disregard medical risk assessment and choose based on social reasons. [Doctors do not let women disregard medical risk and choose vaginal birth for social reasons.]

The collected series over 40 years show a 79.6% VBAC rate. Numerous investigations and data on thousands of patients show TOL is safer than elective repeat cesarean. Routine VBAC would save millions of dollars. "Paradoxically and unintentionally, it appears that an increase in maternal and perinatal morbidity and mortality is being purchased with [the extra dollars spent on elective cesarean]."

Contraindications are classic uterine incision, extensive uterine surgery, T incision, absolute CPD, and patient refusal following full discussion and disclosure. Term lower segment vertical incisions are safe; the safety of preterm vertical incision is unknown. Twins and breeches have been VBACs. Several studies found TOL with multiple scars to be safe. "The diagnosis of [FTP] or [CPD] [generally] has no prognostic value from pregnancy to the next." Women with repeat cesarean for CPD/FTP should not be excluded from TOL. Macrosomia, postterm pregnancy, and unknown scar are not contraindications nor is previously detected asymptomatic scar defect after VBAC. "[I]f [defects] were not large enough and serious enough to require repair in an earlier gestation they probably have healed enough to support a later carefully executed trial of labor." Oxytocin is safe with controlled administration and monitoring. Epidural anesthesia is not contraindicated. EFM should be done and fetal distress is cause for concern, demanding closer study of mother and fetus.

11. Ophir E et al. Trial of labor following cesarean section: dilemma. *Obstet Gynecol Surv* 1989;44(1):19-24.

The following conclusions about the controversies of VBAC management are reached:

- Multiple cesarean should not exclude TOL.

- Oxytocin may be used provided the labor and fetus are closely monitored.

- The risks of using prostaglandin to ripen the cervix are small. Because it may reduce the need for elective cesarean, prostaglandin deserves further investigation.

- Epidural anesthesia is not contraindicated.

- "CPD has no prognostic value from one pregnancy to the next and generally should not exclude a patient from [TOL]."

- Few data exist, but uterine scar does not appear to influence the likelihood of breech VBAC or twins.

- Elective cesarean is riskier for mother and fetus than an appropriately managed labor with a transverse uterine incision.

12. Pridjian G. Labor after prior cesarean section. *Clin Obstet Gynecol* 1992;35(3):445-456.

The review presents documentation that TOL with a low transverse scar(s) is safe and that VBAC is safer for the mother than c-section. Two uncontrolled series on rupture [Scott 1991; Jones et al. 1991] reported poor neonatal outcomes, but controlled studies have not found statistically increased incidence of problems. VBAC rates [seven studies] based on prior indication were: fetal distress 71-75%; breech 84-88%; and FTP/dystocia 65-68% overall, but 79% when diagnosed in latent phase and 61% when diagnosed in active phase [which suggests that cesareans for a diagnosis of FTP/dystocia in latent phase are more likely to be unnecessary cesareans]. "Any institution where obstetrics is practiced has the capability to offer labor after [prior cesarean section]." Contraindications to TOL are vertical fundal scar and T-shaped scar. One prior low segment transverse scar is "very low-risk." Because there are few data, more than one scar, unknown scar, low vertical scar, twin pregnancy, and fetal macrosomia are "higher-risk" labors.

Very low-risk labors generally can be treated like any other labors, with early labor at home, blood sample on admission, continuous EFM or frequent intermittent monitoring, external contraction pressure monitoring, optional IV or Heplock [this is an IV needle containing an anticoagulant that is attached to a stub of tubing. An IV bag can hooked up to it whenever desired], and clear liquids. Higher-risk labors demand IV access on admission, blood sample and two units of blood available, continuous EFM, external contraction pressure measurements with internal monitoring as soon as membranes can be ruptured, and nothing by mouth [see Chapter 11]. If the woman has no prior vaginal births, labor progress should be evaluated by criteria used for nulliparous women. Oxytocin, judiciously administered and carefully monitored, and epidural anesthesia are not contraindicated. Routine scar examination after VBAC is controversial. It may prevent morbidity by diagnosing rupture earlier, but no evidence suggests that asymptomatic dehiscences require repair for healing. Pregnancy after rupture is not contraindicated, but the woman may be at greater risk for repeat rupture. Although women have had VBACs after rupture, planned cesarean is advised.

VBAC Studies Conducted by Obstetricians

(See Tables 4.2, 4.3, and 4.4 for Abstracts 13 through 35.)

Note: I do not include reports from third world countries or reports with 100 or fewer TOLs. I also excluded two reports for idiosyncratic reasons. One had a 56% instrumental delivery rate and a severe perineal tear rate (tears through the anal sphincter, vaginal walls, or cervical tears) of 36%. The authors then used this egregious example of poor care to say the risk of perineal damage should be considered when weighing risks and benefits of labor versus elective cesarean. The other study used forceps prophylactically, had a VBAC rate of only 54%, and failed to distinguish between dehiscence and rupture.

VBAC Studies Conducted by Midwives

(See Tables 4.5, 4.6, and 4.7 for Abstracts 36 through 37.)

Table 4.2: VBAC Reports, Obstetric Studies

STUDY	YEARS	# OF SUBJ	% POP HAVING TOL	VBAC RATE	EFFECT OF OBSTETRIC HISTORY[a]
13. Meier PR and Porreco RP. Trial of labor following cesarean section: A two year experience. *Am J Obstet Gynecol* 1982;144(6):671-678	1980-81	207	—	84.5%	breech 91.2% fetal distress 92.6% CPD/FTP[d] 78.3%
Cook JC. Factors associated with successful vaginal delivery after cesarean section. *J Reprod Med* 1983; 28(1):785-788.	1978-81	194	34%	75%	abnormal presentation 88% fetal distress 82% CPD/FTP 58%[2]
15. Martin JN et al. Vaginal delivery following previous cesarean birth. *Am J Obstet Gynecol* 1983;146(3):255-263.	1981-82	162	22%	62%	malpresentation 61% fetal distress 64% CPD/dystocia 64%
16. Eglington GS et al. Outcome of a trial of labor after prior cesarean delivery *J Reprod Med* 1984;29(1):3-8.	1980	308	35%	78%	breech 86.2% fetal distress 81.6%
17. Graham AR. Trial labor following previous cesarean section. *Am J Obstet Gynecol* 1984;149(1):35-45.	1978-82	242	18%	69%[5]	breech 74% fetal distress 52% CPD/FTP 61%
18. Ngu A and Quinn MA. Vaginal delivery following caesarean section. *Aust NZ J Obstet Gynaecol* 1985;25:41-43.	1978-81	456	44.6%	60%[7]	breech 69% fetal distress 65% obstructed labor/FTP 44%[8] vag birth prior to c-sec 75% prior VBAC 84%
19. Jarrell MA, Ashmead GG, and Mann LI. Vaginal delivery after cesarean section: a five year study. *Obstet Gynecol* 1985;65(5):628-632.	1978-82	216	27%	66%[9]	breech 75% fetal distress 70% CPD 54%
20. Molloy BG, Sheil O, and Duignan NM. Delivery after caesarean section: review of 2176 cases. *Br Med J* 1987;294:1645-1647.	1979-84	1781	82%	90.8%	—

[a]Effect of reason for prior for cesarean or prior vaginal birth on VBAC rate.

[b]Typical eligibility requirements for TOL: documented single low transverse uterine scar, singleton cephalic fetus.

[c] Typical TOL protocol: continuous EFM, intrauterine pressure catheter (IUPC), manual scar exploration. (IV and nothing by mouth were not commonly mentioned, but may be presumed since these are common policies for all laboring women.)

[d]Cephalopelvic disproportion/failure to progress.

[1]Thirteen women who elected a cesarean responded to a questionnaire asking why: nine said fear of labor; two each said easier, more familiar, more controlled, one said avoid risk of rupture. "Neither fear nor convenience constitute justification for cesarean section. Rather these factors identify areas which require further patient education and support." She needs to know she will be closely watched and that pain medication is available.

[2] Sixty-one percent of X-ray documented cases of CPD had a VBAC.

[3] [If these women were excluded, the VBAC rate becomes 70%.]

[4] All had a VBAC.

[5] "The high percentage of labors less than 5 hours in the group with failure reflects the influence of contractions on the patient's desire to continue a trial of labor."

ELEC C-SEC AT MOTHER'S OPTION?	OXYTOCIN ?	EPIDURAL ?	EXCEPTIONS TO TYPICAL PROTOCOL EXCLUSIONS/ INCLUSIONS[b]	EXCEPTIONS TO TYPICAL PROTOCOL[c]
prenatal Y[1] Intrapartum —	19.4%	10.9%	include > 1 c-sec, no "obvious" CPD	none
prenatal Y intrapartum —	N	N	exclude gestation > 42 wks	no mention of EFM or IUPC
prenatal Y Intrapartum 17[3]	Y	17%[4]	exclude suspected fetal weight > 4000 g, allowed > 1 c-sec	none
—	Y	—	some women not meeting protocol were admitted in labor and had VBAC	none
prenatal Y intrapartum Y[5]	—	50%[6]	exceptions: 5 vertical scar had VBAC; 3 > 1 c-sec led to 1 repeat c-sec and 2 VBAC; 3 twin preg, all repeat c-sec	none
—	17%	—	no, but protocol not described in detail	—
prenatal Y Intrapartum 5[10]	N	6%	no, but protocol not described in detail	—
—	induced 23%[11] augmen 17%[11]	4.8%[11]	only stated requirement: one prior c-sec	55 % had continuous EFM, IUPC not used[11]

[6]Fifty percent of those who had VBAC had an epidural.

[7] "Many patients . . . underwent repeat cesarean section without a fair trial of labor as 50% were operated on within 5 hours of labour commencing."

[8]X-ray pelvimetry did not help to predict VBAC.

[9] Percent having TOL went from 9% in 1978 to 36% in 1982. Women admitted in active labor had VBAC 26% more often than women who were in latent phase labor on admission. Three women (out of 74) had a repeat cesarean for abdominal pain suggestive of rupture. All had intact scars.

[10] [If these women were excluded, the VBAC rate would be 68%.]

[11]The maximum oxytocin dose was 36 mU/min. By itself oxytocin did not increase the risk of rupture over spontaneous labor (induced: 0.3%, augmented: 0.4%), nor did epidurals (epidural: 0, non-epidural 0.2%). But more ruptures occurred in women who had both (induced + epidural 5.0%; augmented + epidural 6.7%, $p < 0.05$). The authors theorize using IUPCs could have prevented uterine hyperstimulation.

Table 4.2 continued

STUDY	YEARS	# OF SUBJ	% POP HAVING TOL	VBAC RATE	EFFECT OF OBSTETRIC HISTORY[a]
21. Phelan JP et al. Vaginal birth after cesarean. *Am J Obstet Gynecol* 1987;157(6):1510-1515.	1982-84	1796	65%	81%	breech 89% fetal distress 83% arrest of labor 77%
22. Amir W, Peter J, and Etan Z. Trial of labor without oxytocin in patients with a previous cesarean. *Am J Perinatol* 1987;4(2):140-143.	1982-84	261	46.8%	82.4%[14]	breech 93.3% fetal distress 75% CPD 66.6%
23. Stovall TG et al. Trial of labor in previous cesarean section patients, excluding classical cesarean sections. *Obstet Gynecol* 1987;70(5):713-717	1985-86	272	68.7%[18]	76.5%	nonrecurring 81% dystocia 77%[19]
24. Schneider J, Gallego D, and Benito R. Trial of labor after an earlier cesarean, a conservative approach. *J Reprod Med* 1988;33(5):453-456.	1980-84	339	58.6%	59.6%	breech 87% fetal distress 57% CPD/FTP 33%[21]
25. Duff P, Southmayd K, and Read JA. Outcome of trial of labor in patients with a single previous low transverse cesarean section for dystocia. *Obstet Gynecol* 1988;71(3 Pt 1):380-384.	1984-87	227	81%[22]	74%[23]	c-sec, not dystocia 81% c-sec, dystocia 68%[24,25]
26. Veridiano NP, Thorner NS, and Ducey J. Vaginal delivery after cesarean section. *In J Gynaecol Obstet* 1989;29(4):307-311.	1980-86	194	8.9%[27]	79%	—
27. Meehan FP and Burke G. Trial of labour following prior section; a 5 year prospective study (1982-1987) *Eur J Obstet Gynecol Reprod Biol* 1989;31:109-117.	1982-87	506	54%	78.6%	—

[12]Calculation shows 132 more women had oxytocin in the second time period, but VBAC rates were unchanged (82% versus 81%).

[13]Epidurals did not associate with either increased cesarean rates nor increased morbidity.

[14]Four out of 46 repeat cesareans were for "scar sensitivity," but no rupture was found

[15]"Not a single patient refused TOL when this possibility was offered."

[16]A table comparing other studies with this one shows oxytocin use "has only a limited value in increasing the success rate when used for augmentation." Perhaps a few repeat cesareans for CPD/FTP might have been prevented, but dehiscence rates in oxytocin-using studies tend to be higher compared with this study.

[17]"According to our data, [routine manual scar exploration] has limited, and questionable, clinical value."

[18]Percentage is of those eligible for TOL.

[19]Of those having VBAC after prior c-sec for dystocia, 37.3% had a bigger baby.

[20]VBAC with oxytocin 74% versus 85% without, VBAC with epidural 75% versus 86% without, VBAC with epidural + oxytocin 69% versus 86% with neither. [But did poor progress lead to oxytocin and increased pain to an epidural or did an epidural lead to poor progress and then to oxytocin?]

ELEC C-SEC AT MOTHER'S OPTION?	OXYTOCIN ?	EPIDURAL ?	EXCEPTIONS TO TYPICAL PROTOCOL EXCLUSIONS/ INCLUSIONS[b]	EXCEPTIONS TO TYPICAL PROTOCOL[c]
prenatal Y intrapartum —	1982-83 38%[12] 1983-84 48%[12]	Y[13]	included unknown scar and low vertical incision, 1983-84 included > 1 c-sec	none
N [15]	N[16]	18%	exclude membrane rupture and no labor and postdates because didn't use oxytocin	none[17]
prenatal Y intrapartum —	49%[20]	56%[20]	included > 1 c-sec and low vertical incision, if c-sec not done preterm	none
—	N	N	exclude "gross clinical CPD," membrane rupture and no labor, and prolonged pregnancy [no oxytocin]	2nd stage > 20 min led to assisted delivery under general anesthesia or c-sec, no IUPC.
N[22]	Y[26]	Y	exclude estimated fetal weight > 4500 g	none
prenatal Y intrapartum 6[28]	induced 2.5% augmen 2.5%	15%	include 21 > 1 c-sec, 43 unknown scar, 4 breech, and 2 multiple gestation	bladder catheter inserted
—	induced 25%[29] augmen 7%[29] PGE2 gel 10%	31.2%[29]	exception: 5 > 1 c-sec, 7 twin, 4 breech; exclude "recurring indication for section"	6 hrs active labor before c-sec, no IUPC, but continuous attendance by midwives[30]

[21] This dismal rate is attributed to not using oxytocin. [However, other studies achieved much better rates both overall and with prior CPD/FTP.]

[22] "We have demonstrated that, with appropriate counselling by a physicians who are positively oriented toward [VBAC], virtually all patients will consent to a trial of labor."

[23] Two out of 60 repeat cesareans were for "abdominal pain suggestive of uterine disruption," but the scars were intact.

[24] If the prior c-sec was for FTP in latent phase, the VBAC rate was 79%; if during active labor, it was 61%; if during second stage, it was 65%. [Note that the VBAC rate for latent phase arrest is similar to the rate for nonrecurrent indication. This strongly suggests that cesareans for dystocia in latent phase are highly likely to be unnecessary.]

[25] Even when the current baby exceeded the weight of the prior baby by $\geq$ 200 g, 50% of women had a VBAC.

[26] Oxytocin did not influence the incidence of complications.

[27] Over the time period, 2191 women had an elective cesarean.

[28] [If these women were excluded, the VBAC rate becomes 81%.]

[29] The maximum oxytocin dose was 40 mU/min. Of those having oxytocin, 80.3% had a VBAC. The VBAC rate for oxytocin + epidural was 81.6%.

[30] "We do not use intra-uterine catheters . . . they are invasive and therefore not without inherent risks."

Table 4.2 continued

STUDY	YEARS	# OF SUBJ	% POP HAVING TOL	VBAC RATE	EFFECT OF OBSTETRIC HISTORY[a]
28. Flamm BL et al. Vaginal birth after cesarean delivery: Results of a 5-year multicenter collaborative study. *Obstet Gynecol* 1990;76(5 Pt 1):750-754.	1984-89	5733[31]	38%[32]	74.8% [32,33]	breech 89% fetal distress 73% CPD/FTP 65%
29. Coltart TM, Davies JA, and Katesmark M. Outcome of a second pregnancy after a previous elective cesarean section. *Br J Obstet Gynecol* 1990; 97(12):1140-1143.	1980-87	195[37]	45%	79%	—
30. Nguyen TV et al. Vaginal birth after cesarean section at the University of Texas. *J Reprod Med* 1992;37(10):880-882.	1987-89	242	16.3%	76%[40,41]	breech 86% fetal distress 84% CPD/FTP 66%
31. Arulkumaran S, Chua S, and Ratnam SS. Symptoms and signs with scar rupture—value of uterine activity measurements. *Aust NZ Obstet Gynecol* 1992;32(3):208-212.	1985-90	722	70.9%	70%	—
32. Chua S et al. Trial of labour after previous caesarean section: obstetric outcome. *Aust NZ J Obstet Gynaecol* 1989;29(1):12-17. [subset of Abstract 29]	1985-88	207	68%	69%	nonrecurrent 73.4% recurrent 63.3%
33. Miller M and Leader LR. Vaginal delivery after caesarean section. *Aust NZ J Obstet Gynaecol* 1992;32(3):213-216.	1989-90	125	39%	64%[46]	breech 84% fetal distress 54% CPD 52%
34. Holland JG et al. Trial of labor after cesarean dellivery: experience in the non-university level II regional hospital setting. *Obstet Gynecol* 1992;79(6):936-939.	1987-90	A 85[49] B 52 286 C 149	A 40% B 7% 18% C 23%	A 81% B 79% 71% C 63%	—
35. Brody CZ et al. Vaginal birth after cesarean in Hawaii. Experience at Kapiolani Medical Center for Women and Children. *Hawaii Med J* 1993;52(2):38-42.	1990-91	483	64.6%	73.5%	—

[31]Eleven hospitals participated.

[32]TOL rates at the 11 hospitals ranged from 14%-63%.

[33]VBAC rates at the 11 hospitals ranged from 68%-89%. [Selectivity for TOL did not have much effect on VBAC rate.]

[34]The VBAC rate was 68%.

[35]However, data did not distinguish between epidurals given for pain relief and epidurals given in preparation for c-section.

[36]The VBAC rate was 69%.

[37]All had a prior scheduled cesarean.

[38]Those induced had a 62% VBAC rate versus 86% for those beginning labor spontaneously (OR 3.8, CI 1.9-7.8).

[39]Seventy-five percent of women with an epidural had VBACs.

[40]The incidence of third- and fourth-degree perineal tears was 36%. [!]

[41]With birth weight > 4000 g, the VBAC rate was 73%.

ELEC C-SEC AT MOTHER'S OPTION?	OXYTOCIN ?	EPIDURAL ?	EXCEPTIONS TO TYPICAL PROTOCOL EXCLUSIONS/ INCLUSIONS[b]	EXCEPTIONS TO TYPICAL PROTOCOL[c]
—	29%[34]	18%[35]	include 245 > 1 c-sec[36] and unknown scar	IUPC abandoned in last 3 years; most OBs and midwives no longer do manual scar exam
—	induced 30%[38] augmen 13%	73%[39]	none	—
—	27%[42]	29% [43]	include 7 > 1 c-sec	—
—	—	—	—	IUPC not always used[44]
—	induced 11%[45] augmen 36%[45]	6.2%	none	IUPC only used if oxytocin dose > 2.5 mU/min
prenatal Y intrapartum —	39.2%[47]	48.8%[48]	none	70.4% had continuous EFM
—	Y	Y	7 had low vertical incisions	—
—	induced 9.7%[50]	—	3 breech, 3 twin	—

[42]The VBAC rate with oxytocin was 84.6% versus 72.9% with no oxytocin. [This was an exception to the usual finding that oxytocin use lowered the VBAC rate.]

[43]The VBAC rate with epidural was 94.2% versus 68.6% without.

[44]In five cases of rupture, IUPC diagnosed only two.

[45]The VBAC rate was 70% whether oxytocin was used or not.

[46]VBAC rate with birth weight ≥ 4000 g was 66.6% versus 64.4% without. For 28 women who had X-ray pelvimetry, having adequate versus inadequate pelvic dimensions did not affect VBAC rate either.

[47]Oxtyocin use did not affect VBAC rates (63% with vs 65% without).

[48]The VBAC rate with an epidural was 78.7% versus 56.1% with no epidural.

[49]Three Mississippi Level II hospitals were compared.

[50]The VBAC rate when induced was 63.8% versus 73.7% "without oxytocin." [I think this means not induced but not necessarily not augmented.]

Table 4.3: VBAC Reports, Obstetrician Studies: Maternal Mortality And Morbidity[a] Related to Birth Route or Presence of Scar[b]

STUDY	MORTALITY	HEMORRHAGE[b] (%)	INFECTION[b] (%)	TRANSFUSION[b] (%)
13. Meier and Porreco 1982	0	—	VBAC 0 TOL C-sec 1 (3.1%) Elec C-sec[c] 10 (16.1%)	VBAC 0 TOL C-sec 0 Elec C-sec 1 (1.6%)
14. Whiteside, Mahan, and Cook 1983	—	—	—	—
15. Martin et al. 1983	0	VBAC 0 TOL C-sec 9 (14.8%) Elec C-sec[c] 57 (10.4%)	VBAC 1 (0.9%) TOL C-sec 10 (16.4%) Elec C-sec 54 (9.9%)	—
16. Eglington et al. 1984	Non-TOL 1[1]	—	—	—
17. Graham 1984[3]	0	VBAC 1 (0.6%) TOL C-sec —	—	—
18. Ngu and Quinn 1985	0	—	—	—
19. Jarrell, Ashmead, and Mann 1985	0	—	VBAC 4 (3%) TOL C-sec 39 (6.7%) Non-TOL 39 (6.7%)	—
20. Molloy, Sheil, and Duignan 1987	0	—	—	—
21. Phelan et al. 1987	TOL C-sec 1[7]	—	—	—
22. Amir, Peter, and Etan 1987	0	VBAC 3 (1.4%) TOL C-sec 0	—	0
23. Stovall et al. 1987	0	—	—	—
24. Schneider, Gallego, and Benito 1988	0	—	TOL 8 (2.4%)[11] Non-TOL 25 (10.5%)	—

[a]Placenta previa and accreta associate with presence of scar, and I did not count hysterectomy if it was for sterilization.

[b]Comparisons between studies are difficult because of differing definitions or subjective evaluation.

[c]"Elective C-sec" means the women would have been eligible for TOL.

[d]I presume this in two cases: (1) Other, lesser, maternal and/or infant morbidity were reported so surely these complications would have been reported had they occurred; or (2) the paper makes some general statement about finding no major morbidity.

[1]Placenta previa and accreta caused hemorrhage and then cardiac arrest.

[2]There was one rupture of vertical scar after precipitate preterm vaginal birth, four antepartum c-sec for placenta previa (3) or placenta previa + accreta (1), one for hemorrhage during c-sec.

[3]Morbidity for repeat cesarean was not given.

[4]The indication was "complications of bleeding" (uterine atony, placenta accreta, and broad ligament hematoma).

[5]Uterine ruptures: one baby died intrapartum, the other had severe cerebral palsy and died at 9 mos.

[6]Women who had both epidural and oxytocin were more likely to rupture than women who had neither ($p < 0.05$), but either variable alone did not increase likelihood of rupture.

RUPTURE (%)	SURGICAL INJURY (%)	HYSTERECTOMY (%)	OTHER MAJOR (%)
VBAC 0 TOL C-sec 0 Elec C-sec 0	VBAC 0 (3.1%) TOL C-sec 1 Elec C-sec 1 (1.6%)	VBAC 0 TOL C-sec 0 Elec C-sec 0	VBAC 0 TOL C-sec 1 (3.1%) Elec C-sec 4 (6.5%)
—	—	—	—
TOL 1 (0.6%) Elec C-sec 2 (0.3%)	—	—	VBAC 10 (16.4%) TOL C-sec 11 (10.9%) Elec C-sec 32 (5.9%)
—	—	TOL 0 Non-TOL 6 (1.1%)[2]	—
—	—	—	VBAC 3 (1.8%) TOL C-sec —
—	—	—	—
0	VBAC — TOL C-sec 1 (1.4%) Non-TOL 1 (0.1%)	VBAC 0 TOL C-sec 0 Non-TOL 3 (0.5%)[4]	—
TOL 8 (0.4%)[5,6] Non-TOL —	—	—	—
TOL 5 (0.3%)[8] Non-TOL 4 (0.5%)	—	VBAC 0 TOL 5 (0.3%)[9] Non-TOL 13 (1.5%)[9]	—
0	—	—	VBAC 4 (1.9%)
TOL 1 (0.4%)[10] Elect. C-sec 0	—	—	—
TOL 0[11] Non-TOL 3 (1.2%)[12]	—	TOL 0[11] Non-TOL 2 (0.8%)[12]	TOL 9 (2.7%)[11] Non-TOL 1 (0.4%)

[7]A c-sec for fetal distress led to pulmonary embolus.

[8]A fundal rupture occurred in a woman who had an intact transverse scar, baby died.

[9]Repeat c-sec: five for uterine atony; non-TOL: six for atony, 5 for placenta accreta.

[10]Despite internal EFM and IUPC, diagnosis of rupture was delayed 20 min. The baby recovered, and the rupture was repaired.

[11]Morbidity data did not distinguish between VBAC and repeat c-sec.

[12]Two near-term ruptures of vertical scars; a third rupture was also of vertical scar, but this baby recovered. The two ruptures that led to perinatal death also led to hysterectomies.

Table 4.3 continued

STUDY	MORTALITY	HEMORRHAGE[b] (%)		INFECTION[b] (%)		TRANSFUSION[b] (%)	
25. Duff, Southmayd, and Read 1988	0[d]	VBAC TOL C-sec Non-TOL —	No difference	VBAC 12 (7.2%) TOL C-sec 11 (18.3%) Non-TOL —		—	
26. Veridiano, Thorner, and Ducey 1989	0[d]	VBAC 2 (1.3%) TOL C-sec 0 Non-TOL —		—		—	
27. Meehan and Burke 1989	0	—		—		—	
28. Flamm et al. 1990[15]	Non-TOL 1[16]	—		—		—	
29. Coltart, Davies, and Katesmark 1990	0	—		—		—	
30. Nguyen et al. 1992	0	—		—		VBAC 2 TOL C-sec 1 Non-TOL —	1.2%[18]
31. Arulkumaran, Chua, and Ratnam 1992	0	0[d]		—		0[d]	
32. Chua et al. 1989 (subset Abstract 29)	0[d]	—		—		—	
33. Miller and Leader 1992	0	—		VBAC — TOL C-sec Non-TOL	No difference	VBAC — TOL C-sec Non-TOL	No difference
34. Holland et al. 1992	0	—		VBAC 6 (3%)[22] TOL C-sec 11 (13%) Non-TOL —		—	
35. Brody et al. 1993	0	—		—		—	

[13]An exploratory laparatomy for postpartum bleeding revealed a partial rupture.

[14]The rupture was repaired; the baby was healthy.

[15]The study only reported morbidity and mortality related to uterine rupture.

[16]A TOL was excluded because because the woman had two prior c-sec and was carrying twins. Uterine atony led to shock, disseminated intravascular coagulation, and death.

[17]Rupture rate was not broken down by type of scar. This study allowed both women with multiple c-sec and unknown scar type a TOL.

[18]In the VBAC group, two women had placenta accreta/percreta. One case caused rupture. Both had transfusions and a hysterectomy. One woman in the repeat cesarean group had uterine atonia leading to transfusion and hysterectomy.

[19][The article reported four "scar separations." One was secondary to placenta accreta and led to hysterectomy. Two were found at c-sec for fetal distress. These were symptomatic so I counted them as ruptures. The fourth was found incidentally during c-sec for failed forceps, and I did not count it.]

[20]Incidence of third- and fourth-degree perineal laceration. [I placed this under "Surgical Injury" because all followed an episiotomy, and deep tears rarely occur in the absence of episiotomy. This percentage is substantially higher than generally reported. (See Chapter 14.)]

RUPTURE (%)		SURGICAL INJURY (%)	HYSTERECTOMY (%)	OTHER MAJOR (%)
—		—	—	—
VBAC 1 (0.6%)[13]		—	0[d]	VBAC 1 (0.6%) TOL C-sec 0 Non-TOL —
TOL 1 (0.2%)[14] Non-TOL —		—	—	—
VBAC 2 TOL C-sec 8 Non-TOL —	0.7%[17]	—	TOL 2 (0.03%)[15] Non-TOL —	—
TOL 1 (0.5%) Non-TOL —		—	—	—
VBAC 1[18] TOL C-sec 2 Non-TOL —	1.2%[19]	VBAC 66 (36.1%)[20] TOL C-sec — Non-TOL —	VBAC 2 TOL C-sec 1 — 1.2%[18] Non-TOL —	—
VBAC 3 TOL C-sec 2 Non-TOL —	0.69%[21]	0[d]	0[d]	0[d]
TOL 0 Non-TOL —		—	—	—
TOL 1 (0.8%) Non-TOL 0		—	—	—
VBAC 1 (0.35%) TOL C-sec 0		—	VBAC 1 (0.35%)[23] TOL C-sec 0	—
?[24]		VBAC 29 (8.1%)[20,25]	—	—.

[21]Three women had symptoms only after vaginal birth. One of the repeat cesareans was the case where the baby died; the other was discovered incidentally during a cesarean for FTP.

[22]"Measures of morbidity" between VBAC and TOL c-sec were not different except for infection rates.

[23]Rupture led to hysterectomy.

[24]The article says there were five cases of "scar separation" (1.04%), but it never distinguishes between dehiscence and rupture or says what treatment was required except in one case that did not need repair.

[25]This is the incidence of deep perineal tears.

Table 4.4: VBAC Reports, Obstetrician: Perinatal Mortality and Morbidity[a] Related to Birth Route or Presence of Scar[b]

STUDY	PERINATAL MORTALITY	ADMIT INTENSIVE CARE (%)	BIRTH INJURY (%)	OTHER MAJOR (%)	
13. Meier and Porreco 1982	0	VBAC 0 TOL C-sec 0 Elec C-sec[c] 2 (3.2%)	0	0	
14. Whiteside, Mahan, and Cook 1983	—	—	—	—	
15. Martin et al. 1983	0	—	—	—	
16. Eglington et al. 1984	Non-TOL 2[1]	—	—	—	
17. Graham 1984[2]	0	—	0[d]	0[d]	
18. Ngu and Quinn 1985	0	—	—	—	
19. Jarrell, Ashmead, and Mann 1985	0	—	0[d]	0[d]	
20. Molloy, Sheil and Duignan 1987	TOL 2[3]	—	—	—	
21. Phelan et al. 1987	TOL 1[4] Non-TOL 2[5]	—	—	—	
22. Amir, Peter, and Etan 1987	0	—	0[d]	0[d]	
23. Stovall et al. 1987	0	—	—	—	
24. Schneider, Gallego, and Benito 1988	TOL 0 Non-TOL 2[6]	—	—	—	
25. Duff, Southmayd, and Read 1988	0[d]	—	—	VBAC TOL C-sec Non-TOL —	No difference in infection
26. Veridiano, Thorner, and Ducey 1989	0[d]	—	VBAC 1 (0.6%)[7]	0[d]	
27. Meehan and Burke 1989	0	—	—	—	
28. Flamm et al. 1990[8]	TOL 1[9]	—	—	—	
29. Coltart, Davies, and Katesmark 1990	TOL 1[10]	—	—	—	
30. Nguyen et al. 1992	0	—	—	—	
31. Arulkumaran, Chua, and Ratnam 1992	TOL 1[11]	—	—	—	

STUDY	PERINATAL MORTALITY	ADMIT INTENSIVE CARE (%)	BIRTH INJURY (%)	OTHER MAJOR (%)
32. Chua et al. 1989 (subset Abstract 29)	0[d]	—	—	—
33. Miller and Leader 1992	VBAC 2[12] TOL C-sec 1[12] Non-TOL 1[12]	VBAC 4 (5.1%)[12] TOL C-sec 1 (2.2%)[12] Non-TOL 8 (4.2%)[12]	—	VBAC 1 (1.3%)[12,13] TOL C-sec 1 (2.2%)[12,13] Non-TOL 1 (0.5%)[12,13]
34. Holland et al. 1992	—	—	—	—
35. Brody et al. 1993	—	—	—	—

[a]Placenta previa and accreta associate with presence of scar, and I did not count hysterectomy if it was for sterilization.

[b]Comparisons between studies are difficult because of differing definitions or subjective evaluation.

[c]"Elective C-sec" means the women would have been eligible for TOL.

[d]I presume this in two cases: (1) other, lesser, maternal and/or infant morbidity were reported so surely these complications would have been reported had they occurred; or (2) the paper makes some general statement about finding no major morbidity.

[1] There was one preterm rupture of vertical scar and one nonlabor term rupture of vertical scar.

[2]Morbidity for repeat cesarean was not given.

[3]Uterine ruptures: one baby died intrapartum; the other had severe cerebral palsy and died at 9 mos.

[4]A fundal rupture occurred in a woman who had an intact transverse scar, and the baby died.

[5]These were preterm uterine ruptures.

[6]There were two near-term ruptures of vertical scars;. A third rupture was also of vertical scar, but this baby recovered. The two ruptures that lead to perinatal death also led to hysterectomies.

[7]A midforceps delivery ended in shoulder dystocia and a fractured humerus. The baby recovered.

[8]The study only reported morbidity and mortality related to uterine rupture.

[9]The woman had two prior c-sec, incision type unknown. She arrived at the hospital fully dilated at 39 weeks, with a FHR of 55 bpm. The baby died, and a hysterectomy was necessary. The scar type could not be determined.

[10]The baby died when the scar ruptured during TOL.

[11]Scar pain and prolonged bradycardia occurred, but the c-sec was not done for 40 minutes. The baby had 1- and 5-minute Apgars of 1 and 2 and died on the third day. EFM was standard protocol.

[12][No information was given about the cause of mortality and morbidity so what percentage, if any, is attributable to birth route is unknown.]

[13]This was the neonatal seizure rate.

Table 4.5: VBAC Reports, Midwifery Studies

STUDY	YEARS	# OF SUBJ	% POP HAVING TOL	VBAC RATE	EFFECT OF OBSTETRIC HISTORY[a]
36. Wilf RT and Franklin JB. Six years' experience with vaginal births after cesareans at Booth Maternity Center in Philadelphia. *Birth* 1984;11(1):5-9.	1976-81 1980-81[1]	84 42[2]	44.7%	78.6% 78.6%[1,2]	—
37. Hangsleben KL, Taylor MA, Lynn NM. VBAC program in a nurse-midwifery service. Five years of experience. J Nurse Midwifery 1989;34(4):179-184.	1982-87	53	78%	83%	nonrecurrent 96% FTP 65%

[a]Effect of reason for prior for cesarean or prior vaginal birth on VBAC rate.

[b]Typical eligibility requirements for TOL: documented single low transverse uterine scar, singleton cephalic fetus.

[c] Typical TOL protocol: continuous EFM, intrauterine pressure catheter (IUPC), manual scar exploration. (IV and nothing by mouth were not commonly mentioned, but may be presumed since these are common policies for all laboring women.)

[1]The second set of numbers is a subset of the data that were analyzed in detail.

[2]Twenty-one out of 48 originally hoped for VBAC. Of them, seven were dissuaded by doctor when X-ray pelvimetry showed a small pelvis and three had a c-sec after 12 hours with ruptured membranes and no labor.

[3]If these are excluded, the VBAC rate becomes 84.6%.

Table 4.6: VBAC Reports, Midwifery Studies: Maternal Mortality and Morbitity[a] Related to Birth Route or Presence of Scar[b]

STUDY	MORTALITY	HEMORRHAGE[b] (%)	INFECTION[b] (%)	TRANSFUSION[b] (%)
36. Wilf and Franklin 1984	0	0[c]	TOL 1 (2.4%) Non-TOL —	0[c]
37. Hangsleben, Taylor, and Lynn 1989	0	0[c]	0[c]	0[c]

[a]Placenta previa and accreta associate with presence of scar, and I did not count hysterectomy if it was for sterilization.

[b]Comparisons between studies are difficult because of differing definitions or subjective evaluation.

[c]I presume this in two cases: (1) other, lesser, maternal and/or infant morbidity were reported so surely these complications would have been reported had they occurred; or (2) the paper makes some general statement about finding no major morbidity.

[1]This was a breakdown of episiotomy wound.

ELEC C-SEC AT MOTHER'S OPTION?	OXYTOCIN ?	EPIDURAL ?	EXCEPTIONS TO TYPICAL PROTOCOL EXCLUSIONS/ INCLUSIONS[b]	EXCEPTIONS TO TYPICAL PROTOCOL[c]
prenatal Y intrapartum 3[1,3]	–	–	1 multiple gestation, exclude small pelvis [1]	encourage walking, EFM intermittent, unlimited intake of ice chips, scar exam only in select cases, IV in active labor only
prenatal Y intrapartum –	induced Y[4] augmen 9.4%	none given	none	intermittent EFM, fluids and food allowed, episiotomy avoided,[5] heparin lock an option[6]

[4]The protocol allowed induction for postdates, but they didn't have any cases.

[5]Thirty percent had an intact perineum or first-degree tear, 56% had second-degree tear or episiotomy, and 14% had episiotomy extension.

[6]The emotional and psychological issues of VBAC were addressed in prenatal visits, VBAC classes, and during labor and the postpartum period.

RUPTURE (%)	SURGICAL INJURY (%)	HYSTERECTOMY (%)	OTHER MAJOR (%)
0[c]	0[c]	0[c]	0[c]
0[c]	0[c]	0[c]	VBAC 1 (2.3%)[1]

Table 4.7: VBAC Reports, Midwifery Studies: Perinatal Mortality and Morbidity[a] Related to Birth Route or Presence of Scar[b]

STUDY	PERINATAL MORTALITY	ADMIT INTENSIVE CARE (%)	BIRTH INJURY (%)	OTHER MAJOR (%)
36. Wilf and Franklin 1984	0	0[c]	0[c]	0[c]
37. Hangsleben, Taylor, and Lynn 1989	0	0[c]	0[c]	0[c]

[a]Placenta previa and accreta associate with presence of scar, and I did not count hysterectomy if it was for sterilization.

[b]Comparisons between studies are difficult because of differing definitions or subjective evaluation.

[c]I presume this in two cases: (1) other, lesser, maternal and/or infant morbidity were reported so surely these complications would have been reported had they occurred; or (2) the paper makes some general statement about finding no major morbidity.

EXCLUSIONS

Arguments for Liberal Inclusions When Selecting for TOL

Note: Some studies report TOL with breeches and twins, but the numbers are too small to draw conclusions.

38. Peterson CM and Saunders NJ. Mode of delivery after one caesarean section: audit of current practice in a health region. *BMJ* 1991;303(6806):818-821.

Data were analyzed for 1059 women with a prior history of one cesarean and no other births who had a singleton cephalic term baby during 1988 at one of 17 obstetric units. Of the women, 664 (63%) had TOL (range 35-77%) and 471 (71%) had a VBAC (range 47-87%). No significant correlation was found between the proportion allowed TOL and the VBAC rate. Although taller women and women with smaller babies during the prior pregnancy (average 300 g) were more likely to be allowed TOL, the difference in mean birth weight in the current pregnancy was only 70 g. "[B]irth weight in the previous pregnancy perhaps should not exert undue influence on subsequent management decisions." Units allowing longer labors had higher VBAC rates ($p < 0.05$), and units using more oxytocin for augmentation had a trend toward higher VBAC rates. VBAC rates in spontaneous and induced labors were similar (70.6% versus 74.4%), as were augmented and nonaugmented labors (73% versus 70%). Elective and repeat cesarean were associated with higher infection rates (14.7% and 16.0%) than VBAC (3.4%). One neonatal death occurred after a repeat cesarean for fetal distress. The scar was intact.

39. Rosen MG, Dickinson JC, and Westhoff CL. Vaginal birth after cesarean: a meta-analysis of morbidity and mortality. *Obstet Gynecol* 1991;77(3):465-470.

This meta-analysis analyzed 29 U.S. studies published between 1982 and 1989 to examine the association between prior factors and VBAC rate. A total of 8770 women had TOLs. The percentage accepted for TOL varied from 16% to 81% while VBAC rates varied from 54% to 89%. TOL and VBAC rates did not associate significantly. The average VBAC rate for women with a prior cesarean for CPD/FTP was 67%, prior breech 85%, prior vaginal birth 84%, more than one cesarean 75%, and oxytocin during prior labor 63%. Studies found short labors before the prior cesarean associated with higher VBAC rates. [Cesareans after short labors would be done either for reasons other than labor dystocia or would be labors terminated in latent phase and thus not true diagnoses of dystocia.] One study found dilation of more than 4 cm on admission associated with subsequent VBAC; another study did not. "[F]or almost any indication reviewed herein, there is greater than 50% chance for success. There appear to be no variables studied in this report for which success rates were so low that a [TOL] would be inappropriate patient care."

40. Pickhardt MG et al. Vaginal birth after cesarean delivery: are there useful and valid predictors of success or failure? *Am J Obstet Gynecol* **1992;166(6 Pt 1):1811-1819.**
Data on all women ($N = 312$) who underwent TOL during 1989 at a university hospital were analyzed to determine if variables could be found that would reliably predict VBAC. The VBAC rate was 63.1%. Although some factors significantly associated with VBAC, no clusters could be found that approached a clinically useful positive predictive value in the 80% to 100% range. "[I]t seems appropriate to encourage a [TOL] *in almost all* patients with prior low-segment incisions (transverse or vertical)."

Labor with a Multiple Scar (Review)

41. Roberts LJ. Elective section after two sections—where's the evidence? *Br J Obstet Gynaecol* **1991;98(12):1199-1202.**
Doctors generally assume that the adage "twice a cesarean, always a cesarean" is based on a body of evidence showing that scar rupture is more likely, but no such body exists. Personal opinion has been "quoted, misquoted and paraphrased." Pronouncements have been attributed to authorities who made no mention of the subject, and studies excluding women with more than one cesarean in order to create homogeneous groups were presumed to have done so because of proven concern about rupture. "There is no conclusive proof of an increased risk of scar dehiscence during labour after two caesarean sections and the manner in which we have come to believe that there is should be an embarrassment to all who consider obstetrics to be a scientific specialty." In fact, studies of TOL with more than one cesarean have found no increased risk and high VBAC rates even when one of the cesareans was for CPD.

Studies of Labor with Multiple Scar

(See Table 4.8 for Abstracts 42 through 47.)

Studies of Labor with Unknown Scar

48. Beall M et al. Vaginal delivery after cesarean section in women with unknown types of uterine scar. *J Reprod Med* **1984;29(1):31-35.**
Recent reports reflect a classical scar rate of only 5% to 10%, so offering TOL to

Table 4.8: Trial of Labor After More Than One Cesarean

STUDY	YEARS	# OF SUBJECTS	% POP HAVING TOL	VBAC RATE	VBAC RATE, ONE PRIOR C-SEC[c]
42. Porreco RP and Meier PR. Trial of labor in patients with multiple previous cesarean sections. *J Reprod Med* 1983;28(11):770-772.	1980-82	21 2 C-Sec 20 3 C-Sec 1	—	81%	85%
43. Farmakides G et al. Vaginal birth after two or more previous cesarean sections. *Am J Obstet Gynecol* 1987;156(3):565-566.	"since 1978"	57 2 C-sec 39 3 C-sec 18	—	77%	—
44. Pruett KM et al. Is vaginal birth after two or more cesarean sections safe? *Obstet Gynecol* 1988;72(2):163-165.	1984-86	55 2 C-sec 51 3 C-sec 4	—	45% 2 C-sec 45% 3 C-sec 50%	—
45. Phelan JP et al. Twice a cesarean, always a cesarean? *Obstet Gynecol* 1989;73(2):161-165.	1982-86	501 2 C-sec 501	46%[4]	69%	—
46. Novas J, Myers SA, and Gleicher N. Obstetric outcome of patients with more than one previous cesarean section. *Am J Obstet Gynecol* 1989;160(2):364-367.	1986-87	36 2 C-sec 27 3 C-sec 9	52%[11]	80% 2 C-sec 78% 3 C-sec 89%	71%
47. Hansell RS, McMurray KB, and Huey GR. Vaginal birth after two or more cesarean sections: a five-year experience. *Birth* 1990;17(3):146-150.	1983-87	35 2 C-sec 29 3 C-sec 5 4 C-sec 1	21%	77%[15] 2 C-sec 79% 3 C-sec 60% 4 C-sec 100%	—

[a]Prior indication for cesarean section or previous vaginal birth.

[b]Associated with birth route or the presence of cesarean scar, e.g., placenta previa and accreta associate with presence of scar and I did not count elective hysterectomy for sterilization.

[c]This rate was given for comparison among women at the same institution.

[1] The numbers were too small to analyze for effect of prior indication.

[2]The VBAC rate was 30% with oxytocin versus 64% when oxytocin not used.

[3]Both had a VBAC, postpartum bleeding, and a defective scar; one also had placenta accreta.

[4]The TOL rate rose from 10% in 1982-83 to 60% in 1985-86, but the VBAC was rate unchanged. [Whether cases were more carefully selected or the population was more broad-based did not affect VBAC rates.]

[5]Of 71 women with 2 prior c-sec for CPD/FTP, 56% had VBAC. [!]

[6]The dehiscence rate was 2.1% with oxytocin versus 1.4% with no oxytocin.

[7]The oxytocin rate (94% of which was for augmentation) increased from 22% to 57% over the years of the study, but the VBAC rate was not improved.

EFFECT OF OBSTETRIC HISTORY[a]	OXYTOCIN ?	EPIDURAL ?	MORTALITY[b]	MORBIDITY[b] RUPTURE (%)	HYSTERECTOMY (%)
5 of 17 VBAC had prior vag birth[1]	33%	19%	none	none	none
VBAC not dependent on prior indication	9%	—	none	none	none
—	55%[2]	yes	none	TOL 2 (3.6%)[3] non-TOL —	0
breech 77% CPD/FTP 60%[5] prior vag birth 81% no prior vag birth 67%	57%[6,7]	30%[8]	TOL 1 maternal[9]	TOL 0 non-TOL 1 (0.2%)	TOL 1 (0.2%)[10] non-TOL 7 (1.2%)[10]
4 of 15 with prior c-sec for dystocia had VBAC, 3 with bigger baby	yes	yes	non-TOL 2 perinatal[12]	TOL 1 (2%)[13] non-TOL —	TOL 0 non-TOL 2 (6%)[14]
breech 100% fetal distress 89% CPD/FTP 50%[16] prior vag birth[17] no prior vag birth[17]	—	—	none	TOL 0 non-TOL 1 (0.5%)[18]	TOL non-TOL 2 (1%)[18]

[8]Women having both oxytocin and an epidural had a 54% VBAC rate.

[9]This was a pulmonary embolism during c-sec for fetal distress.

[10]Six done for uterine atony, two for placenta accreta.

[11]Women with unknown scar were allowed TOL.

[12]This was a twin pregnancy in a woman with five prior cesareans. There was one fetal death at 31 weeks, and the doctors did a c-sec; the second baby died subsequently of necrotizing enterocolitis.

[13]The mother had two previous classical incisions. The scar was repaired. The baby was healthy.

[14] These were for placenta previa associated with placenta accreta.

[15]Two of eight c-sec were patient request during TOL. Remove them from the trial, and the VBAC rate becomes 82%.

[16]Three of seven women with a with prior c-sec for CPD had a VBAC with a bigger baby as did four women who had had repeat c-secs for CPD in addition.

[17]Among VBACs, 51.8% had a prior vaginal birth versus seven of eight repeat c-sec had no prior vaginal birth.

[18]There was one for placenta percreta and one for rupture of vertical scar at 33 wks.

women with unknown type of scar seemed reasonable. During 1980, 97 women at a Los Angeles hospital had TOL with one prior cesarean and unknown scar. During that year, of the 406 (48%) women with known scar type, 8% had vertical scars (5% fundal, 3% low vertical). A similar incidence was found at cesarean with unknown scar.

VBAC rates with unknown scar were similar to rates with documented transverse scar. Maternal morbidity and perinatal mortality rates were also similar, whereas women with known fundal (classical) scar had significantly higher rates. Of women with a classical scar, 13% developed a scar abnormality, including one preterm rupture with fetal death. A risk calculation predicts that given a 5% proportion of classical scars in the "unknown scar" population and a 50% fetal death and 5% maternal death rate upon rupture, the increased risks of TOL with unknown scar are similar to those of a planned cesarean over TOL. TOL with unknown scar is reasonable, but the labor must be intensively monitored and take place in a hospital capable of emergency cesarean.

49. Pruett KM, Kirshon B, and Cotton DB. Unknown uterine scar and trial of labor. *Am J Obstet Gynecol* **1988;159(4):807-810.**

Of 393 women undergoing TOL after one or more cesarean, 300 had unknown scar, 88 had documented low transverse incision, and 5 had prior low vertical incision. The VBAC rate (62% versus 52%, overall 59%), maternal and fetal morbidity rates, and scar dehiscence rates were no different compared with known prior transverse incision.

Oxytocin was used at the same rate in both groups (35% versus 33%), and no difference was found in VBAC rates or dehiscence rates between groups; however, the overall VBAC rate was lower compared with nonoxytocin labors (40% versus 70%, $p < 0.0001$). Fewer women who had a VBAC had endometritis ($p < 0.01$). One uterine rupture occurred in a woman at 36.5 weeks gestation being evaluated for labor. Fetal distress led to repeat cesarean. A hemorrhaging rupture of a vertical incision was found and repaired. The mother needed a transfusion; the baby was fine.

Studies of Labor with Macrosomic Baby

50. Phelan JP et al. Previous cesarean birth. Trial of labor in women with macrosomic infants. *J Reprod Med* **1984;29(1):36-40.**

The study group was 311 women with a previous cesarean who gave birth during 1980 or 1982-83 to a baby weighing 4000 g or more (mean birth weight 4308 ± 291 g, range 4000-5000 g). Of that group, 45% had TOL and 67% of women having a TOL had a VBAC compared with 83% of the non-macrosomic TOL group ($p < 0.01$). The VBAC rate for women having oxytocin (40%) was 58% versus 75% in the nonoxytocin group ($p < 0.05$). VBAC rates were increased by having prior VBAC (93%) and decreased by having the prior cesarean done for CPD (54%). Fetal distress rates were similar to the planned cesarean group. Dehiscence rates were similar to both the macrosomic planned-cesarean group and nonmacrosomic groups. One rupture occurred during labor; the scar was repaired, and the baby was fine.

51. Flamm BL and Goings JR. Vaginal birth after cesarean section: is suspected fetal macrosomia a contraindication? *Obstet Gynecol* **1989;74(5):694-697.**

Outcomes were compared among 301 women who had a TOL in 1984-85 with a macrosomic baby (> 4000 g), women having a TOL with a nonmacrosomic baby, and a control group with a macrosomic baby and intact uterus. Of the 301 women, 18 had more than one cesarean. VBAC rates for macrosomic versus nonmacrosomic babies were 55% versus 78% ($p < 0.001$). No significant differences were found in maternal or perinatal morbidity. In all three cases of uterine rupture, the baby was fine. Oxytocin was used in 35% of TOLs with macrosomia and 26% of TOLs with no macrosomia. When oxytocin was used, 45% of the macrosomic group had VBACs versus 69% of the nonmacrosomic TOL group. Significantly more control women [no number given] had vaginal births, but maternal and perinatal morbidity and mortality were similar.

The issue of TOL with a macrosomic baby hinges on the risk of rupture and the likelihood of VBAC. This study found no increased risk of rupture, and the majority of women had a VBAC. Pooling five studies [including Phelan et al., Abstract 50, and this one] shows that for 807 TOLs with macrosomic babies, the VBAC rate was 69%. Moreover, neither ultrasound nor palpation reliably predicted macrosomia. Discouraging women with suspected macrosomia will prevent many women with normal-weight babies from pursuing VBAC.

Study of Labor with Postterm Pregnancy

52. Yeh S, Huang X, and Phelan JP. Postterm pregnancy after previous cesarean section. *J Reprod Med* **1984;29(1):41-44.**
Data from all women with prior cesarean and postdates pregnancy (> 42 wks) during 1979-82 ($N = 112$) were analyzed. Of the 112, 38.4% were judged to have "good obstetric dates" and the rest to have "poor obstetric dates." Thirty-four women (30.4%) had an elective cesarean, and 78 (69.6%) had TOL. All TOLs were spontaneous labor. ("Many obstetricians consider induced labor and forced delivery done solely on the basis of postterm pregnancy to carry more risk than does the postterm condition itself.") Of the TOL group, 57 (73.1%) had a VBAC. For the 25 women whose prior cesarean was for CPD, the rate was 64%. The incidence of macrosomia was 25%, and 46.4% of TOLs with a macrosomic baby ended in VBAC. Perinatal morbidity was similar between TOL and planned cesarean groups. Postterm pregnancy with prior cesarean "can be managed exactly as postterm pregnancy in women who have not had prior C/Ss."

Studies of the Predictability of Pelvimetry

53. Krishnamurthy S et al. The role of postnatal X-ray pelvimetry after caesarean section in the management of subsequent delivery. *Br J Obstet Gynaecol* **1991;98(7):716-718.**
Between 1977 and 1982 331 women who had a cesarean had postnatal pelvimetry and subsequently gave birth in the same hospital; 248 (75%) of them were found to have a "radiologically inadequate pelvis." TOL was planned in 68 women of this group, and in the end eight additional women with inadequate pelvis also had a TOL because the obstetrician "questioned the value of postnatal pelvimetry." The other 180 had planned elective cesareans, and for 139 of these, the decision was made on pelvimetry alone. TOL was also planned for 79 of 83 of the women judged to have an adequate pelvis. The VBAC rate for women with inadequate pelvis (67%) was not significantly different from that of women having TOL with adequate pelvis (77%). "The fallibility of pelvimetry is demonstrated by our study. . . . Pelvimetry . . . is a static examination

which does not take account of changes in pelvic and fetal dimensions during labour and delivery."

54. Thubisi M et al. Vaginal delivery after previous caesarean section: is X-ray pelvimetry necessary? *Br J Obstet Gynaecol* **1993;100(5):421-424.**
Women with one prior transverse cesarean were randomly and evenly allocated to have X-ray pelvimetry at 36 weeks or to have it postpartum (controls) ($N = 288$). Among women undergoing prenatal pelvimetry, 42% were judged to have an "inadequate" pelvis versus 38% among controls. All women in the pelvimetry group with this diagnosis had elective cesareans. Among control women, 60% of those judged inadequate postpartum had vaginal births. "Routine antepartum [X-ray pelvimetry] should . . . be abandoned."

LABOR PROTOCOL ISSUES

Labor Takes Longer

55. Harlass FE and Duff P. The duration of labor in primiparas undergoing vaginal birth after cesarean delivery. *Obstet Gynecol* **1990;75(1):45-47.**
Each woman who had a VBAC after prior cesarean for labor dystocia ($N = 73$) was matched to two control women: a nulliparous woman and a woman who had a prior uncomplicated vaginal birth. Matching factors were maternal age, epidural anesthesia, race, and gestational age. Among study women, 36 had the prior cesarean during latent-phase labor, 29 during active phase, and 8 during second stage. All study women had term labors of spontaneous onset, and none had complications that might influence labor length. Labor was spontaneous among control women, except when oxytocin was needed to correct hypocontractility due to an epidural.
Women who had a prior cesarean during latent phase had longer first-stage labors (765 ± 310 min) compared with women having the prior cesarean in active labor (667 ± 280 min) or second stage (555 ± 366 min). In all cases the length of first stage during TOL was more like nulliparous controls (645 ± 288 min) than multiparous controls (412 ± 211 min). "Accordingly, obstetricians must revise their expectations and not anticipate that these individuals will progress as rapidly in labor as women who previously had vaginal deliveries."

56. Chazotte C, Maden R, and Cohen WR. Labor patterns in women with previous cesareans. *Obstet Gynecol* **1990;75(3 Pt 1):350-355.**
Women having TOL ($N = 68$) were matched to nulliparous and multiparous controls by taking the next birth of the appropriate parity with a birth weight within 200 g of the study infant. When labor curve characteristics were analyzed, women having no history of previous vaginal birth were indistinguishable from nulliparous controls and those with previous vaginal birth were indistinguishable from multiparous contols. In addition, women with no prior vaginal birth had labor disorder frequencies not significantly different from nulliparous women, and women with prior vaginal birth had similar frequencies to multiparous women. Oxytocin and epidural use were not randomly distributed, but excluding these cases yielded similar results. These data are important

because if all women undergoing TOL are judged by multiparous standards, labor dysfunction would be overdiagnosed, which could lead to unnecessary repeat cesareans or oxytocin use.

[The authors also note that of the 13 women who had repeat cesarean for "dystocia," eight "had no labor dysfunctions that could be documented on retrospective review." In most cases, TOL was abandoned in latent labor.]

Labor with Oxytocin

(See Table 4.9 for Abstracts 57 through 62.)

Intrauterine Pressure Catheter Is Unnecessary

63. Rodriguez MH et al. Uterine rupture: are intrauterine pressure catheters useful in the diagnosis? *Am J Obstet Gynecol* **1989;161(3):666-669.**
Of 76 women with uterine rupture (defined as "complete separation of the wall of the ... uterus with or without expulsion of the fetus, which endangered the life of the mother and/or fetus"), 8 women went directly to surgery upon admission (group A), 29 had external tocodynamometry [measurement of contraction pressure using the EFM belt] only (group B), and 39 had IUPC (group C). In one case in group A and two in group C, diagnosis of rupture was made at the time of cesarean for other reasons. The most common sign of rupture was fetal distress (78% of cases). No woman in labor, including those with IUPC, showed loss of uterine tone or cessation of labor, which means IUPC was not useful in diagnosing rupture. Maternal and fetal morbidity were higher in group A but similar for groups B and C, which means that IUPC did not improve outcomes. "The usefulness of the [IUPC] in making the diagnosis of uterine rupture is not supported by this study."

Manual Exploration of Scar Is Unnecessary

64. Gemer O, Segal S, and Sassoon E. Detection of scar dehiscence at delivery in women with prior cesarean section. *Acta Obstet Gynecol Scand* **1992;71(7):540-542.**
The records were reviewed for 1023 women who gave birth between 1985 and 1991 after one or more cesareans. The scar was observed during all cesarean sections and manually examined after all VBACs. Rupture was defined as a scar separation accompanied by fetal distress or hemorrhage. One woman had a rupture (0.15%). Routine transcervical examination revealed two suspected cases, but only one was confirmed at laparotomy [which means the other woman had unnecessary surgery].

As has been found elsewhere, more dehiscences were found during surgery, which implies that transcervical examination misses some dehiscences. Others, too, have failed to confirm scar separation at laparotomy in more than half the cases. [Therefore, manual examination is neither sensitive nor specific.] Asymptomatic defects have been left untreated, with no apparent problems. Routine manual examination has questionable prognostic value for future pregnancies. Moreover, transcervical examination is invasive and may increase the risk of infection or convert a dehiscence into a true rupture. "Thus, when viewed with respect to the yield and potential benefits, the value of routine examination becomes doubtful."

Table 4.9: Trial of Labor Using Oxytocin

STUDY	YEARS	# OF SUBJECTS (%)[a]	VBAC RATE WITH OXYTOCIN
57. Horenstein JM et al. Oxytocin use during trial of labor in patients with previous cesarean section. *J Reprod Med* 1984;29(1):26-30.	1980	58 (20%) induc 21% augmn 79%	53% – –
58. Horenstein JM and Phelan JP. Previous cesarean section: The risks and benefits of oxytocin usage in a trial of labor. *Am J Obstet Gynecol* 1985;151(5):564-569.	1982-83	289 (40%) induc 11% augmn 89%	69%[2] induc 72% augmn 69%
59. Lao TT and Leung BF. Labor induction for planned vaginal delivery in patients with previous cesarean section. *Acta Obstet Gynecol Scand* 1987;66(5):413-416.	1980-83	137 (21%)[3] induc 100% augmn 0%	82%
60. Silver RK and Gibbs RS. Predictors of vaginal delivery in patients with a previous cesarean section, who require oxytocin. *Am J Obstet Gynecol* 1987;156(1):57-60.	1983-85	98 (?%) induc 35% augmn 65%	59%[5] induc 53% augmn 63%
61. Flamm BL et al. Oxytocin during labor after previous cesarean: results of a multicenter study. *Obstet Gynecol* 1987;70(5):709-712.	1984-85	485 (27%)[7] induc 35% augmn 65%	64%[8] induc 56% augmn 69%
62. Sakala EP et al. Oxytocin use after previous cesarean: Why a higher rate of failed labor trial? *Obstet Gynecol* 1990;75(3):356-359.	1984-86	73 (31%) induc 66% augmn 34%	68%[10] induc 58% augmn 88%

[a]The number in parenthesis shows what percentage of all women having TOL this number of subjects represents.

[1]The increase was significant, but the *p* value was not given.

[2]The VBAC rate was higher in women who had a prior vaginal birth. If a woman had a prior cesarean for CPD/FTP or fetal distress, VBAC was less likely if she required oxytocin.

[3]If the Bishop score [a scoring system for cervical readiness] was less than 4, vaginal prostaglandin gel was used. The overall hospital induction rate was 31.1% [!]. The most common indication for induction was postmaturity (43.1%).

[4][There was no discussion of whether the difference was significant.]

[5]A nonrecurrent indication for the prior cesarean favored VBAC among both augmented and induced women. Prior vaginal birth favored VBAC only among augmented women (86% VBAC). Of 62 women carrying larger infants than

REFERENCES

ACOG. Vaginal birth after cesarean section. Report of a 1990 survey of ACOG's membership. 1990.

———. Guidelines for vaginal delivery after a previous cesarean birth. *ACOG Committee Opinion* 1988; No 64.

Enkin M. Labour and delivery after previous caesarean section. In *A guide to effective care in pregnancy and childbirth.* Enkin M, Keirse MJNC, and Chalmers I, eds. Oxford: Oxford University Press, 1989.

Feldman GB and Freiman JA. Prophylactic cesarean section at term? *N Engl J Med* 1985;312(19):1264-1267.

VBAC RATE NO OXYTOCIN	MAXIMUM OXYTOCIN RATE	INCREASED MORBIDITY COMPARED WITH NO OXYTOCIN ?
84%	22 mU/min	increase in postpartum hemorrhage (32% vs 16%) and transfusion (16% vs 4%) not related to scar separation[1]
89%	22 mU/min	increase in dehiscence (3.1% vs 1.4%, NS), more c-sec for fetal distress in no oxytocin group (P < 0.05), more hemorrhage during repeat c-sec in no oxytocin group
87%	64 mU/min	increase in postpartum hemorrhage (6% vs 0)[4]
—	64 mU/min[6]	no comparison group of no oxytocin TOLs
78%[9]	20 mU/min	no difference in rates of rupture, dehiscence, or hysterectomy
89%	24 mU/min	no difference in rates of dehiscence, rupture, transfusion, or infection

in the prior delivery, 30 had VBACs.

[6]In 26% of cases, oxytocin was stopped or reduced because of hypercontractility, abnormal fetal heart rate, or both.

[7]Induction with oxytocin is recommended for postdates or rupture of membranes instead of elective c-section. [Why not just watch and wait for spontaneous labor (see Chapter 9?)]

[8]The VBAC rate was higher if the prior cesarean was for breech and lower if it was for FTP.

[9]If the prior cesarean was for FTP, 54% had a VBAC with oxytocin and 70% had a VBAC if no oxytocin was used.

[10]When cesareans for failed induction were excluded, the proportions of other indications for repeat cesarean were the same as in the no oxytocin group. "Successful trial of labor may be enhanced by awaiting spontaneous labor or inducing with a favorable cervix."

Flamm BL. *Birth after cesarean: The medical facts.* New York: Simon and Schuster, 1990.

Flamm B, MacDonald D, Shearer E, Mahan CS. Roundtable discussion: Should the electronic fetal monitor always be used for women in labor who are having a vaginal birth after a previous cesarean section? *Birth* 1992;19(1):31-35.

Jones RO et al. Rupture of low transverse cesarean scars during trial of labor. *Obstet Gynecol* 1991;77(6):815-817.

Joseph GF, Stedman CM, and Robichaux AG. Vaginal birth after cesarean section: the impact of patient resistance to a trial of labor. *Am J Obstet Gynecol* 1991;164(6 Pt 1):1441-1447.

Kirk EP et al. Vaginal birth after cesarean or repeat cesarean section: medical risks or social realities? *Am J Obstet Gynecol* 1990;162(6):1398-1405.

Kline J and Arias F. Analysis of factors determining the selection of repeated cesarean section or trial of labor in patients with histories of prior cesarean delivery. *J Reprod Med* 1993;38(4):289-292.

Laufer A et al. Vaginal birth after cesarean section. Nurse-midwifery management. *J Nurse Midwifery* 1987;32(1):41-47.

Lomas J, et al. Opinion leaders vs audit and feedback to implement practice guidelines. *JAMA* 1991;265(17):2202-2207.

McClain CS. Patient decision making: the case of delivery method after a previous cesarean section. *Cult Med Psychiatry* 1987;11(4):495-508.

NACC. Standards Committee Opinion on Vaginal Birth After Cesarean Section. 1992.

"News." *Birth* 1994;21(2):114.

Norman P, Kostovcik S, and Lanning A. Elective repeat cesarean sections: how many could be vaginal births? *Can Med Assoc J* 1993;149(4):431-435.

Porreco RP. Commentary: the twice-wounded uterus. *Birth* 1990;17(3):150-151.

Scott JR. Mandatory trial of labor after cesarean delivery: an alternative viewpoint. *Obstet Gynecol* 1991;77(6):811-814.

Shapiro MC et al. Information control and the exercise of power in the obstetrical encounter. *Soc Sci Med* 1983;17(3):139-146.

Shearer E. Interview with author. 1989.

Taffel SM et al. 1989 U.S. cesarean section rate steadies—VBAC rate rises to nearly one in five. *Birth* 1991;18(2):73-77.

U.S. Department of Health and Human Services. Rates of cesarean delivery—United States, 1991. *MMWR* 1993;42(15):285-289.

5

Labor Dystocia, Failure to Progress, Cephalopelvic Disproportion, and Active Management

> Myth: *I'm afraid labor just isn't progressing the way it should.*
>
> Reality: *"[I]t does not appear that liberal use of oxytocin augmentation in labour is of benefit....This does not imply that there is no place for oxytocin augmentation in slow progress of labour. It does suggest, however, that other simple measures, such as allowing the woman freedom to move around, and to eat and drink as she pleases, may be at least as effective and certainly more pleasant for a sizeable proportion considered to be in need of augmentation of labour."*
>
> Crowther et al. 1989

In a western movie parody on Sid Caesar's "Show of Shows" the stagecoach is being pursued by a band of marauding Indians. It looks as if the passengers are doomed when suddenly the cavalry charge rings out. "We're saved!" rejoice the passengers. Sid Caesar looks out the window. "Nope," he deadpans, "it's just an Indian with a bugle."

American women are like the stagecoach passengers when it comes to labor dystocia (difficult labor)* the major reason for the rise in primary [first-time] cesareans. Obstetricians are pursuing women with scalpels, and "active management of labor," the proposed solution, far from rescuing them, is an Indian with a bugle.

The principles of active management were developed in the 1970s at the National Maternity Hospital in Dublin, Ireland (O'Driscoll and Meagher 1986). It encompassed the following protocol:

---

*In the interest of brevity I will use *labor dystocia* to encompass cephalopelvic disproportion (CPD) and failure to progress (FTP). All mean the baby is not coming out within someone's idea of a reasonable time.

- Diagnosis of labor is based on either painful contractions and complete cervical effacement or rupture of membranes. Painful contractions alone are not enough. Women deemed not in labor are not admitted to the labor unit.

- One hour after admission, progress is assessed and amniotomy (artificial rupture of membranes) performed.

- Thereafter cervical dilation must advance by at least 1 cm per hour. Otherwise, providing amniotic fluid is clear and the fetus correctly positioned, an oxytocin intravenous (IV) drip is started and the number of drops per minute is increased until the mother has 5 to 7 contractions every 15 minutes.

- Maximum labor length is 12 hours (10 hrs to dilate 10 cm, 2 hrs to push out the baby), although a cesarean is not mandatory at the cutoff point.

- A midwife stays with each woman throughout labor to monitor the labor and encourage the mother.

- The midwives manage labor; senior staff are available for consultation; residents do not make decisions.

- Induction of labor is rare. Labor is induced by amniotomy. If labor does not begin spontaneously within 24 hours, an oxytocin drip is started and labor is managed as above.

- Pain medication is available but is discouraged. (The doctors decided women can bear the pain if they know labor length is limited.)

The cesarean section rate with this program hovers around 4%, although, as a graph shows but the text omits, this is slightly higher than the preprotocol rate.

A rising cesarean rate for dystocia was not at issue, but the Maternity Hospital physicians were frustrated by waiting out "the tedious hours" of slow labors. "Efficient uterine action," they decided, "was the key to normality." Any woman who did not progress at the statistical mean of 1 cm per hour dilation should be given oxytocin to correct her problem. At one stroke, mere deviation from average became pathological, and a philosophical basis was created for devising a protocol to force all primiparous labors to conform to the average (multiparous women laboring slowly were perceived to have problems with fit rather than drive).

Achieving this goal meant giving 40% of women oxytocin (Boylan 1989). Of course, if 40% of women need oxytocin to progress normally, then something is wrong with the definition of normal, but this point escaped the Dublin doctors and all advocates of active management since.

The Dublin Maternity Hospital doctors were delighted with a program that gave them the ability to control what they saw as a disconcertingly haphazard and uncertain process. They presumed mothers to be equally delighted because they were guaranteed labor would not exceed 12 hours and they would never be left alone. They never tested their theory, though, and clearly they have no idea what women want. They were, for example, "surprised" when one of their studies revealed women prefer vaginal to rectal exams to check labor progress.

They might have been more surprised if they had asked women whether they liked active management or would rather be left in peace to have less painful, albeit longer, labors. Crowther et al. (1989) report that a study of women's opinions of oxytocin augmentation found 80% of mothers said labor hurt more and over half would not want it again. Penny Simkin (1986) surveyed 159 new mothers and found that 76% of them said oxytocin drips were stressful and 46% said the same of amniotomy. Vaginal exams were rated "stressful" by 56% of the women. Rectal exams, the norm in Dublin, would presumably be worse. For 55% and 61%, respectively, external and internal electronic fetal monitoring (EFM), standard in the U.S. when giving oxytocin, was stressful. Restriction to bed stressed 64% of women, and restricting movement in bed, sometimes required with external EFM or IVs, stressed 77%.

In any case, it never mattered what women thought. Women rank as "privates" in the Dublin scheme of "military efficiency with a human face." They are to take orders, not make a fuss, and not disrupt the labor unit by making "the degrading scenes that occasionally result from the failure of a woman to fulfill her part of the contract" (O'Driscoll and Meagher 1986). Indeed, one reason given for tying the oxytocin drip to number of contractions is to prevent soft-hearted nurses from turning down the drip when women complain of the pain. The real boon of active management accrues to the hospital: "The newfound ability to limit the duration of stay has transformed the previously haphazard approach to planning [staffing] for labor."

Unlike Dublin, where the cesarean rate remained low, in the U.S., as we have seen, the cesarean rate soared from 5% in 1970 to 24% by 1986. Dystocia was responsible for 29% of the increase (Taafel, Placek, and Kosary 1992; Wolfe and Jones 1991).

As we have seen, American obstetricians came to believe that cesareans were safe and necessary, guaranteed good infant outcome, and would protect them if they were sued (Rosen and Thomas 1989), whereas dystocia plus oxytocin plus bad outcome was likely to equal successful malpractice suit (Cetrulo and Cetrulo 1987). Furthermore, cesareans were time efficient and (usually) more remunerative.

Consider how these factors subtly affect decision making: Let us say it is evening. The patient arrived in labor this morning; she has not progressed beyond 3 cm dilation since having her epidural; and one hour on an oxytocin drip has not helped. If the doctor ends up doing the delivery in the middle of the night, he or she will be tired for tomorrow's surgeries and office hours. Guess what happens next.

Still, even diehard cesarean apologists do not try to defend a 24% cesarean rate, so when active management appeared, American doctors jumped at it. Here was a protocol that promised to allow them to continue business as usual without paying for it with a high cesarean rate.

Unfortunately, the only pieces of the program that survived the Atlantic crossing were routine amniotomy, the liberal use of oxytocin, and the time limit on labor. Other parts—the continuous support of an experienced woman, that residents did not make decisions, the minimal use of epidurals (5%), the minimal use of induction (< 10%), not using painful contractions as the sole diagnosis of labor—did not make it, and all of these elements are likely to contribute to better labor pattern and/or fewer cesareans. Moreover, the Dublin doctors expected women to give birth vaginally, a belief they imparted to their patients. With one in four American women having a cesarean, clearly neither American obstetricians nor their patients had this same confidence.

Does active management reduce the cesarean rate for dystocia outside Dublin? Yes (Boylan 1989) and no. Obviously, when more labors are forced to fit unrealistic notions of labor length, fewer cesareans will be performed for labors exceeding the time limit. And if doctors believe active management works and convince their patients of that, the placebo effect and their bias will make it a self-fulfilling prophecy.

However, as the abstracts show, active management is not always successful—or as successful as it has been in Dublin—and it has risks. Turner, Brassil, and Gordon (1988) report a neonatal death caused when, contrary to protocol, an oxytocin drip was continued despite fetal distress. In fact, quite unnoticed by themselves or anyone else, the Dublin doctors hang active management with their own evidence (MacDonald et al. 1985). The Dublin randomized controlled trial of EFM reported that three babies delivered by forceps for prolonged second stage died of their forceps injuries. They also found that neonatal seizures associated both with labor longer than five hours and oxytocin use. In 19 of 24 longer labors that resulted in newborn seizures, oxytocin was used.

Active management may be better than what it replaces, but that proves nothing but how injurious typical obstetric management is. It does not mean something else will not work equally well. Even among proponents of active management, waiting one more hour before starting an oxytocin drip led to an equally low cesarean rate and half the number of augmentations (Arulkumaran et al. 1987, abstracted below). Based on their study of amniotomy and oxytocin, Seitchik, Holden, and Castillo (1985) argue that 1 cm per hour progress is too rigid a standard and that oxytocin should not be used until two hours with no progress. *But the real point is active management is not needed at all.* Midwives also maintain 4% cesarean rates simply by leaving most women alone (Rooks et al. 1989).

Obstetricians do not take a leaf from the midwives' book because passive management does not appeal to them. As one obstetrician sniffed of watchful waiting during slow labors, "[T]he authorities . . . are preaching a gospel of obstetric conservatism that is not much more than midwifery" (Wright 1983). The average obstetrician will always choose doing something over doing nothing or having the mother do something. It is telling that *not one study* looking to reduce the cesarean rate for dystocia (other than one small pilot study of walking versus oxytocin—Read, Miller, and Paul 1981, abstracted below) compared active management to an approach advocating patience, allowing women freedom of activity and behavior, offering supportive rather than interventive care, and discouraging pain medication.

Sheila Kitzinger (1990), commenting on active management, offered insight into its hidden agenda. The medicalization of birth, she said, denies and suppresses female sexuality, which obstetricians perceive to be dangerous, threatening, and disruptive. By viewing women as defective machines to be managed on the fetus's behalf, by draining the warmth and sensuality out of the experience, by converting it to a timetable-driven mechanical process, by becoming the central figure in the drama and controlling every aspect of the mother's behavior and activities down to the sounds she may make, birth comes to feel safe to the doctor.

Kitzinger pleads for the midwifery approach: help women find their own way. Help them confront their fears and master them. Let them experience this powerful, creative female force. The greatest obstacle to this process and the most invasive and potentially dangerous technology (because from it proceeds all the others) is not a new invention. It is the clock.

SUMMARY OF SIGNIFICANT POINTS

- True cephalopelvic disproportion (the baby too big to pass through the mother's pelvis) is rare. (Abstracts 1-4, 15)

- The diagnosis of dystocia and the decision to perform a cesarean are highly subjective and are influenced by many factors that have nothing to do with the mother. (Abstracts 3, 5, 9, 12, 15, 17-19, 21-22, 37)

- Mismanagement and callousness play a role in some cesareans for dystocia. They may be covered up by lying. (Abstracts 8, 15, 18, 22)

- Induction leads to cesareans. (Abstracts 8, 14-15, 17-19, 28)

- Longer than average labor does not cause fetal distress. (Abstracts 4, 23)

- The indiscriminate use of oxytocin does no good and may harm the baby. Active management is overkill. (Abstracts 3-4, 8, 14, 20, 23-28)

- (Barring medical problems), if contractions are not getting longer, stronger, and closer together as well as being painful, women should stay home. Once the woman is admitted to hospital, impatience if progress is not made can lead to unnecessary intervention and possibly a cesarean section for dystocia. (Abstracts 13-14, 16)

- Excessive stress (which may be caused by the atmosphere, interruptions, and procedures of typical hospital management) inhibits labor. (Abstracts 13, 30, 36)

- Mobility and avoidance of supine (on the back) positions help rotate posterior presentations (baby facing mother's belly), thus improving labor progress. (Abstracts 29, 31)

- Upright positions improve contraction quality and promote progress without fetal risk or additional pain. They also reduce the need for pain medication and oxytocin. Oxytocin works too, but it increases pain. (Abstracts 31-33, 35-37)

- Varying position improves contraction quality. (Abstract 34)

- Upright positions for pushing shorten second stage, increase spontaneous birth rate, increase comfort, and protect the perineum from injury. (Abstracts 37-39)

- Epidural anesthesia associates suspiciously with delayed progress, oxytocin, and cesarean for dystocia.* (Abstracts 6, 10, 21)

ORGANIZATION OF ABSTRACTS

Note: Because cesarean rates vary markedly from country to country, I have added the country of origin in the citation.

Dystocia as a State of Mind

Birth Weight Does Not Matter
Factors Having Nothing to Do with the Mother Matter
The Convenience Factor
The Role of Impatience

Induction Leads to Cesarean Section

High-Dose Oxytocin Augmentation Is Not a Panacea

It Does Not Always Work
Other Regimens Work Equally Well

*According to report, the cesarean rate at Dublin Maternity Hospital has risen concomitant with an increase in the use of epidurals.

DYSTOCIA AS A STATE OF MIND

Birth Weight Does Not Matter

1. Sokol RJ, et al. Risks preceding increased primary cesarean birth rates. *Obstet Gynecol* **1982;59(3):340-346.** (U.S.)

Looking at the risks associated with cesarean birth for 2744 women, neither birth weight over 4000 g (8 lb 13 oz) nor birth weight over 4500 g (9 lb 14 oz) increased the relative risk of cesarean. Ninety percent of babies weighing 4001-4500 g were born vaginally as were 87% of babies weighing over 4500 g. Nineteen percent of labors were augmented. The total cesarean rate was 13.9%, and the primary cesarean rate was 9.3%.

2. Turner MJ et al. The influence of birth weight on labor in nulliparas. *Obstet Gynecol* **1982;76(2):159-163.** (Ireland)

An analysis of the influence of birth weight on delivery route among 1000 term nulliparas with a single cephalic fetus showed that increasing birth weight associated with cesarean section for dystocia. Even so, 91.7% of babies weighing 4000 to 4499 g were born vaginally, as were 86.4% of babies weighing over 4500 g. The overall cesarean rate was 5.2%.

Factors Having Nothing to Do with the Mother Matter

Note: Whether the cesarean benefits the doctor (more money or sleep) or the mother (fewer emergency services at night), the result for the mother is the same: a cesarean instead of more time for labor.

3. Sheehan KH. Caesarean section for dystocia: a comparison of practices in two countries. *Lancet* **1987;1(8532):548-551.** (Ireland and the U.S.)

Outcomes were compared between Irish ($N = 569$) and American ($N = 471$) populations of nulliparous, white, low-risk women for the years 1980-82. The Irish had more amniotomies (51.6% versus 44.8%, $p < 0.03$), more oxytocin augmentations (48.8% versus 24.0%, $p < 0.001$), and less epidural anesthesia (0 versus. 15.0%, [no p given]). This resulted in shorter mean labor length (6.8 hr versus 9.3 hr, $p < 0.001$), fewer labors exceeding 12 hours (8.1% versus 24.7%, $p < 0.001$), fewer cesareans (5.6% versus 12.3%, $p < 0.01$), and fewer cesareans for CPD (1.7% versus 11.0%, $p < 0.001$). The cesarean rate nearly doubled (20%) for American women who went beyond 41 weeks gestation, but postdates had little effect on the Irish rate (8.5%). Possible explanations for the higher American cesarean rate were the expectation that prolonged labor should lead to cesarean, financial incentives, and fear of malpractice suits over improper use of oxytocin.

Despite the different percentages of women diagnosed with CPD, mean birth weights were similar. "The six-fold higher rate of diagnosis of cephalopelvic disproportion in the American group supports earlier suggestions that there is a strong subjective element in the differential diagnosis between inefficient uterine action and cephalopelvic disproportion." Apgar scores did not differ, which suggests the high cesarean rate was not benefiting the babies.

4. Bottoms SF, Hirsch VJ, and Sokol RJ. Medical management of arrest disorders of labor: a current overview. Am J Obstet Gynecol 1987;156(4):935-939. (U.S.)

This study reviewed the records of 4573 women who had arrest of labor disorders with no medical complications. Although cesarean rates were five times higher among women with an arrest disorder, 86.7% still gave birth vaginally. No infant death was associated with the arrest disorder; low Apgar scores were not more frequent; and although admission to neonatal intensive care was more frequent after oxytocin stimulation, that was also true after cesarean birth. The authors comment that older studies consigned as many as 37% of women to cesarean section for CPD on the basis of X-ray pelvimetry, a test now known to have "little predictive value."

5. Carpenter MW et al. Practice environment is associated with obstetric decision making regarding abnormal labor. Obstet Gynecol 1987;70(4):657-661. (U.S.)

Responders to a 1984 survey of Maine obstetricians (59 of 86 responded) were grouped according to whether their cesarean rate exceeded or was less than the median percentage. The median cesarean rates among the 59 responders were: total rate, 21%; primary rate, 14%; and the percentage of women who had a cesarean after a diagnosis of dystocia, 65%. Analysis revealed the following a significantly higher total cesarean rate associated with fewer than two other doctors sharing night call, which suggests physician fatigue played a role. More doctors with privileges at more than one hospital fell into the higher-than-average group, but the trend did not reach significance. A higher cesarean rate for dystocia associated significantly with "hospital less able to do a stat cesarean section" (no 24-hour in-house anesthesia or blood bank availability).

6. Neuhoff D, Burke MS, and Porreco RP. Cesarean birth for failed progress in labor. Obstet Gynecol 1989;73(6):915-920. (U.S.)

The study compares outcomes for 192 healthy nulliparous women at term with a singleton vertex fetus managed by clinic obstetricians with 415 similar women with private physicians at the same hospital. The total cesarean rate on the clinic service was 5.2% versus 17.1% on the private service ($p < 0.001$), and the cesarean rate for FTP was 0.5% versus. 13.7% ($p < 0.001$.)

For women in spontaneous labor, cesarean rates were similar on both services (5.2% versus 7.9%). Epidural anesthesia and oxytocin use were the key variables associated with cesarean section.

Epidural rates were identical (42%), but while having an epidural did not change either the total cesarean rate (5.0%) or the rate for FTP (1.2%) on the clinic service, both the total rate (24.9%) and the FTP rate (20.2%) were significantly affected by epidural use on the private service ($p < 0.001$ for both comparisons). The relative risk of an epidural but no oxytocin leading to cesarean for FTP on the private service was 4.3 times that on the clinic service ($p = 0.05$).

Oxytocin was used more often in the absence of an epidural by the private service (31.8% versus 19.6%, $p < 0.02$), yet the relative risk of a cesarean was 13.6 ($p = 0.001$). Oxytocin was used equally often (about 70%) in conjunction with an epidural. Despite this, the relative risk of a cesarean on the private service was 14.0 ($p < 0.001$).

The authors concluded that the difference lay in the amount of oxytocin given and that clinic patients, especially clinic patients with epidurals, were more "aggressively" treated. They propose aggressive use of oxytocin to solve the problem of "the psychology of prolonged and nonprogressive labor dominat[ing] management strategies, as *physicians*, patients, and families become exhausted and frustrated with lack of progress [emphasis mine]."

7. Berkowitz GS et al. Effect of physician characteristics on the cesarean birth rate. *Am J Obstet Gynecol* 1989;161:146-149. (U.S.)

The authors correlated physician characteristics with cesarean section rate among 48 private doctors at a single hospital attending 6327 mostly low-risk women. The overall cesarean rate was 23.7%. For the [presumably higher-risk] clinic patients at the same hospital, the total cesarean rate was 18.2%, and the primary cesarean rate was 17.8%. Physician age and experience correlated significantly with higher operative vaginal delivery rates and lower cesarean section rates.

8. Perez P. The patient observer: what really led to these cesarean births? *Birth* 1989;16(3):130-139. (U.S.)

Perez, a monitrice [professional labor attendant], presents the discrepancies between the nurse's notes, physician's notes, and mothers' recall on her previous cesarean for five of her VBAC clients. The deliveries took place after 1982 and are "typical" of those in her files.

Patient 1: Perez was "dismayed by the discrepancy between 6 cm dilatation and -2 station charted by the physician and 10 cm dilatation and +1 station recorded by the nurse. . . . Why, if the mother was pushing well and at +1 station, was she taken to the delivery room after only 35 minutes?" The mother recalls that while her husband was waiting to join her in the delivery room, he overheard the doctor telling someone over the telephone to go on to the party. He would be there in 45 minutes.

Patient 2: The mother reports that the doctor told her during pregnancy she was too short (5 ft 1 in) to deliver vaginally. In labor he said she was not progressing and insisted she have an epidural in case he had to do a c-section. Perez writes, "The nurse noted that . . . she started the patient pushing at 9 cm dilatation, and that pushing continued for 37 minutes. The doctor recorded that the mother was completely dilated, yet that she had a rim of cervix, and that she pushed for two hours. . . . Did the nurse have the mother push at 9 cm to try to help her deliver vaginally before the physician came to do a cesarean section?"

Patient 3: The doctor's notes are incoherent, containing such comments as "there is some confusion as the patient never even separated." He notes "fetal distress" as well as CPD as a diagnosis. The only distress occurred when the oxytocin drip was increased, and it disappeared when the drip was turned down. The nurse notes the baby was at +1 station. The doctor writes the baby was at -1, and that even pushing on the uterus did not bring the baby down. The mother pushed with an epidural [well known to slow descent] for one hour before the cesarean.

Patient 4: This mother presented with contractions but a "hard, thick, closed" cervix. She was given an enema and then oxytocin. The doctor notes the mother dilated to 3 to 4 cm. The mother commented, "I agreed to the C section with the understanding that I had . . . made absolutely no progress since my admission." She was given pain medication, of which she says, "I was shocked to find out later that they had given me pain medicine against my wishes."

Patient 5: The mother recalls, "I wanted to walk around but they told me I had to sit in a rocker. . . . They told me I needed [pain] medication but I refused. They gave it to me anyway. . . . They kept asking me if I felt like pushing and I kept saying no. They finally held me up and told me to push anyway. . . . When they sat me up for the epidural, I really felt like pushing and kept saying, 'Wait, wait a minute. I need to push.' They ignored me and gave me the epidural." The doctor then tried forceps, which failed, and proceeded to a cesarean.

9. Guillemette J and Fraser WD. Differences between obstetricians in caesarean rates. Br J Obstet Gynecol 1992;99(2):105-108. (Canada)

Nulliparas in spontaneous term labor (N = 546) who gave birth from 1988 to 1990 were grouped according to whether their doctor's cesarean rate for dystocia was low (6.0-6.5%) or high (9.4-15.0%). Both groups were similar with respect to infant birth weights, dilation at admission, and whether membranes were intact. Intrapartum care was similar with respect to epidural use (76.5% versus 82.2%), amniotomy (52.7% versus 52.8%), oxytocin (49.7% versus 56.1%), use of EFM (81.6% versus 85.5%), and percentage of cesareans performed at 5 cm or less dilation (33.3% versus 26.7%). Although the only significant difference was for cesareans for dystocia in second stage (2.4% versus 7.9%, p = 0.0025), doctors in the high group were more likely to perform a cesarean for dystocia in first stage (3.9% versus 6.1%) or fetal distress (3.0% versus 4.7%). Outcomes for babies were similar except five babies had clavicular fractures [broken collarbone] and four had facial palsies [nerve injury]. All were from the low group and 8 of 9 were forceps or vacuum extractions. The risk of trauma might be lessened without increasing cesarean rates by "more judicious timing" of instrumental delivery. Mean second-stage duration was less than the recommended two hours (79 min versus 92 min, p < 0.006) [and most had epidurals!].

10. McCloskey L, Petitti DB, and Hobel CJ. Variations in the use of cesarean delivery for dystocia: lessons about the source of care. Med Care 1992;30(2):126-135. (U.S.)

The likelihood of cesarean delivery was compared for low-risk primiparous women (so that dystocia would be the main indication) giving birth at a single hospital that had private doctors, clinic doctors, and salaried doctors (working for a health maintenance organization, HMO) who worked shifts. The cesarean rate was 21% for private, 17% for clinic, and 15% for HMO patients. [Recall that these were low-risk women.]

After controlling for demographic and biologic variables, compared with a private doctor, women with HMO physicians were 66% as likely to have a cesarean but only if aged 25 to 29 years. Otherwise, a cesarean was equally likely. The relative risk of cesarean with epidural anesthesia was 2.5 times those without. After adjusting for epidural use, HMO women were only 46% as likely to have a cesarean compared with private physicians. Again, this was true only for women aged 25 to 34 years. HMO patients delivering within 12 hours of labor were 49% as likely to have a cesarean compared with private patients, but by 20 hours, the difference disappeared. However, clinic patients in labor longer than 20 hours were 66% as likely to have cesareans.

The authors speculate on why cesarean rates vary: physician age may affect rates (HMO doctors were older than those in private practice), and institutional culture may be important (most doctors at this hospital were in private practice). Data presented here were gathered one year after formation of the HMO. Two years later, there had been a "marked" increase in cesarean rate among HMO physicians. Similarly, another study found that only an HMO with its own hospitals (Kaiser Permanente) had lower than average cesarean rates. Other HMOs did not.

The Convenience Factor

11. Evans MI et al. Cesarean section: assessment of the convenience factor. *J Reprod Med* **1984;29(9):670-676.** (U.S.)

An analysis of time of day and day of week for primary cesarean section was undertaken at three Chicago hospitals with private physicians and compared with Chicago Lying-In (CLI), a hospital with salaried physicians working shifts. The primary cesarean rate was 5.8% at CLI and 11.0%, 8.8%, and 11.0% at hospitals A, B, and C, respectively.

Acute and semiacute cesareans showed no periodicity, but significantly fewer nonacute cesareans (CPD, dystocia, prolonged rupture of membranes, failed induction) were done between 12 a.m. and 8 a.m. at hospitals A and C ($p < 0.001$), but not hospital B or CLI. No significant differences for birth weight, gestational age, Apgar score, or parity were found to account for the variation. Fewer cesareans were performed on weekends, probably reflecting weekday inductions of women at risk for cesarean (i.e., postdates, preeclamptics, growth-retarded fetuses).

One explanation is "the primary C-section ratio at CLI is lowest when the economic incentives to perform surgery are the least." Another is the availability of staff and services at CLI around the clock.

12. Fraser W et al. Temporal variation in rates of cesarean section for dystocia: does "convenience" play a role? *Am J Obstet Gynecol* **1987;156(2):300-304.** (Canada)

This study of 4232 nulliparous women in spontaneous labor found that more cesareans were performed for dystocia in the evening than at night (during sleep hours) or during the day (when office hours and surgeries are scheduled). The difference persisted when the results were stratified by length of labor to adjust for the fact that labors usually start at night and so will be considered "prolonged" by the following evening. Nighttime ancillary services were available and doctors were paid the same for vaginal and cesarean deliveries.

The Role of Impatience

13. Hemminki E and Simukka R. The timing of hospital admission and progress of labour. *Eur J Obstet Gynecol Reprod Biol* **1986;22:85-94.** (Finland)

After compensating for the intrinsic speed of labor, healthy, nulliparous Finnish women in uncomplicated labor (N = 591) laboring slowly who arrived later in labor (contractions $\geq$ 4 hrs) were less likely to have diagnosis of difficult delivery (3.3% versus 11.7%, p < 0.05), oxytocin augmentation (30% versus 45%, p < 0.05), amniotomy (72% versus 84%, p < 0.05), pain medication (67% versus 80%, p < 0.05), instrumental delivery (14.3% versus 8.8%, NS), and cesarean section (4.4% versus 16.5%, p < 0.01) than similar women arriving earlier in labor. For women progressing rapidly, early or late arrival made no difference. "Protracted labor" was the cesarean indication for seven early comers but no latecomers, regardless of progress rate. "If the results . . . reflect the negative consequences of early admission, then the stress caused by the hospital admission in a sensitive part of labour or the longer time spent at risk for various interventions could be the mechanisms."

14. Arulkumaran S et al. Obstetric outcome of patients with a previous episode of spurious labor. *Am J Obstet Gynecol* **1987;157(1):17-20.** (Singapore)

Outcomes were compared between women having an episode of spurious labor at term (painful, regular contractions at least once every 10 minutes but no established labor within the next 24 hours) (N = 168) and women who established spontaneous labor within 24 hours (N = 1041). The induction rate for study women was 15.5%. Augmentation rates were 35.7% versus 19.7% (p < 0.001), and cesarean rates were 20.2% versus 8.0% (p < 0.001). The fetal distress rate was 25.6% versus 8.9% (p < 0.001) when oxytocin was used and 7.3% versus 2.6% (p < 0.05) when it was not. The cesarean rate was 27.9% versus 8.9% (p < 0.001) when oxytocin was used and 12.2% versus 7.8% (NS) when it was not. The authors conclude that women with an episode of spurious labor constitute a group at high risk for fetal distress and obstetric intervention. [False labor may signal problems with effective labor, but the cause of the increased cesarean and fetal distress rates seems likely to be the use of oxytocin, especially for induction.]

15. Stewart PJ et al. Diagnosis of dystocia and management with cesarean section among primiparous women in Ottawa-Carleton. *Can Med Assoc J* **1990;142(5):459-463.** (Canada)

Outcomes were examined at two Level III and two community hospitals in 1984 for 3887 primiparous women of whom 3781 had "some" labor. Of women allowed to labor, 30.1% were diagnosed as having dystocia. Women with no fetal heart sounds on admission, prolapsed cord, or antepartum or intrapartum hemorrhage were excluded. "Almost one-third of the women in our study were given a diagnosis of abnormal progress or disproportion. This proportion is so high that one wonders whether the criteria used to define 'normal' adequately reflect the actual variations in labour patterns among women." The cesarean rate among hospitals ranged from 11.8% to 19.6%, and 75% were done for dystocia, CPD, or failed induction. Labor was induced in 21%, of whom 14% had a cesarean in latent phase (< 4 cm dilation). Only 3% had a cesarean in latent phase with labor of spontaneous onset. "Cesarean section is being done for disproportion without a trial of labour beyond the latent phase and for dystocia in the absence of fetal distress. If these practices were modified the [primary] cesarean section rate could be reduced from 16% to about 8%."

16. Summers PR et al. Pregnancy outcome in patients with repeat visits to the labor observation area near term. *South Med J* 1991;84(4):436-438. (U.S.)

Entry criteria were term cephalic singleton gestation presenting at the hospital at least twice during three consecutive days ($N = 71$). Analysis showed the subgroup making more than one visit within 24 hours complaining of labor was more likely to have a cesarean for "failure to progress" [percentages not given] ($p < 0.05$). The authors conclude that women with repeat visits have a high potential for abnormal labor. [An equally plausible explanation is that impatience leads to inappropriate intervention, a diagnosis of prolonged labor, and cesarean section.]

17. DeMott RK and Sandmire HF. The Green Bay cesarean section study. II. The physician factor as a determinant of cesarean birth rates for failed labor. *Am J Obstet Gynecol* 1992;166(6 Pt 1):1799-1810. (U.S.)

In order to determine how physician practices ($N = 11$) influence cesarean rates, all nulliparous term pregnancies between 1986 and 1988 where a cesarean was done for FTP were analyzed. Total cesarean rates ranged from 6.0% to 19.5%. Cesarean rates for FTP ranged from 2.7% to 16.0%. Doctors were grouped into low, medium, and high rates of operative delivery. Maternal and fetal characteristics, in particular infant birth weights and head circumference, were similar among groups. Compared with the medium and high group, doctors in the low group were more likely to start oxytocin later (dilation 5.3 cm versus 4.0 cm and 4.7 cm, $p < 0.01$), use it more often (43% versus 30% and 31%, $p < 0.04$), and in higher doses (18.3 mU/min versus 12.0 mU/min and 11.9 mU/min, $p < 0.001$). They were less likely to induce than the high group (16% versus 15% versus 21%, NS). More women in the low group achieved full dilation before cesarean section. Neonatal outcomes were similar. All six cases of endometritis occurred in women who had cesareans. "To reduce the need for cesarean section in nulliparous patients, administer more oxytocin to more patients for longer time periods." [Great article; wrong conclusion. Midwives have shown that oxytocin is not necessary to achieve low cesarean rates.]

INDUCTION LEADS TO CESAREAN SECTION

18. Macer JA et al. Elective induction versus spontaneous labor: a retrospective study of complications and outcome. *Am J Obstet Gynecol* 1992;166(6 Pt 1):1690-1697. (U.S.)

A hospital with a 30% elective induction rate compared outcomes for 253 women induced electively with 253 matched controls who began labor spontaneously. Seventy percent of the population were multiparas. In the induction group, 83.8% had an epidural versus 55.7% among controls, which is ascribed to agreeing to induction together with planning for pain control [not because induced labor was more painful]. Cesarean rates were similar (14.6% induced versus 11.1% spontaneous) [dystocia is rarely an issue among multiparas, and most of the population was multiparous]. The cesarean rate among induced nulliparas was 33.8% versus 22.1% (NS). [This trend is dismissed. However, failure to achieve significance is probably due to small population size.] Among nulliparas with an unfavorable cervix (Bishop score ≤ 5), the cesarean rate was

50%. The article concludes that except for these women, elective induction poses no hazard and is therefore fine.*

19. Jarvelin MR, Hartikainen-Sorri AL, and Rantakallio P. Labour induction policy in hospitals of different levels of specialisation. *Br J Obstet Gynaecol* **1993;100(4):310-315.** (Finland)

Data came from singleton births excluding elective cesareans ($N = 8606$) occurring in two administrative districts during 1985-86. Induction rates varied from 17.7% to 29.4% among hospital types, of which 51.3% were elective. Induced women were more likely to be parous (31.6% of nulliparas versus 49.1% with one or two prior births). The cesarean rate among women induced for indication was 15.0% versus 8.1% among those electively induced versus 5.9% with spontaneous onset. The risk of cesarean with elective induction was 1.5 times that with spontaneous onset (CL 1.1-1.9). The most common reason was dystocia (dysfunctional labor 1.4% versus 2.8%, $p < 0.01$; CPD 1.0% versus 2.0%, $p < 0.05$).

HIGH-DOSE OXYTOCIN AUGMENTATION IS NOT A PANACEA

It Does Not Always Work

20. Cohen GR et al. A prospective randomized study of the aggressive management of early labor. *Am J Obstet Gynecol* **1987;157(5):1174-1177.** (U.S.)

Term primigravidas ($N = 150$) with inadequate contractions (< 40 sec long, < 3 contractions in 10 min) were randomly assigned to two equal-sized groups. (Labor was defined as contractions and dilation > 3 cm or contractions and ruptured membranes.) The "early aggressive management" group had an internal catheter and oxtocin drip within 30 minutes of admission. The control group was not given oxytocin unless they had arrest of dilation lasting longer than two hours or arrest of descent in second stage for longer than one hour. The cesarean rates were similar (13% versus 15%). "In our population early intervention failed to reduce the incidence of cesarean birth as a result of dystocia or to affect the duration of labor. We recommend careful consideration before the widespread use of such methods." In a letter following, the Dublin doctors deplore the use of the word aggressive instead of active. ["A rose by any other name . . ."]

21. Lopez-Zeno JA et al. A controlled trial of a program for the active management of labor. *N Engl J Med* **1992;326(17):450-454.** (U.S.)

Nulliparous patients in spontaneous term labor with a singleton vertex fetus (medical complications were not excluded) were randomly assigned to active ($N = 351$) or traditional management ($N = 354$). Despite similar epidural (72.1% versus 72%) and augmentation (71.2% versus 66.1%) rates, the cesarean rate was 10.5% for active management versus 14.1% for controls, a significant decrease after controlling for confounding variables ($p < 0.05$). [Augmentation rates in other active management studies have

---

*According to *Unnecessary Cesarean Sections: Halting a National Epidemic* (VanTuinen and Wolfe, 1992), this hospital had a 36.9% cesarean rate in 1989.

been around 40%, and the cesarean rate for primiparas in Dublin is 5%.] The difference was greater for private patients (11.1% versus 16.1%) leading the authors to comment, "This method of labor management was especially effective for private patients, a group recognized as being at increased risk for dystocia." [Private patients are at increased risk of being diagnosed as having dystocia, quite a different matter.] Since the cesarean rate for nulliparas during the year before the study was 22.4% [!], the authors believe there was a drift toward active management of control group women.

22. Rothman BK. The active management of physicians. *Birth* **1993;20(3):158-159.** (analysis of Abstract 21)

Carrying out the study meant a 30.3% drop in cesarean rate from the previous year for private patients who were not in the active management arm, a greater drop than for active versus control groups. If the contribution of private patients is extracted, then the cesarean rate among actively managed clinic patients was 8.9% versus 8.8% among controls, or no different. However, the previous year the cesarean rate was 17.0% for clinic patients. Therefore, carrying out the study halved the rate for clinic patients, whether they were actively managed or not. The fact that the lowest rate is found for clinic patients during a trial and the highest rate for private patients when there is no trial "argues that the cesarean section rate is partly a product of how tightly watched physicians feel they are (with less attention paid, more unnecessary cesareans are done) and partly a product of the well-documented bias toward overtreatment of private patients. . . . I suggest the cesarean rate is more a product of the management of physicians than the management of labor."

Other Regimens Work Equally Well

23. Hunter JS et al. The outcome of prolonged labor as defined by partography and the use of oxytocin: a descriptive study. *Am J Obstet Gynecol* **1983;145(2):189-192.** (Canada)

This study looked at management and outcome as it related to rate of progress for 300 term primigravidas who had reached 3 cm dilation without oxytocin. Group 1 consisted of women with no delay in dilation, group 2 of women with less than 2 hours delay, group 3 of women with 2 to 4 hrs delay, and group 4 of women with greater than 4 hrs delay. The epidural rate rose from 59% of group 1 to 95% of group 4 ($p < 0.001$), with an overall rate 74.6%. The oxytocin rate rose from 0 to 41%, with an overall rate 16.7%. The cesarean rate rose from 3.2% to 34.2%, with overall rate 13% ($N = 39$). Of the 23 cesareans done for dystocia, there were none in group 1, two each in groups 2 and 3, and 19 in group 4.

Equal numbers of cesarean sections for fetal distress were performed in all groups. Apgar scores did not decline with prolonged labor, suggesting earlier intervention would not benefit babies.

The authors compare their outcomes with another study in which all women with 2 hours or more delay had oxytocin. Both studies yielded similar cesarean rates (23% versus 22% in this study for women with ≥ 2 hours delay), but here only one-third of such women had oxytocin, suggesting that oxytocin could be used less liberally with no loss of benefit. To the contrary, only nine of the women having cesareans for dystocia in this study had oxytocin. Giving more of them oxytocin might have helped. [The authors discount the role of epidural anesthesia in slowing dilation rate, but see

Chapter 13.]

24. Arulkumaran S et al. Augmentation of labour—Mode of delivery related to cervimetric progress. *Aust N Z J Obstet Gynaecol* **1987;27(4):304-308.** (Singapore)

This study of term women in spontaneous labor (nulliparas 1158, multiparas 1360) looked at oxytocin treatment and cesarean rate among women (nulliparas 19% multiparas 7.3%) in dysfunctional labor (defined as delayed progress for $\geq$ 2 hours after dilating to 3 cm). The epidural rate was 2%. The overall augmentation rate was 12.7%. Among nulliparas, the cesarean rate for dystocia was 3.6%, and the augmentation rate was 18.2%. [Thus, waiting one hour longer than the Dublin protocol before treatment resulted in one-third the augmentation rate overall and halved the augmentation rate in nulliparas without increasing the cesarean rate.]

Problems with High-Dose Oxytocin

25. Bidgood KA and Steer PJ. A randomized control study of oxytocin augmentation of labour. 1. Obstetric outcome. *Br J Obstet Gynecol* **1987;94:512-517.** (England)

Primiparous women in spontaneous term labor making poor progress were prospectively randomized into three groups: group 1, defer oxytocin eight hours ($N = 20$); group 2, give oxytocin based on intrauterine pressure catheter readings ($N = 21$); group 3, give oxytocin according to Dublin high-dose regimen ($N = 19$). Diagnosis of labor was based on painful contractions, complete cervical effacement, and dilation 3 cm or more. Inadequate progress was defined as four or more hours at a dilation rate of less than 0.5 cm per hour. All but two women had epidural anesthesia. One had a contraindication; the other asked for and got [!] a cesarean despite progressive labor.

The cesarean rates were: group 1, 45% [40%, subtracting the elective cesarean]; group 2, 33%; group 3, 26%. Differences among cesarean rates were not significant, but that may be because study size was small. Seven women (37%) in the high-dose group suffered uterine hyperstimulation, one of which led to a cesarean for fetal distress. The authors concluded the high-dose regimen is hazardous.

26. Seitchik J. The management of functional dystocia in the first stage of labor. *Clin Obstet Gynecol* **1987;30(1):42-49.**

Here are some points from this clinical management paper relevant to dystocia and oxytocin regimens:

- "Artificial rupture of the membranes (AROM) is a time honored but highly overrated method for the management of functional dystocia."

- Oxytocin regimens are based on the belief that oxytocin has a half-life of five minutes and that maximum effect of any given dose will be seen by 20 minutes or so. The half-life is actually ten minutes, and it takes 40 minutes to see maximum effect. [You need to wait longer before increasing the dose or risk overdosing.]

- The rate of oxytocin absorption from the blood and the sensitivity of uterine muscle are independent characteristics with wide individual variation. Rapid response indicates overdosing. [Dose should be titrated to maternal response, not given by formula.]

- Because of technical difficulties, 10% of uterine pressure catheter readings are worthless.

- The number of contractions is a more sensitive indicator of inadequate contractions than strength.

For these reasons Seitchik recommends waiting 40 minutes to see if the contraction pattern is adequate before increasing the dose. If it is, wait an hour to see if the mother makes at least 1 cm progress before increasing the dose further. If oxytocin has any effect, use arithmetic rather than geometric progression when increasing the dose to minimize the chance of overdosing.

27. Akoury HA et al. Oxytocin augmentation of labor and perinatal outcome in nulliparas. *Obstet Gynecol* **1991;78(2):227-230.** (Canada)

Of 1080 nulliparas subjected to active management, 456 had oxytocin augmentation for nonprogressive labor (42%). The cesarean rate was 5.9%. Uterine hyperstimulation (defined as ≥ 5 contractions within 10 min or contraction length ≥ 90 sec) occurred in 14% of nonstimulated labors and 21% of augmented labors. Hyperstimulation did not harm the babies. [However, hyperstimulation can cause fetal distress.] In 16 cases of hyperstimulation, protocol was not followed and oxytocin infusion was not decreased. [If hyperstimulation is ignored 4% of the time in a hospital with a standardized protocol, what might the percentage be in a less controlled environment?]

28. Satin AJ et al. High- versus low-dose oxytocin for labor stimulation. *Obstet Gynecol* **1992;80(1):111-116.** (U.S.)

A high-dose (6 mU/min increment) and low-dose (1 mU/min increment) oxytocin regimen were compared. The low-dose regimen was used for five months in 1990 ($N = 1251$) and the high-dose regimen for the next five months ($N = 1537$). Overall, 1676 women were augmented, of whom 732 had low-dose and 944 had high-dose oxytocin. All women had EFM. Amniotomy was routine. Few women had epidurals (< 8%). Uterine hyperstimulation was more common during high-dose augmentations (52% versus 39%, $p < 0.0001$), but the cesarean rate for fetal distress was 4% in both groups. [Still, if hyperstimulation is not promptly managed, it can cause fetal distress.] High dose oxytocin reduced the cesarean rate for dystocia (9% versus 12%, $p = 0.04$) and shortened labor. [This trial was not blinded and diagnosing dystocia is highly subjective.] Fewer infants were septic in the high-dose group (2% versus 0.3%, $p < 0.002$), which is attributed to shorter labors with high-dose oxytocin. [Neonatal sepsis varies with length of time after membrane rupture and number of vaginal exams. If they did not rupture membranes or do exams, would there be a difference?]

Oxytocin induction (519 low dose versus 593 high dose) associated with an increase in cesarean rate for fetal distress in the high-dose group (6% versus 3%, $p < 0.05$) and higher rates for dystocia compared with augmented labors (16% versus 13%). The failed induction rates (undelivered) were 19% versus 14%. [Apparently this meant induction was discontinued. In most protocols it means a cesarean.]

EVIDENCE SUPPORTING NONINTERVENTIVE MANAGEMENT

Why It Works

29. Andrews CM and Andrews EC. Nursing, maternal postures and fetal position. *Nursing Res* **1983;32(6):336-341.** (U.S.)

[Posterior position—baby facing the mother's belly—slows or halts progress because the fetal head fits poorly into the pelvis and neither descends well nor acts as an effective wedge against the cervix.] The authors theorized that the force of gravity in the hands-and-knees position together with abdominal stroking and/or pelvic rocking would coax the fetal back downward into the mother's belly, shifting the baby into the favorable anterior position.

Healthy primiparas at 38 weeks or more gestation [not in labor] with posterior babies ($N = 100$) were randomly assigned in groups of 20 to do the following for 10 minutes: (1) assume hands-and-knees position (HK), (2) HK with pelvic rocking, (3) HK with the mother stroking the baby downward, (4) HK with pelvic rocking and stroking, (5) (the control, a neutral position with respect to gravity) sit upright. No significant differences were found among the four study alternatives. The number of successful rotations ranged from 12 to 18 of 20. None of the control fetuses rotated. [One can infer that, conversely, lying supine, even with shoulders propped, would inhibit rotation.]

30. Simkin P. Stress, pain, and catecholamines in labor: part 1. A review. *Birth* **1986;13(4):227-233.**

Simkin concluded:

> From all these studies one can see a picture emerging. A reasonable amount of stress is harmless to the mother and to labor progress, and actually benefits the fetus by promoting adaptation to labor and birth. Excessive stress (as yet undefined in perinatal medicine) causes increased maternal catecholamine production which may be related to dysfunctional labor and fetal and neonatal distress and illness.
>
> Much of the stress of labor is preventable because many of the stressors are not inherent to labor; they are imposed in the form of thoughtless routines, unfamiliar personnel, and technological interventions. Benefits will be gained by exploring non-interventive ways to preserve the normal maternal-fetal adaptive responses to labor by minimizing stress and pain in the laboring mother. Among the most promising are improved childbirth education, better labor support, more judicious use of medications and interventions, and the most comfortable possible environment for birth.

31. Fenwick L and Simkin P. Maternal positioning to prevent or alleviate dystocia in labor. *Clin Obstet Gynecol* **1987;30(1):83-89.** (U.S.)

Citing numerous studies, this clinical practice paper describes the physiologic benefits of upright positions, especially when tilting forward from the waist, squatting, walking, and pelvic rocking. These positions and activities help guide the fetal head into the pelvis, put the fetus and pelvis in line with the directional force of contractions, increase contraction force, increase pelvic diameters, reduce pain and stress, and rotate posterior fetuses into the favorable anterior position. Supine positioning has the opposite effect and, in addition, can cause fetal distress by putting pressure on major maternal blood vessels. "[M]aternal positioning provides a valuable, non-invasive and acceptable intervention."

Freedom of Movement (Review)

32. Lupe PJ and Gross TL. Maternal upright posture and mobility in labor—a review. *Obstet Gynecol* **1986;67(5):727-734.**
This review paper analyzes the methodology and conclusions of seven articles. Four studies concluded that ambulation shortened labor and two that it had no effect. Four studies that measured contraction intensity all concluded that contractions were stronger. All studies had methodological weaknesses. Still, although unequivocal benefits of ambulation and upright posture have yet to be established, especially in the case of delayed progress, no study reported any adverse effects, and "most studies" reported greater maternal comfort and satisfaction. Therefore, in the absence of specific medical exclusionary factors, laboring women should not be denied this option.

Freedom of Movement (Studies)

33. Caldeyro-Barcia R. The influence of maternal position on time of spontaneous rupture of the membranes, progress of labor and fetal head compression. *Birth* **1979;6(1):1.** (South America)
Low-risk women in spontaneous labor with intact membranes were randomly assigned to recumbency during first-stage labor ($N = 225$) or to do as they pleased ($N = 145$). Only 5% chose to lie down. Women were matched with respect to parity and maternal weight and height, as well as infant birth weight, length, loops of umbilical cord [around the neck or body?], and circumference of head, abdomen, and chest. No woman had pain relief medication or oxytocin.
Contractions became stronger but less frequent as a woman went from supine to lying on her left side. Contractions were stronger and equally frequent when she went from supine to standing. (Gravity alone adds 35 mm Hg to contraction pressure.) For primigravidas, active first-stage labor (4-5 cm dilation to 10 cm) was shortened by a median length of 78 minutes (36%). The additional pressure on the fetal head when the mother stood did not increase the incidence of fetal head molding, caput succedaneum [a pressure-caused swelling on the fetal head], or heart rate decelerations. "Thus, in upright positions, labor is effectively shortened. . . . The upright positions are reported to be associated with less pain during labor and are preferred by women when they are given their choice of position in labor."

34. Roberts JE, Mendez-Bauer C, and Wodell DA. The effects of maternal position on uterine contractility and efficiency. *Birth* **1983;10(4):243-249.** (U.S.)
[A table in the introduction summarizes nine studies between 1963 and 1981 on the effect of maternal positioning.] Nineteen nulliparous women in term spontaneous labor alternated sitting upright with side lying for 30-minute periods beginning in early labor. Eleven women alternated lying supine with head and shoulders propped with side lying.

Uterine efficiency (UE) [a formula incorporating contraction strength and frequency and dilation] significantly favored side lying over sitting ($p < 0.01$).

When side lying, contractions were more intense than when propped supine ($p < 0.01$), but because they were less frequent, UE was not significantly different. Efficiency also varied with the comparison position. Integrating earlier work measuring supine/standing, supine/sitting, and standing/sitting reveals that supine was most efficient when alternated with side lying, sitting had a higher UE alternated with standing than side lying, side lying had a higher UE alternated with sitting than supine, and standing had a higher UE alternated with sitting than supine. This suggests that varying position may be even more beneficial than assuming any one particular position.

Walking

35. Read JA, Miller FC, and Paul RH. Randomized trial of ambulation versus oxytocin for labor enhancement: a preliminary report. *Am J Obstet Gynecol* **1981;139(6):669-672.** (U.S.)

Women who had made no progress for one hour and "whose contractions were deemed to be inadequate" were randomly assigned to ambulation ($N = 8$) or oxytocin ($N = 6$). Pain medication was not permitted during the study period. A baseline period of 30 minutes while side lying preceded the two-hour study period, and no changes in dilation or station [descent of the fetal head] were observed.

During the first hour all ambulant women made progress in descent and dilation, whereas only three women in the oxytocin group made progress. During the second hour, one ambulant woman gave birth, the other seven made additional progress, and four of six in the oxytocin group made progress. However, neither the mean dilation change (ambulant 2.2 cm versus oxytocin 1.63 cm) nor the mean station change (ambulant +1.48 cm versus oxytocin +0.67 cm) were significantly different, probably because the study size was small. All oxytocin patients reported more pain whereas four ambulant patients said pain was lessened and three said it remained the same.

36. Andrews CM and Chrzanowski M. Maternal position, labor and comfort. *Applied Nursing Res* **1990;3(1):7-13.** (U.S.)

Forty nulliparas in active-phase uncomplicated labor with intact membranes and a singleton, vertex, anterior fetus were randomly and evenly allocated to upright and recumbent groups. Upright women could stand, walk, sit, squat, or kneel upright. Recumbent women could lie on their backs, sides, or assume the hands-and-knees position. Fifteen upright women chose to lie down after receiving medication. Of them, five immediately got back up, saying contractions were more painful lying down. Ten rested on their sides for up to one hour. Maternal comfort was assessed by a scoring system based on the mother's behavior.

Mean length of active labor differed by 90.25 minutes (recumbent 324.75 min versus upright 234.50 min, $p = 0.003$). [This is as good as or better than amniotomy achieves. (See Chapter 12.)] "Rapid cervical dilation is promoted by fetal descent; it is likely that gravitational forces assisted fetal descent in the upright group." Upright women were not less comfortable, though contractions were stronger and more frequent. Upright women received less narcotic analgesia possibly because nurses, judging them to be more comfortable, did not offer it. Recumbent women were more likely to have external EFM (13 versus 1, $p = 0.085$), which was associated with increased discomfort, probably because they were in bed and more accessible.

[T]he upright labor positions have the distinct advantages of facilitating efficient uterine contractions and reducing the duration of the phase of maximum slope in labor with no adverse effect on the pain experienced. . . . For the most part, hospital environments and health care personnel encourage laboring women to be recumbent, [but] the woman who chooses to ambulate can [gain a] sense of control over her own body. She can work with her body to accomplish a marathon event with little or no assistance from medicinal or mechanical interventions.

Sitting

37. Chen S et al. Effects of sitting position on uterine activity during labor. *Obstet Gynecol* **1987;69(1):67-73.** (Japan)

Healthy women in spontaneous labor with a singleton vertex fetus ($N = 183$) were randomized to sit throughout labor, lie down during the first stage and sit during the second stage, or lie down throughout. Sitters used a couch during the first stage and a birth chair for pushing. Women were excluded ($N = 67$) after allocation for various reasons, including oxytocin augmentation, cesarean for CPD, or epidural anesthesia. [Among nulliparas, 6% of the sit-sit group had oxytocin versus 12% of the recumbent groups, and 3% of the sit-sit group had cesareans for CPD versus 9% of the recumbent groups. Epidural rates were the same (9% versus 10%).]

Among nulliparas, first-stage labor was 23% shorter for sitting versus recumbent women (NS, probably because the study size was so small) and second stage was 48% shorter ($p < 0.05$.) Among multiparas, active phase was 42% shorter for sitters ($p < 0.05$), and second stage was the same length. Nulliparas who pushed in the recumbent position were more likely to have a forceps delivery (7 of 23 versus 1 of 37, $p < 0.05$).

Gravity Positive Position and Pushing

38. Gardosi J, Sylvester S, and B-Lynch C. Alternative positions in the second stage of labour: a randomized controlled trial. *Br J Obstet Gynaecol* **1989;96:1290-1296.** (England)

Laboring term nulliparous women with no epidural anesthesia were randomized into upright (squatting, kneeling, sitting upright, or standing) ($N = 73$) and recumbent (side lying or supine, propped about 30 degrees) ($N = 78$) pushing positions. In the upright group, 74% completed the protocol. Fifteen women chose recumbency, and four were asked to lie on their sides to facilitate hearing fetal heart tones or improve progress. In the recumbent group, 81% remained recumbent. Six women chose to be upright; nine were advised to do so to improve progress. The trial was ended after three months because the midwives, who had no preferences before the study began, increasingly perceived upright positioning to benefit progress.

Upright women adopted more postures during second stage than recumbent women. Kneeling facing the raised head of the bed was favored as the most comfortable and easiest to maintain. The mean length of second stage did not differ (upright 48.8 min versus recumbent 47.1 min), but the time from perineal bulging to the birth did (upright

9.8 min versus recumbent 16.2 min, $p < 0.01$). More upright women had an intact perineum or first-degree tear [a nick of the skin only, which does not need repair] (37% versus 26%, $p < 0.05$), and kneeling was especially protective for 17 of 30 women (57%). Possible reasons were less pressure on the perineum, shorter end stage resulting in fewer episiotomies to expedite delivery, and lying on the back with flexed thighs tightens the perineum and narrows the vaginal opening.

39. Gardosi J, Hutson N, and B-Lynch C. Randomized controlled trial of squatting in the second stage of labour. *Lancet* **1989;2(8654):74-77.** (England)

This randomized controlled trial allocated nulliparous women with no epidural either to upright ($N = 218$) or recumbent ($N = 209$) positions for second stage. Upright women could kneel, assume all fours, sit upright, or squat using a thick, foam, U-shaped cushion with side handle-grips. Recumbent women could lie on either side or propped on their back. Among the upright group, 82% remained upright, of whom 71% squatted using the cushion. Among the recumbent group, 89% remained recumbent. The rest had heard about the squatting cushion from other women.

Upright women had fewer instrumental deliveries (8.7% versus 16.3%, $p < 0.05$), shorter mean length of second stage (39 min versus 50 min, $p < 0.001$), and more intact perineums (46% versus 32%, $p < 0.01$). The babies were equally healthy, and upright positioning did not lead to increased postpartum blood loss (which has been documented with birth chairs).

Women using the squatting cushion were sent a questionnaire two months later and 78% responded. They reported they could push more easily, they felt more involved and in control, and backache was relieved. Ninety-five percent of responders would request the cushion again.

REFERENCES

Boylan PC. Active management of labor: results in Dublin, Houston, London, New Brunswick, Singapore, and Valparaiso. *Birth* 1989;16(3):114-118.

Cetrulo CL and Cetrulo LG. Medicolegal dystocia. *Clin Obstet Gynecol* 1987;30(1):106-113.

Crowther C, et al. Prolonged Labour. In *A guide to effective care in pregnancy and childbirth.* Enkin M, Keirse MJNC, and Chalmers I, eds. Oxford: Oxford University Press, 1989.

Kitzinger S. The desexing of birth; some effects of professionalization of care; the godsibs; what matters to women—their words. Paper presented at Innovations in Perinatal Care: Assessing Benefits and Risks, ninth conference presented by *Birth,* San Francisco, November 1990.

McDonald D et al. The Dublin randomized controlled trial of intrapartum fetal heart rate monitoring. *Am J Obstet Gynecol* 1985;152(5):524-539. (abstracted in Chapter 7)

O'Driscoll K and Meagher D. *Active management of labour.* 2d ed. London: Bailliere Tindall, 1986.

Rooks JP et al. Outcomes of care in birth centers. The National Birth Center Study. *N Engl J Med* 1989;321(26):1804-1811. (abstracted in chapter 16)

Rosen M and Thomas L. *The cesarean myth.* New York: Penguin Books, 1989.

Seitchik J, Holden AE, and Castillo M. Amniotomy and the use of oxytocin in labor in nulliparous women. *Am J Obstet Gynecol* 1985;153(8):848-854. (abstracted in Chapter 12)

Simkin P. Stress, pain and catecholamines in labor: part 2. Stress associated with childbirth events: a pilot survey of new mothers. *Birth* 1986;13(4):234-240.

Taafel SM, Placek PJ, and Kosary CL. U.S. cesarean section rates 1990: an update. *Birth* 1992;19(1):21-22.

Turner MJ, Brassil M, and Gordon H. Active management of labor associated with a decrease in the cesarean section rate in nulliparas. *Obstet Gynecol* 1988;71(2):150-154.

Wolfe SM and Jones RD. *Women's health alert.* Reading, MA: Addison-Wesley, Inc., 1991.

Wright CH. The active management of prolonged labor. *J Nat Med Assoc* 1983;75(2):223-226.

6

Breech Presentation

Myth: *Now that your baby is breech, the only safe thing to do is schedule a cesarean.*

Realities: *"External version, near term, of the breech presentation can safely increase the [number of vertex fetuses] . . . and reduce the need for cesarean birth."*

Morrison et al. 1986

"[R]outine cesarean delivery of the near-term or term breech fetus increases maternal morbidity, maternal mortality, and the cost to society, but it does not provide a foreseeable benefit to the near-term and term breech fetus."

Weiner 1992

Medical fashion changes. In the past some doctors deliberately reached inside at the delivery to turn head down babies breech and pull them out feet first. Now most doctors believe that vaginal breech [baby presents buttocks or feet first] birth is so dangerous that it should not be permitted. Breech babies do suffer higher mortality and morbidity rates, but the two cures—external cephalic version [turning the baby by manipulating it from the outside] (ECV) and universal cesarean section—are not so straightforward a cure as they would seem.

ECV is an old technique. Anthropologist Brigitte Jordan (1984) documents that midwives and doctors throughout the world have long practiced it with few complications. But always they have stressed that problem-free success depends on a gentle, patient manipulator and a comfortable, relaxed mother.

Unfortunately, some not-so-gentle doctors, using general anesthesia and brute force, caused placental abruptions (detachment from the uterine wall), hemorrhages, and fetal distress. Some babies died. Predictably, doctors condemned ECV instead of their technique.

Recently, ECV has been revived as a high-tech procedure using tocolytics (uterine relaxant drugs), ultrasonography, and electronic fetal monitoring (EFM). As with traditional ECV, no anesthesia is used, and gentleness is advised. To minimize the presumed dangers, version is performed only on women who meet strict eligibility requirements and is often restricted to one attempt late in pregnancy.

These restrictions limit its benefits. The side effects of tocolytic drugs exclude women with certain medical complications. The later in pregnancy the procedure is done, the lower the success rate is because the baby is bigger; there is less amniotic fluid; and membranes are more likely to rupture or labor begin before the procedure is performed. Allowing only one attempt also lowers success rates. Even so, numerous studies document that high-tech ECV safely and effectively reduces the number of babies born breech.

Nonetheless, despite the data, few American women have ECV. The incidence of breech at term is 3% to 4%. According to VanTuinen and Wolfe (1992), consistent use of ECV could lower this incidence to as little as 0.6%, yet 2.9% of all births in 1989 were cesareans for breech.

The reluctance to perform high-tech version is puzzling. Opponents point to major complications, but only one study since 1980 has reported any (Kasule, Chimbira, and Brown 1985). That study was of black African clinic patients, and neither tocolytics, ultrasound scanning, nor fetal heart monitoring were used. Technique and possibly poor maternal health were likely culprits for the poor outcomes, although, as happened with ECV earlier, the authors blame the procedure. *William's Obstetrics* (Cunningham, MacDonald, and Gant 1989) refers to a maternal death reported in Stine et al. (1985, abstracted below), implying that the death related to ECV. In fact, the mother died during a cesarean section unconnected with ECV.

Furthermore, high-tech ECV is the only technique obstetricians offer. High success rates are reported anecdotally for postural remedies and alternative medicine techniques such as acupuncture, acupressure, and moxibustion (stimulating acupressure points with heat), but little research has been done. Nonetheless, these techniques are unlikely to do harm so they are worth trying.*

This returns us to the other alternative: avoiding vaginal breech birth. *William's Obstetrics* provides a classic example of American obstetric thinking. It acknowledges that breech babies do worse primarily because of prematurity and congenital problems, lists the numerous fetal injuries caused by hasty or forceful manipulations during vaginal birth, and admits that birth injuries occur during cesareans. Yet it recommends "liberal use of cesarean section"

---

*See *The Birth Partner* by Penny Simkin (Boston: Harvard Common Press, 1989), for a postural technique.

because "spontaneous complete expulsion of the fetus who presents as a breech . . . is seldom successfully accomplished." As does *William's,* U.S. obstetricians ignore this gap in logic. Because cesarean for breech is all but universal, despite the rarity of breech presentation, it is the third most common reason for cesarean section (VanTuinen and Wolfe 1992).

Does cesarean section improve breech outcomes? The major reasons why breech babies have more problems than vertex babies have nothing to do with birth route. Breech babies are more likely to be premature or growth retarded. They are more likely to have congenital anomalies, genetic defects, or neuromuscular deficits or problems such as hip dysplasia or cerebral palsy (Claussen and Nielssen 1988; Hytten 1982). This is because size, weight, shape, and normal movements guide the baby into the vertex position. In most cases vaginal breech birth did not cause the problem, and cesarean section will not cure it.

In many other cases, as happened with ECV, doctors blame breech injuries on vaginal birth instead of their own mismanagement. So, for example, Weiner (1992, abstracted below) favors epidurals despite the fact that data from his own hospital show that the baby is more likely to be injured when the mother has one. Why? An epidural keeps the woman from becoming "uncooperative" when a doctor pushes on her belly to deliver the baby's head. This illustrates perfectly the harm done by the "just in case" mentality. Obstetricians say, "Because we might have trouble, we'll give an epidural, put the mother on her back in stirrups, and extract the baby manually or with forceps," thereby maximizing the odds of having trouble because they have disrupted every mechanism facilitating easy birth. The lithotomy position is the worst position because it increases the incidence of fetal distress, the mother pushes the baby uphill, and her pelvis, made flexible by the influence of pregnancy hormones, is fixed in position by the delivery table (Mahmood 1990; Fenwick and Simkin 1987). Epidural anesthesia diminishes contraction strength and impedes maternal pushing efforts. Add the obstetrician's impatience and unnecessary or overly forceful manipulation, and the stage is set for birth injury or asphyxia. The baby may be damaged, but vaginal birth was not at fault.

Moreover, universal cesarean section does not eradicate iatrogenic injuries and asphyxia. Breech babies have been injured as doctors maneuver them through the cesarean incision, and with general anesthesia, asphyxia rates are as much as tripled (Bodmer et al. 1986). Babies have also been cut badly enough to need suturing.

In fact, with one exception (Thorpe-Beeston, Banfield, and Saunders 1992), studies have consistently found that while breech babies do worse than their cephalic counterparts, cesarean section did not help. That study's very uniqueness suggests there may be other explanations for its findings.

Certainly some breech babies should be delivered by cesarean section, but which ones? Cesarean section is usually advised if the fetal neck is hyperextended (tipped back) because of the risk of spinal cord injury during the birth, but there agreement ends. Some experts recommend restricting vaginal birth to frank breech presentations (buttocks down). They reason that umbilical cord prolapse (the cord comes down ahead of the baby) is unlikely (0.5%, similar to vertex; Confino et al. 1985, abstracted below), and because the buttocks are almost as big as the head, the cervix will dilate far enough to pass the head as well. Other studies that include nonfrank breeches find no excess mortality or morbidity. They argue that although a cesarean may be necessary, with proper monitoring a cord prolapse should not cause asphyxia because unlike prolapse in vertex positions, the prolapsed cord is protected from compression by the soft fetal legs (Cruikshank 1986, abstracted below). And while few studies allow vaginal birth after cesarean with a breech, one study found no reason to treat such women differently (Ophir et al. 1989).

A woman with a small pelvis and a big baby risks head entrapment because the largest, most unyielding part of the baby comes last, but where do you draw the line? Pelvimetry (measuring the pelvis) has poor predictive value for head-down babies, and there is no reason to think it does any better for breech (Mahmood 1990; Hofmeyr 1989). Pelvimetry also assumes, incorrectly, that the pregnant woman's pelvis is rigid and that no other factors besides pelvic dimensions affect her ability to push out the baby.

Finally, although I will focus on term singleton breech, preterm breech management is equally muddy. More and more doctors are delivering the tiniest babies by cesarean based on statistics from retrospective studies, an inadequate data source. In one of many examples of obstetric minds being made up ahead of the facts, doctors sabotaged one attempt at a randomized controlled trial of cesarean versus vaginal birth (for both vertex and breech preterm infants) by refusing to enroll their patients (Lumley 1985). Retrospective data from the time period that the trial was supposed to be taking place showed that vaginally born babies were smaller and younger than cesarean born babies. This suggests that vaginally born babies in nonrandomized studies may be disadvantaged. In other words, women are undergoing the risks of surgery and having their future reproductive lives blighted by a scarred uterus without firm evidence that a cesarean improves outcomes. Worse yet, because the lower segment of the uterus does not develop until close to term, these women will usually have vertical incisions made in the uterine muscle and will not be candidates for vaginal birth after cesarean (VBAC).

Some guidelines emerge from the confusion. The woman with a breech fetus should try self-help strategies to turn it starting in the eighth month, then ECV, and if ECV fails, she should seek evaluation for vaginal breech birth from someone experienced, ideally someone whose practices promote spontaneous birth. Optimal management for a preterm or twin breech or when no one is experienced with vaginal breech is unclear. Women should insist on a sonogram to rule out anomalies incompatible with life before agreeing to a cesarean. And whatever she decides, she must understand that no matter what is done (or not done), good outcome cannot be guaranteed—and that includes delivering the baby by cesarean.

Note: Here are the breech types:

- *Frank breech*: bottom down in pike position, flexed at the hips with legs straight.

- *Complete breech*: bottom down, flexed at both hips and knees. A complete breech may convert to an incomplete breech during labor.

- *Incomplete breech*: usually a footling breech—has one or both feet or knees presenting to the birth canal.

SUMMARY OF SIGNIFICANT POINTS

- Rotating a posterior baby to anterior (by assuming the hands-and-knees position; see Abstract 29 in Chapter 5) will increase the odds of successful ECV. (Abstracts 22-23)

- Tocolytic use excludes women with certain medical problems from ECV, but tocolytics are not essential. (Abstracts 6, 8-9, 20-21)

- ECV significantly reduces the number of breech babies. Success rates range from 41% to 77% and average 63%. Because the presenting part engages late in black African women, success rates averaged 89%. (Abstracts 6-21)

- ECV studies have shown no fetal morbidity among a collective population of 1419 women. (Abstracts 6-21)

- Experience is not a factor in ECV success rates. (Abstract 6)

- Labor is not too late to try ECV. (Abstracts 4, 12, 19, 42)

- Computed tomography (CT) scans provide better pelvimetry pictures at one-third to one-eleventh the X-ray radiation exposure. (Abstracts 4, 35, 42)

- There is no evidence that radiation pelvimetry has better predictive value than clinical pelvimetry, and ultrasound can be used to look for anomalies and rule out hyperextended neck. (Abstracts 1, 3, 5, 43)

- Most breech morbidity is unrelated to birth route. (Abstracts 1-3, 24, 26, 28-29, 32-33)

- Vaginal breech birth is a viable option. Cesarean rates have safely been as low as 20%. (Abstracts 1-5, 19, 34, 36-43)

- Increased cesarean rates have not improved breech outcomes. (Abstracts 1, 3, 25-34)

- Primiparas, nonfrank breeches, and VBAC candidates should not be routinely excluded from vaginal birth. (Abstracts 1-3, 5, 41-43)

- Cesarean section carries risks for both mother and baby, including birth injuries. (Abstracts 1-2, 4-5, 11, 24-25, 36, 39-42)

- Epidural anesthesia increases the odds of birth injury. (Abstract 5)

- Forceps are not always required. (Abstracts 4-5, 38, 42-43)

ORGANIZATION OF ABSTRACTS

Review Papers

External Cephalic Version Is Safe and Effective

Randomized Controlled Trials
Reports
Tocolytics Are Not Necessary
Factors Affecting ECV Success Rates

Cesarean Section Does Not Improve Breech Outcomes

Long-Term Follow-Up (Review Paper)
Long-Term Follow-Up (Studies)

Vaginal Breech Is Safe

Pelvimetry: CT Scan Versus X Ray
Frank Breech
Nonfrank Breech
All Types of Breech

REVIEW PAPERS

1. Confino E et al. The breech dilemma. A review. *Obstet Gynecol Surv* **1985;40(6):330-337.**
Sources of morbidity are explored. Injury or anoxia comes from mechanical trauma—either from the birth process itself or from efforts to extract the baby.

Hyperextension of the fetal head (about 5%) is particularly dangerous and requires a cesarean. Cord prolapse is more likely among multiparas, premature babies, and non-frank presentations, but EFM allows timely diagnosis so that intervention can avert harm. More breeches are preterm (30% born by 34 weeks gestation versus 5% of vertex babies). Congenital anomalies are also more frequent (6.3% versus 2.4%). Breech may cause musculo-skeletal problems because the baby cannot move freely. Uterine malformations and placental implantation site also may cause a breech.

Despite cesarean rates as high as 90%, asphyxia rates still exceed rates in vertex infants and long-term prognosis has not improved. Damage and trauma have occurred during cesarean extraction. In addition, maternal morbidity is increased.

As for vaginal breech management, primiparity is not an indication for cesarean. X-ray pelvimetry can be useful but exposes the fetus to cancer-causing radiation, and predictability for birth problems is poor. "The . . . belief, that dysfunctional labor could be masked [by oxytocin], is not supported by any controlled prospective studies." Epidural anesthesia permits ease of intrauterine manipulations. While guidelines help with selection, "miraculous prescriptions do not exist for a safe breech delivery. Individualization and sound clinical judgement are indispensable."

2. Cruikshank DP. Breech presentation. *Clin Obstet Gynecol* 1986;29(2):255-263.
Predisposing factors are malformations, uterine anomalies, uterine overdistension, high parity, and pelvic obstruction. Prematurity strongly associates partly because a smaller fetus is freer to be breech and partly because the factors that predispose to breech also predispose to preterm labor. Only one-third of perinatal deaths are potentially preventable.

Routine cesarean section is not recommended because "1) cesarean delivery does not guarantee an atraumatic or nonasphyxiating birth [and] 2) cesarean holds a much greater risk of both maternal morbidity and mortality." In addition, many breech infants have nonsurvivable anomalies.

We have no evidence that primiparous women or incomplete breeches should routinely have cesareans. Umbilical cord prolapse occurs more often in footling breeches, but with EFM, it is not a disaster because the legs protect the cord from compression. "Nonetheless, it is difficult in today's medicolegal climate to argue too vociferously with those who wish to deliver all incomplete breeches abdominally." [In other words, it is OK for the doctor's interest to supersede the patient's.] With prior cesarean, a repeat cesarean is recommended, although no evidence supports this. Hyperextended neck is a cesarean indication; neck straight up is not.

X-rays are recommended for pelvimetry and to rule out hyperextended neck and malformations. X ray or ultrasound should be done after labor onset because babies turn spontaneously and because the baby may move its head.

As for labor management, membrane rupture is not recommended except for internal EFM. Arrest of dilation or descent is an indication for cesarean, and oxytocin should not be used. Primiparas should not exceed one hour to push out the baby and parous women 30 minutes. Epidural anesthesia is "excellent" but not "mandatory" if the mother is "cooperative" and can refrain from pushing until full dilation. The "conservative course" is to allow the epidural to wear off because it slows pushing [it would not wear off in the time allotted]. A "generous" episiotomy is necessary, preferably mediolateral, and the baby's body should be extracted by hand and the head with forceps.

With the premature breech, a vertical cesarean incision is best because the lower uterine segment is poorly developed, although this "seriously compromises future child-bearing." With a mature breech, the transverse incision may need to be extended to a J-shape [which could also cause problems later].

3. Myers SA and Gleicher N. Breech delivery: why the dilemma? *Am J Obstet Gynecol* 1986;156:6-10.

When prematurity and cord prolapse are accounted for, nonfrank breeches do no worse than frank breeches. One study showed reduced mortality when forceps were routinely applied to the head, but no other data exist. No study has found that babies weighing more than 1500 g (30-31 weeks gestation) do better with cesareans. Studies showing benefits for babies weighing less than 1500 g have significantly more infants weighing less than 1000 g in the vaginal group. One study that accounted for confounding variables found no differences in long-term outcomes. The argument that inexperience with breech managment dictates cesarean section is specious; trauma can also occur during a cesarean. "Inexperience should never be the reason for a surgical solution." A woman in labor with a breech should have an ultrasound examination to exclude anomalies, check placental location, evaluate fetal weight, and rule out hyperextended neck. She should have continuous EFM and make normal progress in labor. "The need for abdominal delivery should . . . not exceed 20% to 25% of all breech deliveries."

4. Gimovsky ML and Schifrin BS. Breech management. *J Perinatol* 1992;12(2):143-151.

Because many breeches are not identified until late in labor, all doctors should know how to manage vaginal breech birth safely. The highest injury rates occur when birth is imminent and there is no protocol [probably partly because the doctor panics]. Even to perform a safe cesarean, a doctor must be "facile with total breech extraction, an inherently more dangerous procedure than the assisted breech delivery that we anticipate in the majority of vaginal deliveries." Studies have shown that when vaginal breech is managed by protocol, outcomes are comparable to elective cesarean.

In the past, using force during ECV led to hemorrhage and isoimmunization, a risk when RhoGAM [a globulin injected into Rh-negative mothers that prevents antibody formation to an Rh-positive fetus] was not available. Tocolysis, ultrasound, and nonstress testing contribute to ECV's safety today. ECV may be attempted in labor unless membranes are ruptured. Then success is unlikely and the cord may prolapse.

Pelvimetry must be done to confirm an average-size term fetus (3500-4000 g is the upper limit). CT scans give more accurate information at one-third the radiation exposure of X rays. Pelvic diameters are not rigid guidelines because "maternal position alone during labor may affect pelvic diameters. . . . [I]t is important to maximize the effect of pelvic diameters by careful maternal placement and positioning during labor and delivery." Head hyperextension contraindicates vaginal birth. Even during a cesarean, these infants demand an adequate incision and great care to avoid spinal cord injury.

Women may elect a cesarean at any time [!]. Oxytocin induction is permitted, but augmentation should be used rarely, if at all, "given the current medicolegal atmosphere." EFM is essential because of the hazard of umbilical cord prolapse. Since this is more likely in second stage, second stage should be conducted in the delivery room.

If prolapse occurs during the second stage and the EFM tracing remains normal, spontaneous birth can be allowed. Pudendal blocks are routine. When available, regional anesthesia is preferred because it reduces the urge to push before full dilation. Investigators, primarily anesthesiologists, have noted "the ease with which breech labor and delivery can be conducted under epidural anesthesia." (In one case a woman became hysterical, efforts to place her under anesthesia [presumably forcibly] in order to deliver the baby were prolonged, and the baby died.) "Vaginal . . . breech . . . requires watchful waiting and gentle manipulation. . . . A 175-lb obstetrician can exert great force on a 7-lb neonate." Forceps are not always required. "Haste is dangerous and usually unnecessary. . . . In two thirds of cases, delivery of the infant by C/S takes significantly longer than vaginal delivery." This protocol has achieved a 35% to 45% vaginal birth rate.

5. Weiner CP. Vaginal breech delivery in the 1990s. *Clin Obstet Gynecol* 1992;35(3):559-569.

Based on the difference between the cost of vaginal and cesarean birth at the University of Iowa ($8600), a 50% vaginal breech rate would save $718 million annually in the U.S. Focusing on studies after 1979 of the term and near-term breech, this review examines whether routine elective cesarean for breech is justified.

Retrospective studies ($N = 13$) of vaginal birth for selected breeches usually found outcomes to be equivalent to cesarean delivery and that c-section did not eliminate birth injuries. Two studies reported increased perinatal mortality for vaginal birth. One was small (68 neonates), and the seemingly high rate is due to one baby's dying of respiratory distress. The linkage to birth route is unclear. The second report is exceptional for two reasons: vaginal birth rate was among the highest (79%), and birth injuries were unusually severe and frequent. Neonatal trauma rates were slightly increased for vaginal birth, but most cases resolved without sequelae.

The University of Iowa database provides additional data on morbidity. X-ray pelvimetry was done in only 35% of women and changed the plan in only 19%. "X-ray pelvimetry for the vertex does not predict vaginal delivery. . . any better than does clinical pelvimetry. . . . In light of the vertex studies, we must question its predictablity for the breech fetus." Overall 69% of women had a trial of labor (TOL) (316 of 458), of whom 63% had vaginal births (43% overall). Vaginal birth increased the incidence of acidosis [an indicator of oxygen lack] (6.3% versus 1.1%, $p = 0.02$), but this would also be true for vertex vaginal births versus elective cesareans. Head entrapment occurred during cesareans (vaginal 2.6% versus cesarean 0.8%, $p = 0.3$). Neonatal trauma happened more often during vaginal birth (45% versus 8%, $p < 0.0001$), but significant trauma did not (2.1% versus 3.3%, NS). No trauma resulted in permanent damage. Epidurals were used in 45% of vaginal births, and their use was associated with increased total trauma (50% versus 38%) but not significant trauma [no numbers given]. C-section increased maternal morbidity and length of hospital stay ($p < 0.001$). Moreover, three large retrospective reports have not found that route of delivery had an impact on neonatal morbidity.

Only two randomized trials have been done. Although they were small, their results agree with the retrospective studies. Long-term follow-up studies include 5000 near-term breeches. They, too, confirm the safety of selected vaginal breech birth. "[A] 40-60% cesarean rate for the near-term and term breech fetus can be justified."

The University of Iowa protocol uses X ray or ultrasound to search for anomalies and rule out neck hyperextension ("stargazers"). Breeches should be either frank or complete. Epidural anesthesia eliminates premature pushing and fears of an "uncooperative" patient during delivery when an assistant will push on the mother's belly to guide the head through the pelvis. [Notice that the mother is not trusted to give birth, and an epidural is used to keep her from reacting to the pain of someone pushing on her belly. Meanwhile, epidurals increase the incidence of neonatal trauma.] Forceps are not often needed. "Often the hardest part of a vaginal breech delivery is doing nothing while the breech crowns." "I do not expect obstetricians to change their practice patterns based on this review. [Why not? Shouldn't evidence change practice?] Rather, those doing vaginal breech deliveries of selected patients should not doubt that the clinical practice has a solid foundation."

EXTERNAL CEPHALIC VERSION IS SAFE AND EFFECTIVE

Note: Except where noted, ECV was preceded by a nonstress test and a sonogram and tocolytics were given. The version itself took about five minutes. Severe pain was a reason to stop. ECV occasionally caused complications, but no morbidity resulted.

Randomized Controlled Trials

Note: All randomized controlled trials except Hofmeyr 1983 (Abstract 7) excluded uterine scar, antepartum bleeding, and placenta previa.

6. Van Dorsten JP, Schifrin BS, and Wallace RL. Randomized control trial of external cephalic version with tocolysis in late pregnancy. *Am J Obstet Gynecol* 1981;141(4):417-424.

	Control ($N = 23$)	Study ($N = 25$)
success rate	—	68%
spontaneous version rate	17%	—
spontaneous reversion rate	—	0
c-section rate	74%	28%

Exclusions: Heart disease, diabetes, thyroid dysfunction "because of possible adverse effects with beta-mimetic [tocolytic drug]," conditions predisposing to placental insufficiency such as hypertension, premature labor or ruptured membranes, intrauterine growth retardation (IUGR), oligohydramnios, and fetal anomaly or nuchal cord [umbilical cord wrapped around the baby's neck].

Time period when attempted: 37-39 weeks.

Miscellaneous: Only 1 of 17 women with a successful ECV had a cesarean versus 6 of 8 of the failures. Experience did not improve the success rate (69% in the first half of the study versus 67% in the latter half).

7. Hofmeyr GJ. Effect of external cephalic version in late pregnancy on breech presentation and caesarean section rate: a controlled trial. *Br J Obstet Gynaecol* **1983;90:392-399.**

	Control (N = 30)	Study (N = 30)
success rate	—	97%
spontaneous version rate	33%	—
spontaneous reversion rate	—	0
c-section rate	20%	43%

Exclusions: Contracted pelvis, Rh-negative blood, obesity.
Time period when attempted: after 36 weeks.
Miscellaneous: Engagement hinders spontaneous version. The high spontaneous version rate is probably because the presenting part tends to engage late among black Africans.

8. Brocks V, Philipsen T, and Secher NJ. A randomized trial of external cephalic version with tocolysis in late pregnancy. *Br J Obstet Gynaecol* **1984;91:653-656.**

	Control (N = 56)	Study (N = 74)
success rate	—	41%
spontaneous version rate	14%	9%
spontaneous reversion rate	—	3%
c-section rate	46%	27%

Exclusions: Uterine anomalies, signs of placental insufficiency, maternal contraindications to beta-mimetics [tocolytic drugs], and conditions favoring premature labor (hypertension, Rh-negative mother).
Time period when attempted: 37 weeks.
Miscellaneous: The ECV was successfully repeated on both spontaneous reversions. Cesarean rate for breech was 50%. Only one vertex baby (2%) was a c-section. ECV success rate in multiparas was 62%.

9. Van Veelen AJ et al. Effect of external cephalic version in late pregnancy on presentation at delivery: a randomized controlled trial. *Br J Obstet Gynaecol* **1989;96(8):916-921.**

	Control (N = 90)	Study (N = 89)
success rate	—	48%
spontaneous version rate	26%	—
spontaneous reversion rate	—	6%
c-section rate	9%	14%

Exclusions: Congenital malformations, oligohydramnios, uterine abnormalities, ruptured membranes, fetal growth retardation.

Time period when attempted: 33-40 weeks.

Miscellaneous: *No tocolytics were used.* Five minutes of auscultation were done
instead of a preceding nonstress test. Assuming a spontaneous version rate of 20% and
a successful ECV rate of 45%, the study had the power to show a significant difference.
Attempts could be repeated up to four times at subsequent visits. The cesarean rate for
breech was 16%. [Therefore, even though more study women had vertex presentations,
cesarean rates for study and controls were similar because the cesarean rate for breech
was so low. Also, spontaneous version rates were high because the study began at 33
weeks.]

**10. Mahomed K, Seeras R, and Coulson R. External cephalic version a term. A
randomized trial using tocolysis. *Br J Obstet Gynaecol* 1991;98:8-13.**

	Control ($N = 105$)	Study ($N = 103$)
success rate	—	86%
spontaneous version rate	17%	—
spontaneous reversion rate	—	3%
c-section rate	33%	13%

Exclusions: Severe hypertension, diabetes, cardiac disease, ruptured membranes.

Time period when attempted: After 37 weeks.

Miscellaneous: The sample size could demonstrate a reduction in breech presentation
from 80% to 30% with 95% certainty. The cesarean rate for breech was 39%. This
study, like Hofmeyr 1983 [see Abstract 7], was of black African women, and like
Hofmeyr's study, ECV success rates and spontaneous version rates were high. Hofmeyr
attributed high spontaneous version rates to a tendency toward late engagement of the
presenting part among African women. [This would also explain high ECV success
rates.]

Reports

Note: All took place under tocolysis. Exclusions in common were oligohydramnios
and fetal anomaly. Except where noted, ECV was done at 36 to 37 weeks or later.

**11. Stine LE, et al. Update on external cephalic version performed at term. *Obstet
Gynecol* 1985;65(5):642-646.**

($N = 148$)

Exclusions: same as Van Dorsten, Schifrin, and Wallace 1981 [Abstract 6].

ECV success rate: 73%.

Spontaneous version rate: 17% controls, 0% ECV failures.

Spontaneous reversion rate: 7%.

Cesarean rate: 24% successes versus 74% controls versus 85% failures.

Miscellaneous: This study incorporates Van Dorsten, Schifrin, and Wallace 1981.

Controls were 23 eligible women randomized to a control group. The overall cesarean rate at this California hospital was 8%. The authors do not know why the cesarean rate is so high among ECV successes. One woman died during a cesarean for fetal distress (unconnected with her ECV). A hemorrhage led to a hysterectomy, and she died of cardiac arrest from an amniotic fluid embolus.

12. Ferguson JE and Dyson DC. Intrapartum external cephalic version. *Am J Obstet Gynecol* 1985;152(3):297-298.

ECV under tocolysis was tried on 15 women in active labor with intact membranes and succeeded in 11 (73%) "without untoward maternal or fetal outcomes." ECV failed in all women with ruptured membranes.

13. Dyson DC, Ferguson JE, and Hensleigh P. Antepartum external cephalic version under tocolysis. *Obstet Gynecol* 1986;67(1):63-68.

($N = 158$)

Exclusions: Conditions predisposing to placental insufficiency such as hypertension, antepartum bleeding, vertical uterine scar, diabetes, cardiac disease, hyperthyroidism, placenta previa, or IUGR.

ECV success rate: 77%.

Spontaneous version rate: 12% controls, 0% ECV failures.

Spontaneous reversion rate: 0%.

Cesarean rate: 14% successes versus 80% controls versus 92% failures.

Miscellaneous: The control group was 40 women similar to the study group on whom ECV was not attempted.

14. Rabinovici J et al. Impact of a protocol for external cephalic version under tocolysis at term. *Isr J Med Sci* 1986;22(1):34-40.

($N = 58$)

Exclusions: Antepartum bleeding; hypertension; diabetes, cardiac, or thyroid disease; more than 5 prior pregnancies; uterine scar or anomaly; contractions and more than 3 cm dilation; placental insufficiency or abruption; IUGR,; placenta previa; ruptured membranes.

ECV success rate: 67%.

Spontaneous version rate: 5% ECV failures.

Spontaneous reversion rate: 3%.

Cesarean rate: 8% vertex versus 61% breeches.

Miscellaneous: The two reversions were successfully reconverted to vertex. [Cesarean rates were not broken down by ECV success versus failure.]

15. O'Grady JP et al. External cephalic version: a clinical experience. *J Perinat Med* 1986;14(3):189-196.

($N = 85$)

Exclusions: Fixed, engaged presenting part; serious pregnancy medical disorder; pregnancy complications such as membrane rupture, abruptio placenta.

ECV success rate: 62.5%.

Spontaneous version rate: 10% ECV failures.

Spontaneous reversion rate: 2%.

Cesarean rate: 9.8% success versus 50.0% failures.

<u>Miscellaneous</u>: The version was attempted at 35 weeks or more.

16. Morrison JC et al. External cephalic version of the breech presentation under tocolysis. *Am J Obstet Gynecol* 1986;154(4):900-903.
(*N* = 304)
<u>Exclusions</u>: Cardiac disease, hypertension, ruptured membranes, IUGR, uterine scar, placenta previa.
<u>ECV success rate</u>: 68%.
<u>Spontaneous version rate</u>: 0% ECV failures.
<u>Spontaneous reversion rate</u>: 3%.
<u>Cesarean rate</u>: 10% success versus 62% failures.

17. Marchik R. Antepartum external cephalic version with tocolysis: a study of term singleton breech presentations. *Am J Obstet Gynecol* 1988;158(6 Pt 1):1339-1346.
(*N* = 65; 53.7% of term breech presentations)
<u>Exclusions</u>: Only those held in common.
<u>ECV success rate</u>: 60%.
<u>Spontaneous version rate</u>: 0% ECV failures.
<u>Spontaneous reversion rate</u>: 0%.
<u>Cesarean rate</u>: 23% success versus 95% failures.
<u>Miscellaneous</u>: The cesarean rate at this California hospital was 28.9% [!]. In 72% of cases where ECV was not attempted, the reasons were patient refusal [which the authors admit meant the obstetrician was not enthusiastic], version not offered, or breech was undiagnosed before labor. A discussant of the paper says that while version decreases the cesarean rate for breech, "we may find ourselves at increased legal risk, should a serious complication arise." [In other words, judge the procedure not on its merits for mother and baby but on its risks for the doctor.]

18. Hanss JW. The efficacy of external cephalic version and its impact on the breech experience. *Am J Obstet Gynecol* 1990;162(6):1459-1464.
(*N* = 96)
<u>Exclusions</u>: None listed.
<u>ECV success rate</u>: 48.9%.
<u>Spontaneous version rate</u>: 2% ECV failures.
<u>Spontaneous reversion rate</u>: 2%.
<u>Cesarean rate</u>: 17.2% success versus 77.5% failures.
<u>Miscellaneous</u>: One success took two attempts.

19. Cook HA. Experience with external cephalic version and selective breech delivery in private practice. *Am J Obstet Gynecol* 1993;168(6 Pt 1):1886-1890.
(*N* = 60)
<u>Exclusions</u>: Ruptured membranes, oligohydramnios, placenta previa, abnormal antepartum test, previous cesarean.
<u>ECV success rate</u>: 53%.
<u>Spontaneous version rate</u>: 0?.
<u>Spontaneous reversion rate</u>: 0.
<u>Cesarean rate</u>: 28% success versus 86% failures.

Miscellaneous: One successful ECV was done in early labor. Among five additional women who had no ECV attempt, four had vaginal birth. Overall, 31 of 65 fetuses (48%) were born vaginally. Of the 33 term breeches, only 2 of 25 cesareans done for breech presentation were done intrapartum. The rest were scheduled. The most common reason was refusal of TOL (10). "The trend toward [cesarean for breech] has become so entrenched in the minds of the public that many patients expressed surprise at the possibility of vaginal delivery."

Tocolytics Are Not Necessary

20. Robertson AW et al. External cephalic version at term: is a tocolytic necessary? *Obstet Gynecol* **1987;70(6):896-899.**
The ECV protocol was typical except that women were randomized to tocolytic ($N = 30$) or no tocolytic ($N = 28$). The success rate was 66.7% in the tocolytic group versus 67.8% among controls. Of the nine control group failures, only one was successful after tocolytic administration. Although the numbers are small, success rates are similar to other studies, and failures acted as their own controls in that subsequent tocolytic use did not appreciably increase success. Insulin-dependent diabetes, hyperthyroidism, and some forms of heart disease contraindicate tocolytics.

21. Scaling ST. External cephalic version without tocolysis. *Am J Obstet Gynecol* **1988;158(6 Pt 1):1424-1430.**
Sixty-six women underwent 90 ECVs without use of tocolytics. The success rate at 34 weeks gestion or less was 74.3% versus 45.5% at beyond 35 weeks. The overall success rate was 60.6%. Five women had spontaneous reversions after successful ECV earlier than 34 weeks. All were successfully reconverted. No maternal or fetal morbidity resulted. One infant had a one to two minute bradycardia that reverted to normal without treatment. Advantages of early ECV are more room in utero, less need for tocolytics since the uterus is less irritable, less discomfort, and the fetus has not dipped into the pelvis so less force is required. "The essence of success without complications appears to be *gentle* manipulation of the fetus and nonpersistence if version is not readily accomplished."

Factors Affecting ECV Success Rates

Note: Many studies, including these two, evaluated what factors affected ECV success, but except for posterior lie, none were factors that could be changed (see Abstract 29 in Chapter 5).

22. Ferguson JE, Armstrong MA, and Dyson DC. Maternal and fetal factors affecting success of antepartum external cephalic version. *Obstet Gynecol* **1987;70(5):722-755.**
For anterior versus posterior fetuses ($N = 158$), the odds were 14 to 1 for successful ECV ($p = 0.003$), by far the strongest association. The next strongest was multiparity versus nulliparity at 5 to 1.

23. Donald WL and Barton JJ. Ultrasonography and external cephalic version at term. *Am J Obstet Gynecol* **1990;162(6):1542-1547.**

Among 65 fetuses, only frank breech ($p < 0.05$) and anterior position ($p < 0.01$) associated significantly with successful ECV.

CESAREAN SECTION DOES NOT IMPROVE BREECH OUTCOMES

24. Gimovsky ML and Paul RH. Singleton breech presentation in labor: experience in 1980. *Am J Obstet Gynecol* **1982;143(7):733-739.**

Of 330 pregnancies, 74.2% were cesareans. Preventable mortality was limited to infants weighing less than 1300 g and morbidity was largely confined to low-birth-weight babies. Brachial plexus injury [injury to a network of nerves serving the arm, shoulder, and chest] occurred in four infants, of whom two were cesareans and two were assisted vaginal births. Neonatal morbidity did not differ between vaginal and cesarean birth. However, of 245 women who had cesarean sections, one had a hysterectomy for hemorrhage, two had aspiration pneumonia, and nine had serious wound infections. There was no morbidity among women giving birth vaginally.

25. Green JE et al. Has an increased cesarean rate for term breech delivery reduced the incidence of birth asphyxia, trauma, and death? *Am J Obstet Gynecol* **1982;142(6 Pt 1):643-648.**

The study compares outcomes for healthy term breeches and mothers with a similar vertex population during two time periods at the same hospital: 1963-73, when the breech cesarean rate was 22%, and 1978-79, when it was 94%. Neither deaths nor birth injuries decreased significantly. "Rates of asphyxia have remained the same and continue to be much higher than rates in vertex deliveries, which emphasizes the fact that the risk inherent to the maneuvers of extracting a breech by cesarean section is similar to that associated with the delivery of a breech via the vaginal route [or that the causes of asphyxia are not related to birth route]."

26. Petitti DB and Golditch IM. Mortality in relation to method of delivery in breech infants. *Int J Gynaecol Obstet* **1984;22:189-193.** (See Abstract 27 for morbidity.)

This study analyzed method of delivery with respect to mortality for 1593 breech infants weighing 1000 g or more born in 1976-77 at northern California Kaiser hospitals. Compared by birth weight, neonatal death rates between cesarean and vaginal birth were similar. Neonatal plus intrapartum death rates were not consistently higher in one group. By contrast, perinatal mortality was significantly higher for vaginal breeches. Thus, the differences were entirely due to antepartum deaths. "[W]e conclude that routine cesarean delivery for breech infants at any birth weight is not justified considering the risk of mortality."

27. Croughan-Minihane MS et al. Morbidity among breech infants according to method of delivery. *Obstet Gynecol* **1990;75(5):821-825.** (See Abstract 26 for mortality.)

Using the same population as Abstract 26, outcomes were compared for cesarean versus vaginal birth for 1240 singleton breech infants born who were free of congenital neurologic abnormalities and alive at hospital discharge. The cesarean rate was 75%.

The analysis focused on perinatal asphyxia, intracranial hemorrhage, skull fractures, neonatal seizures, cerebral palsy, developmental delay, mental retardation, and spasticity. After adjustment for birth weight, all of these outcomes, whether considered individually or in groups of multiple factors, were similar for vaginal versus cesarean-born babies. Of the three malpractice suits over cerebral palsy, two were cesarean-born infants. One of the cesarean infants was a term baby weighing 4830 g, and the other two were preterm. "This study and others provide support for the notion that proper selection of cases of breech presentation does not increase the risk of childhood morbidity in those delivered vaginally."

28. Rosen MG and Chik L. The effect of delivery route on outcome in breech presentation. *Am J Obstet Gynecol* **1984;148(7):909-914.**
A series of 17,667 births, of which 403 were breech, was analyzed. Multiple births, footling breech, major fetal anomalies, planned cesareans, and antepartum deaths were excluded. Delivery route did not significantly associate with neonatal death or neurologic morbidity. The raw mortality figures suggested vaginal birth to be riskier than cesarean section, but stratification into birth weight categories revealed a disproportionate number of breech infants weighing less than 1000 g were born vaginally, probably in an attempt to spare mothers of nonviable infants a cesarean section. Birth weight and maturity explained the largest proportion of variance in outcome.

29. Schutte MF et al. Perinatal mortality in breech presentations as compared to vertex presentations in singleton pregnancies: an analysis based upon 57819 computer-registered pregnancies in the Netherlands. *Eur J Obstet Gynecol Reprod Biol* **1985;19(6):391-400.**
Data represent 70% of all hospital births since 1982 ($N = 57,819$). After correcting for the higher proportion of low gestational age and birth weight among breech infants and excluding congenital anomalies (also higher among breech infants), breech mortality exceeded vertex mortality at every gestational age ($p < 0.01$). However, cesarean section did not improve outcomes. At 37 weeks or more, the neonatal death rate (this excludes prenatal deaths as a confounding factor in vaginal birth) among breeches was 1.0% for c-section versus 0.7% for vaginal birth. "If the higher neonatal mortality in breech presentation were due to the risk of vaginal delivery, neonatal mortality should be lower in those delivered by caearean section. However, although the incidence of caesarean section was higher in the breech group than in the vertex group at any gestational age, the neonatal mortality after caesarean section was higher in the breech than in the vertex group and there was no statistical evidence that neonatal mortality was lower after caesarean section."

Long-Term Follow-Up (Review Paper)

30. Westgren M and Ingemarsson I. Breech delivery and mental handicap. *Ballieres Clin Obstet Gynaecol* **1988;2(1):187-194.**
More breeches than cephalic babies are born preterm, a difference intrinsic to breech because the difference persists when cases are stratified by week of gestation. Congenital anomalies are more common, as are complications of pregnancy that pose fetal risk (abruptio placentae, placenta previa, oligo- and hydramniosis). "[I]t seems prudent to consider the possibility that the causes of breech presentation may play a more impor-

tant role in the final outcome than the mechanisms at delivery."

Five recent studies (infants born in the 1970s and 1980s) found no difference in breech outcomes for vaginal versus cesarean birth. A sixth [Svenningsen NW, Westgren M, and Ingemarsson I, Abstract 34] concluded that vaginal birth of infants with hyperextended head accounted for the difference. "Vaginal delivery in strictly selected cases of breech presentation can be performed with minimal risk for the infant, and the rate of neurodevelopmental handicap will not be higher than in abdominally delivered breech infants or in cephalic presentations. It is not possible to give the ideal rate of cesarean section for full-term infants . . . [but] several authors have reported excellent long-term outcome with a caesarean section rate of 20-40%."

Long-Term Follow-Up (Studies)

31. Huchcroft SA, Wearing MP, and Buck CW. Late results of cesarean and vaginal delivery in cases of breech presentation. *Can Med Assoc J* 1981;125:726-730.

The study compared functioning at ages 2½ to 8½ for 281 vaginal breech births with 106 breech intrapartum cesarean deliveries and 16 planned cesareans. Cognitive and motor abilities, behavior, and health problems were evaluated. "The difference between children delivered vaginally and those delivered by cesarean section with labour are negligible in size and not statistically significant. The results were unaltered by gestation-specific analysis." The numbers were too small for statistical analysis, but the babies born by planned cesarean did worse.

32. Faber-Nijholt R et al. Neurological follow-up of 281 children born in breech presentation: a controlled study. *Br Med J* 1983;286:9-12.

This Dutch study compared 256 breech-born children with vertex matched controls who underwent neurologic examination at 18 months or at 3 to 10 years. Matching criteria were sex, birth weight, gestational age, and age, parity, and blood pressure of the mother. The study excluded birth weights below 1000 g but included twins. Perinatal mortality was high (13.2%) among the breeches, but deaths were "almost exclusively" due to causes unrelated to birth route. The cesarean rate was 20%. While breeches tended toward more neurologic dysfunction, the difference was not significant. "[T]he main danger of breech presentation is in the associated complications of pregnancy and . . . there is no reason to advocate a higher frequency of abdominal delivery than the 20% found in this study."

33. Rosen MG et al. Long-term neurological morbidity in breech and vertex births. *Am J Obstet Gynecol* 1985;151(6):718-720. (subset of same data as Abstract 24)

Seventy frank breech vaginal births with no congenital anomalies and for whom records could be obtained for two years after birth were matched by birth weight and race with a similar breech infant born by cesarean, a vertex vaginally born infant, and a vertex cesarean-born infant. Only major brain damage was evaluated because it is less subject to socioeconomic variables. No significant differences were found between breech populations or between breech and vertex presentations. The change to cesarean section has not benefited frank breeches. Studies of the effect of birth route on breeches are often confounded by the high incidence of low birth weight and congenital anomalies, variables controlled for here.

34. Svenningsen NW, Westgren M, and Ingemarsson I. Modern strategy for the term breech delivery—A study with a 4-year follow-up of the infants. *J Perinat Med* **1985;13:117-124.**

Two time periods were compared: 1971-74 (period A), when the cesarean rate was 17% (N = 300), and 1974-77 (period B), when pelvic measurement criteria were stricter and estimated birth weight greater than 4000 g and hyperextended neck became cesarean indications, and the cesarean rate was 37% (N = 339). Preterm and anomalous infants, multiple births, and antenatal deaths were excluded. Neurologic examinations were performed at two and four years old. The 4-year examination was compared with a control group of vaginally born, full-term singletons.

At two years, the handicap rate was 4.6% in period A versus 1.5% in period B, with most of the difference in vaginally born babies. At four years the rates were 5.3% in period A, 2.4% in period B, and 1.5% for vertex infants. The difference between period A and vertex infants was significant ($p < 0.05$). Five of the 14 problem children in period A would have been cesareans under the later criteria. Two of the five problem children in period B had vaginal births with hyperextended heads despite the criteria. Had these been cesareans, the difference between period B and vertex infants would disappear. "Vaginal delivery in strictly selected cases of breech deliveries can be performed with minimum risk to the infant."

VAGINAL BREECH IS SAFE

Pelvimetry: CT Scan Versus X Ray

35. Kopelman JN et al. Computed tomographic pelvimetry in the evaluation of breech presentation. *Obstet Gynecol* **1986;68(4):455-458.**

CT scans consistently take better-quality pictures at one-third the radiation exposure of conventional X rays.

Frank Breech

Note: All are term, singleton, frank breech. I list only birth-route-related complications.

36. Collea JV, Chein C, and Quilligan EJ. The randomized management of term frank breech presentation: a study of 208 cases. *Am J Obstet Gynecol* **1980;137(2):235-244.**

N = 208; 115 women randomized to trial of labor, 93 to cesarean.

Cesarean rates: 52% of women allocated to vaginal birth, 18% of the 60 women with adequate pelvimetry.

Management: Oxytocin augmentation permitted. Forceps for aftercoming head in 57 of 60 vaginal births; three were spontaneous. Birth anesthesia was pudendal block, 38; epidural, 1; general, 10; none, 6.

Infant morbidity: Vaginal (3%): two brachial plexus injuries, one resolved and the other resolving when lost to follow-up and two with depressed 5-minute Apgar scores, one due to narcotics. Cesarean (1%): two with depressed 5-minute Apgars.

Maternal morbidity: Vaginal (2%): one transfusion. Cesarean (13%): three wound infections resulting in 21- and 18-day hospital stays in two cases and eventual hysterectomy in the third; another hysterectomy for hemorrhage when an artery was nicked; 14 additional cases of transfusion; one inhalation pneumonia from general anesthesia.

Miscellaneous: Five women allocated to cesarean had vaginal births. Sixty women allocated to vaginal birth had cesareans either because they were disqualified by pelvimetry or during labor. Brachial plexus injuries occur when there are nuchal arms [arms behind baby's neck]. "[O]bstetricians performing breech extraction carefully and without haste should be able to avoid the occurrence of nuchal arms."

37. Watson WJ and Benson WL. Vaginal delivery for the selected frank breech infant at term. *Obstet Gynecol* **1984;64(5):638-640.**

$N = 91$ actually entered into the trial. Out of 254 term breeches, 91 (35.8%) were nonfrank breech (all but three were cesareans). Of the remaining 165 frank breech presentations, 12 gave birth vaginally before pelvimetry was done, leaving 151 eligible for protocol management. Of these, 24 had cesareans because the doctor did not want the patient in the protocol, there was no time for pelvimetry, or it was an elective repeat cesarean. Five babies had a hyperextended neck, there were miscellaneous medical reasons in four cases, and 27 women had a contracted pelvis.

Cesarean rates: 24% among women allowed to labor, 36% among all frank breeches, 67% (including the additional reasons above) among the total population.

Exclusions: Hyperextended neck, estimated weight more than 4000 g, complications such as placenta previa, abruption, distress, or contracted pelvis

Infant morbidity: 0

Miscellaneous: This study assigned women to three groups: (1) adequate pelvic measurements, (2) borderline, and (3) contracted. Group 1 had a 21% cesarean rate, group 2 a 33% cesarean rate [no p value given], and group 3 had scheduled cesareans. Oxytocin was used in group 1. "[T]he absence of reliable capability for rapid cesarean section at the authors' institution has led to the current policy of cesarean section for nonfrank breech presentations." [This is an admission that the hospital provides inadequate care to all women and subjects women with nonfrank breeches to the risks of cesarean surgery unnecessarily.]

38. Stein A. A cooperative nurse-midwifery medical management approach. *J Nurse-Midwifery* **1986;31(2):93-97.**

$N = 89$; 62 met criteria for labor (14 had footling breech).

Cesarean rates: 64% overall, 48% of women meeting criteria for labor.

Exclusions: Maternal health problems, uterine scar, hyperextended neck, "unusually large" fetus, inadequate pelvic measurements, postdates, abrupted placenta, membranes ruptured and no labor.

Management: EFM, IV, no oxytocin or amniotomy. Birth position sitting on delivery table with feet in or out of stirrups. Midwife helps guide baby, but expulsive force is mother's. All births spontaneous.

Infant morbidity: 0

Miscellaneous: Births were attended by midwives.

39. Bingham P, Hird V, and Lilford RJ. Management of the mature selected breech presentation: an analysis based on the intended method of delivery. *Br J Obstet Gynaecol* 1987;94(8):746-752.

$N = 313$; 149 trial of labor, 164 planned cesarean.

Cesarean rates: 40% among women allowed to labor, 71% among the total group.

Infant morbidity: Vaginal (1%): one fractured clavicle. cesarean (0.4%): one laceration.

Maternal morbidity: Vaginal: 0. Cesarean (0.4%): one hysterectomy for hemorrhage.

Miscellaneous: Nine percent of breeches were first diagnosed in labor. No relation found between birth weight, pelvimetry, and birth route. Ten scheduled cesareans were performed on eligible women at their request. "The higher the rate of failed trial of labour, the less desirable a policy of allowing a trial of labour becomes . . . because the risks of emergency caesarean are greater than those of elective operations." [Nonetheless, vaginal birth is the safest of all.]

40. Christian SS et al. Vaginal breech delivery: a five-year prospective evaluation of a protocol using computed tomographic pelvimetry. *Am J Obstet Gynecol* 1990;163(3):848-855.

$N = 159$ met study criteria (40.4% of all breeches), 122 had CT pelvimetry (77% of 159 eligible cases), and 85 had adequate measurements (70% of 122 having CT scan).

Cesarean rates: 18.8% among 85 women allowed to labor, 43% among 122 women having CT scan.

Exclusions: Estimated birth weight less than 2000 g or more than 4000 g, congenital anomalies, placenta previa, hyperextended head, inadequate pelvis.

Infant morbidity: Umbilical cord pH was lower among vaginal births ($p < 0.05$), but the difference was clinically insignificant..

Maternal morbidity: Vaginal: four intrapartum fever, one postpartum fever, postpartum anemia. Cesarean: five intrapartum fever, 8 postpartum fever, one wound separation, anemia. [The text says significantly more anemia among planned cesarean compared with vaginal birth, but a chart shows more among vaginal births.]

Miscellaneous: ECV is performed and has a 67% success rate [see Abstract 20]. CT scan radiation exposure about 82 mrad versus X ray at 500-1100 mrad. Compared with vaginal birth, uterine infection after cesarean was more common in women who labored (43.8%, $p < 0.01$) and anemia more common among nonlabor cesareans ($p < 0.01$), probably due to "unlabored lower uterine segment and resultant greater intraoperative blood loss."

Nonfrank Breech

41. Gimovsky ML et al. Randomized management of the nonfrank breech presentation at term. *Am J Obstet Gynecol* 1983;146(1):34-40.

$N = 105$; 70 randomized to trial of labor, 35 to cesarean.

Cesarean rate: 56% among women allowed to labor.

Exclusions: Severe hypertension, more than 1 prior cesarean, history of stillbirth or infertility, Class B or greater diabetes, IUGR, abnormal antepartum tests, abnormal amniotic fluid volume, inadequate pelvic measurements.

Management: EFM, oxytocin allowed, "generous" midline episiotomy or episioproctotomy [through the rectal sphincter, which leads to serious long-term problems; see Chapter 14], 22 assisted delivery with forceps, six assisted manually, three spontaneous

Infant morbidity: Vaginal (6.7%): one death (3.2%) (the woman became hysterical during birth, was anesthetized with difficulty), one 5-minute Apgar less than 7 (no sequelae). Cesarean (3%): one laceration, one 5-minute Apgar less than 7.

Maternal morbidity: Vaginal (3%): one fever. Cesarean (64%): 37 fever, six transfusion, two wound infections.

Miscellaneous: Four women allocated to cesarean had vaginal births. Three cases of cord prolapse and two cases of body prolapse in first-stage labor were delivered by cesarean; all did well.

All Types of Breech

Note: Except where noted, all are term pregnancies.

42. Flanagan TA, et al. Management of term breech presentation. *Am J Obstet Gynecol* **1987;156(6):1492-1502.**
N = 623; 244 trial of labor, 379 planned cesarean.
Cesarean rate: 28% of women allowed to labor, 72% overall.
Exclusions: Inadequate pelvic measurements, hyperextended head, estimated weight more than 3850 g.
Management: 17% oxytocin use, 66% pudendal, 24% epidural (the authors like epidural because it "allows a slow, controlled delivery"), 3% general, 7% no anesthesia, 18% spontaneous, 74% assisted or partial extraction, 8% complete extraction.
Infant morbidity: Vaginal (6%): nine bruising, one buttock laceration. Cesarean (1%): three bruising, three buttock laceration.
Maternal morbidity: Vaginal: 6.3% transfusion, 2.3% wound infection, 0.6% endometritis. Planned cesarean: 7.7% transfusion, 1.3% wound infection, 13.7% endometritis. Cesarean after labor: 4.3% transfusion, 14.5% endometritis.
Miscellaneous: Only 61% of breeches were identified before labor, of which 48% underwent ECV. Of these, only 48% were successful, but ruptured membranes, uterine scar, and anterior placenta were not excluded. Of planned cesareans, in 42% the indications were "patient's choice," "breech," or "previous cesarean section." One of the authors observes that although umbilical artery pH was lower [more acidic] among vaginal births, this was not clinically significant, and "If you do not know how to deliver a breech vaginally, you do not know how to do it by cesarean either."

43. Roumen FJ and Luyben AG. Safety of term vaginal breech delivery. *Eur J Obstet Gynecol Reprod Biol* **1991;40(3):171-177.**
N = 247; 234 trial of labor, and 13 planned cesareans.
Cesarean rate: 15.4% among women allowed to labor, 20.6% overall.
Exclusions: Hyperextended neck, gross obstruction of birth canal, gross anomalies.
Management: *No pelvimetry was done*, EFM, oxytocin used, no epidural anesthesia. Spontaneous birth in 109 (44.1%), assisted delivery in 87 women (35.2%), total extraction in two cases, and forceps for aftercoming head in four cases.
Infant morbidity: Vaginal (1.5%): one death when head was trapped (0.5%), one

Erb's palsy (recovered), one clavicular fracture. In all breech groups umbilical cord pH was lower compared with a vertex, vaginal birth group, but the findings were not clinically significant (the lower values were unrelated to Apgar scores or neurologic morbidity).

[No maternal morbidity given.]

Miscellaneous: "[A] trial of labor in carefully selected patients with a healthy child in breech presentation at term is a safe procedure, that can be successfully completed in almost 80% of cases." [This is a Dutch study. In Holland cesarean rates are very low, and one third of the population has home births.]

REFERENCES

Bodmer B et al. Has use of cesarean section reduced the risks of delivery in the preterm breech presentation? *Am J Obstet Gynecol* 1986;154(2):244-250.

Clausen I and Nielsen KT. Breech position, delivery route and congenital hip dislocation. *Acta Obstet Scand* 1988;67(7):595-597.

Cunningham FG, MacDonald PC, and Gant N, eds. *William's Obstetrics*. 18th ed. Norwalk, CT: Appleton and Lange, 1989.

Fenwick L and Simkin P. Maternal positioning to prevent or alleviate dystocia in labor. *Clin Obstet Gynecol* 1987;30(1):83-89. (abstracted in Chapter 5)

Hofmeyr GJ. Suspected fetopelvic disproportion and abnormal lie. In *A guide to effective care in pregnancy and childbirth*. Enkin M, Keirse MJNC, and Chalmers I, eds. Oxford: Oxford University Press, 1989.

Hytten FE. Breech presentation: is it a bad omen? *Br J Obstet Gynaecol* 1982;89(11):879-880.

Jordan B. External cephalic version as an alternative to breech delivery and cesarean section. *Soc Sci Med* 1984;18(8):637-651.

Kasule J, Chimbira THK, and Brown McL. Controlled trial of external cephalic version. *Br J Obstet Gynaecol* 1985;92:14-18.

Lumley J et al. A failed RCT to determine the best method of delivery for very low birth weight infants. *Controlled Clin Trials* 1985;6:120-127.

Mahmood TA. The influence of maternal height, obstetrical conjugate and fetal birthweight in the management of patients with breech presentation. *Aust N Z J Obstet Gynaecol* 1990;30(1):10-14.

Ophir E et al. Breech presentation after cesarean section: always a section? *Am J Obstet Gynecol* 1989;161(1):25-28.

Thorpe-Beeston JG, Banfield PJ, and Saunders NJ. Outcome of breech delivery at term. *BMJ* 1992;305:746-747.

VanTuinen I and Wolfe SM. *Unnecessary cesarean sections: halting a national epidemic*. Washington, D.C.: Public Citizen's Health Research Group, 1992.

7

Fetal Distress and Electronic Fetal Monitoring

Myth: *Electronic fetal monitoring allows us to rescue babies from death or brain damage.*

Reality: *"Twenty-five years after electronic fetal monitoring became part of intrapartum care, . . . it is yet to be proved of value in predicting or preventing neurologic morbidity."*

Rosen and Dickinson 1993

H.L. Mencken is supposed to have said, "For every complex problem there is a solution that is simple, neat—and wrong." Electronic fetal monitoring (EFM) is a perfect example of that truth. The reasoning behind EFM goes like this (Freeman 1990): Asphyxia (inadequate oxygen) during labor causes many perinatal deaths and cases of mental retardation and cerebral palsy (CP). Auscultation (listening to the fetal heart rate) picks up abnormal patterns preceding these outcomes, but intervening rarely averts them. The problem must be too little information too late. Surely a machine that continuously monitors the fetal heart rate (FHR), making a tracing for analysis, will give doctors a reliable means of diagnosing fetal distress and preventing damage. However, none of the links in this chain of reasoning is sound.

One grave misapprehension is that labor events are a significant source of neurologic damage. Few instances of brain damage originate during labor. Among the 20 to 40 cases of CP and 40 cases of mental retardation that occur per 10,000 births (Hall 1989, abstracted below), asphyxia is implicated in only about 8% of the CP cases (1.6-3.2/10,000) (Hall 1989) and 5% of the severe mental retardation cases (2/10,000) (Rosen and Hobel 1986, abstracted below). Thus, at most, eradicating asphyxia would prevent three cases of CP and two cases of severe retardation per *10,000* babies. Moreover, in many cases of asphyxia, asphyxia was not the only insult, and it is by no means clear what portion of the damage can be attributed to it. Commenting on malpractice suits arising from brain damage, a *Lancet* editorial (1989) remarked, "In light of the evidence . . . , the continued willingness of doctors to reinforce the fable that intrapartum care is an important determinant of [CP] can only be regarded as shooting the specialty of obstetrics in the foot."

A second, equally grave error is the belief that abnormal FHR patterns are reliable predictors of markers of asphyxia. Studies in this chapter show that while a normal pattern predicts good outcome (high specificity), the reverse is not true (low sensitivity). The high false-positive rate has led EFM zealots to think EFM effective. Fetal distress appears; a prompt cesarean or forceps delivery is performed; voilá—the baby is fine. Conclusion: EFM saved the baby—only the baby was fine all along.

Furthermore, low short-term Apgars and acidosis (low blood pH, a symptom of oxygen lack) are themselves poor predictors of brain damage. Again, false negatives are rare, false positives common. If the link between abnormal FHR and asphyxial symptoms is weak and the tie between asphyxia and brain damage is weak, then the link between fetal distress and damage is weak indeed.

Some have argued that doctors do not interpret tracings properly (ACOG 1989; Parer 1986), but even experts disagree on the same set of tracings (interobserver variability) (Nielsen et al. 1987; Beaulieu et al. 1982). What is more, no expert does a good job at predicting which babies will be born asphyxiated (Murphy et al. 1990). The latest research wrinkle is computer analysis of tracings, but if no distress pattern ties closely with outcome, neither computer analysis nor refinements of EFM technology can help.

Others argue that follow-up tests of a suspect fetus will reduce the number of false alarms, but follow-up tests—fetal scalp-blood sampling, vibro-acoustic or tactile stimulation, or looking at FHR variability (small increases and decreases over time)—can be done in conjunction with auscultation. Also, as with all other measures of fetal well-being, good news reassures, but bad news does not unequivocally confirm problems.

Another mistaken belief is that information from a machine is more reliable than information from people. With external monitoring, which uses ultrasound to pick up the FHR through the mother's abdomen, electronics may cause halving or doubling of the heart rate (Amato 1983). Sometimes the transducer picks up the maternal pulse instead of the fetus's resulting in a false diagnosis of bradycardia (abnormally slow heart rate) and a possible emergency cesarean, unless someone compares the monitor with the mother's pulse.

In fact, the widespread use of EFM has not improved outcomes. Yes, three of the ten randomized controlled trials (RCTs) of EFM versus ausculation (all abstracted below) have found EFM beneficial. However, Thacker (1987, abstracted below) gave one of those two trials (Renou et al. 1976) a dismal 29% quality rating on a scale where more than 80% was considered good. The second trial found more seizures among the EFM group (9 versus 16 among

10,094 babies), but follow-up at one year showed no difference in disability (MacDonald et al. 1985). The third trial also suffered serious methodological problems and reported results widely discrepant from any other RCT.

On the contrary, EFM is doing harm. All of the trials except one showed significant increases in cesarean, instrumental, or operative delivery rates (a combination of both) among electronically monitored women. Between 1980 and 1985 "fetal distress" contributed 16.1% to the rise in cesarean rate, and by 1989, 9.9% of all births were cesareans for this diagnosis, up from 1.2% in 1980. (VanTuinen and Wolfe 1992).

In addition, studies of women's preferences have found that depersonalized care is a concern although one of EFM's so-called advantages, especially with the newer central stations, is less patient contact (Hansen et al. 1985; Garcia et al. 1985). It is telling that in one study ascertaining women's preferences before randomization and after labor, substantially more women (three to two) originally preferring EFM were converted to auscultation by their labor experience than vice versa. And while not to disparage the importance of women's preferences, hands-on care may affect outcomes. Several studies have found that personal contact reduces complication and intervention rates (Sosa et al. 1980; Klaus et al. 1986; Hodnett and Osborn 1989; Kennell et al. 1991).

Theoretically, a new test should prove itself better than the old before it becomes widely accepted, but as Freeman (1990) put it, "The story of [EFM] . . . illustrates the need for proper randomized clinical trials before new forms of technology are introduced that may become the standard of practice without clearly demonstrated benefit." As EFM repeatedly failed comparisons with auscultation, it should have withered away, but it did not. The percentage of U.S. women undergoing EFM rose from 45% in 1980 to 62% in 1988, and 73% of women had EFM in 1990 (U.S. Department of Health and Human Services 1993). The increase was greater among low-risk women, who were least likely to benefit, than high-risk women (Albers and Krulewitch 1993).

Doctors tell us that EFM protects against malpractice suits or hospitals have too few nurses to auscultate often enough (*Ob Gyn News* 1988). The malpractice argument rests on beliefs that tracings are valuable courtroom evidence and that not using EFM renders doctors liable because it is standard practice. As to the first, Sandmire (1990, abstracted below) trenchantly observes that a tracing "leaves a permanent record for hindsight interpretation by expert witnesses" who will claim that mild deviations indicate fetal distress. As for the liability issue, Gilfix (1984) reviewed the law pertaining to EFM and informed consent and concluded that using auscultation over EFM did not render a doctor liable because of the abundant evidence that auscultation is equally good. Indeed, Gilfix continued, informed consent demands that women be informed of risks and benefits of proposed tests and treatments, which would mean a duty to inform women that EFM has not been shown to improve outcomes but increases operative delivery rates. Finally, "too few nurses to auscultate" really means too few nurses to provide optimum care. Gilfix thinks doctors may be obliged to inform women of this too.

Meanwhile, what about "first do no harm"? Both of these defenses of EFM are predicated on benefits to doctors and hospitals at the expense of mothers and babies.

Judith Lumley (1982), quoting J.B. McKinley, paints yet a darker picture of the forces driving EFM:

> The success of an innovation has little to do with its intrinsic worth ... but is dependent upon the power of the interests that sponsor and maintain it. . . . *The power of such interests is also evident in their ability to impede the development of alternative practices . . .* that could conceivably threaten an activity in which there is already considerable investment. [italics added]

> The "need" for universal EFM legitimates so many other contentious decisions on the place, style and management of labor that it will not be discarded in favor of [auscultation] but only displaced when another new, equally unevaluated procedure arrives on the obstetric scene.

This would explain why only one study has looked at whether auscultation was feasible in a big, busy unit—finding, by the way, that it was (Sandmire 1990, abstracted below).

To Lumley I add that EFM fits what obstetricians want to believe. When doctors call normal labor "asphyxiating" (Nageotte 1985; Parer and Livingston 1990), they can then cast themselves as heroes—ever vigilant, using special knowledge and the miracles of technology to rescue infants unable to withstand the rigors of labor from the clutches of their mother's bodies. This fantasy may be preferable to the painful truth: that doctors must make their best guess, that EFM does not eliminate the guesswork, and that in most cases harm cannot be averted, yet inaction may mean fetal death or damage. Moreover, the unnecessary operative deliveries generated by EFM may injure or kill healthy mothers or babies.

SUMMARY OF SIGNIFICANT POINTS

- Infant neurologic morbidity rarely correlates with labor events. (Abstracts 1-7, 9, 32)

- Markers of asphyxia correlate poorly with brain damage. Even when asphyxia precedes brain damage, it may be a result, not the cause. (Abstracts 1, 3-4, 7-12, 16, 32)

- Abnormal FHR correlates poorly with markers of asphyxia and brain damage. (Abstracts 3, 13-19, 25, 34)

- Compared with auscultation, EFM benefits neither high-risk nor low-risk infants. RCTs that found that EFM improved outcomes either had serious methodological flaws or found only short-term benefits. (Abstracts 4-5, 13, 20-24, 27-30, 32, 33-36)

- EFM increases the odds of cesarean or instrumental delivery. (Abstracts 13, 20-24, 26-31, 33-34)

- EFM may increase the risk of CP, possibly because internal EFM increases infection rates. (Abstracts 4, 32, 36)

- Oxytocin increases fetal morbidity rates. (Abstracts 10, 21, 31)

- The "cure" for fetal distress—cesarean or forceps delivery—can itself be asphyxiating or traumatizing. (Abstracts 2, 14, 16, 18, 26-27, 31)

- Auscultation is feasible in a big, busy unit. (Abstract 23)

- Rubbing the fetal head or holding a buzzer against it can be used as a follow-up test for abnormal FHR instead of fetal scalp-blood sampling. (Abstracts 38-39)

- By diminishing FHR variability, narcotic analgesia can falsely indicate fetal compromise and perhaps confound the reassurance test. (Abstracts 38-39)

- More babies have abnormal FHR patterns with EFM than with auscultation. Is this an artifact or might EFM be *causing* it? (Abstracts 28, 33-34, 37)

ORGANIZATION OF ABSTRACTS

Fetal Distress and Brain Damage

Intrapartum Events a Rare Cause of Brain Damage (Reviews)
Intrapartum Events a Rare Cause of Brain Damage (Studies)
Measures of Asphyxia Predict Brain Damage Poorly
Abnormal FHR Predicts Asphyxial Signs Poorly

EFM and Fetal Distress

EFM (Review Papers and Analyses)
EFM (Randomized Controlled Trials and Follow-up Studies)
Alternatives to Fetal Scalp Blood Sampling

FETAL DISTRESS AND BRAIN DAMAGE

Intrapartum Events a Rare Cause of Brain Damage (Reviews)

1. Paneth N and Stark RI. Cerebral palsy and mental retardation in relation to indicators of perinatal asphyxia. *Am J Obstet Gynecol* **1983;147(8):960-966.**

Among school-aged children, 3 to 4 per 1000 are severely mentally retarded. About 8% of the retardation is of perinatal origin, which includes causes other than asphyxia. Therefore two to three cases of severe retardation of perinatal (but not necessarily asphyxial) origin occur per 10,000 school-age children. Excluding congenital anomalies, 2 to 2.5 per 1000 school-aged children have CP.

Studies found that "anoxia" (defined by low Apgar scores or a need for resuscitation) associated only weakly with lowered IQ or CP among term infants. For example, 18 of 22 "apparent stillbirths" had normal IQ. The four who did not took more than 30 minutes to establish respirations. Term infants with a 5-minute Apgar of 3 or less had more than a 95% chance of being free of CP, and the "overwhelming majority" had normal IQ. Perinatal asphyxial indicators account for less than 1% of the variance in IQ at age seven. "[T]he role of perinatal events in the genesis of severe mental retardation and cerebral palsy is not as large as popularly thought. . . . The majority of even quite severely asphyxiated babies suffer no detectable neurologic or intellectual sequelae."

2. Rosen MG and Hobel CJ. Prenatal and perinatal factors associated with brain disorders. *Obstet Gynecol* **1986;68(3):416-421.** (summary of a 1985 report of the same title)

CP, mental retardation, and epilepsy arise from many causes, and asphyxia rarely plays a role. Even when it does, it is often found with other complications. The asphyxial response may be occurring in an already damaged fetus. Conversely, most severely asphyxiated infants will be normal. "Most dismaying," only rarely can asphyxia be prevented. Even suboptimal obstetric care did not result in more cases of CP.

Mental retardation not associated with epilepsy or CP associates with hypoxia in less than 5% of cases. Socioeconomic status has far stronger associations. Epilepsy with no other neurologic deficits may not be due to birth injury at all. The incidence of CP has not changed in the past decade [despite the rise in EFM].

[A discussion of implications for obstetric care remarks that the reduction in complicated forceps deliveries has reduced trauma-caused deaths and injuries, a damning indictment of the harm doctors do—harm now shifted mostly to mothers by the increased cesarean rate.] If 3.38 babies per 1000 live births develop CP, how can we prevent that without overtreating the other 996 mothers? "Even if all infants were born by cesarean, at least half of [CP] cases would still exist, because in at least this proportion, the causes antedate the labor period."

3. Hall DMB. Birth asphyxia and cerebral palsy. *BMJ* **1989;299:279-282.**

Two to four cases of CP occur per 1000 births and 3.7 cases of mental retardation per 1000 births. There is little evidence that the incidence of either has declined despite improved obstetric standards or that the most reliable predictors of damage—seizures or hypoxic-ischemic encephalopathy [neurologic symptoms believed due to oxygen deprivation]—have declined either. Most mental retardation unaccompanied by CP is prenatal in origin. About 8% of CP cases associate with (but may not be caused by) birth asphyxia. Identifying which cases of CP are asphyxial is difficult because FHR abnormalities, acidosis, meconium staining, and low Apgar scores do not reliably predict CP. Hypoxic-ischemic encephalopathy and neonatal seizures are more reliable, but both may have causes other than asphyxia. Asphyxia is unlikely to begin in labor because prompt delivery rarely prevents adverse outcome. Asphyxia in most cases may be a chronic or subacute process in pregnancy rather than an acute insult in labor, but difficulty with resuscitation leads to the erroneous diagnosis of birth asphyxia.

"[N]either the traditional signs of fetal distress nor the use of electronic monitoring permit the reliable recognition of the asphyxiated infant during labour. . . . Even when fetal distress is recognised and leads to speedy delivery the damage may already have been done. . . . [W]hen the infant is found to be suffering from cerebral palsy [or mental retardation] it is unwise to assume that more prompt action would have avoided it."

4. Nelson KB and Emery ES. Birth asphyxia and the neonatal brain: what do we know and when do we know it? *Clin Perinatol* 1993;20(2):327-344.

The review is limited to term, singleton infants free of malformations and to characteristics identifiable after labor onset. CP occurs in 1 or 2 per 1000 births, and of these, 10% or fewer (1 or 2/10,000) experienced severe birth asphyxia. Because of this rarity, even tests with 90% specificity and sensitivity rates will produce primarily false positives.

Meconium: Meconium staining is common. Its major predictor is advanced gestational age. Thick meconium results from low amniotic fluid volume, a risk in its own right. Meconium alone is not associated with a significant increase in CP. A small increase in risk is found for the few cases who also had low 5-minute Apgars.

FHR: Marked fetal bradycardia (< 60 beats per minute) somewhat increases risk of CP. In two trials (Grant 1989; Shy et al. 1990, Abstracts 32 and 36) EFM associated with increased risk of later neurologic abnormality, especially in low-birth-weight children. This may be because internal EFM predisposes to chorionitis [infection], a risk factor for CP. EFM has not been shown to predict long-term neurologic outcome.

Low Apgar scores: Most low Apgars are related to prenatal events. Moderately and briefly low Apgar scores do not relate to neurologic outcome, although very low long-term Apgars do predict CP. Apgar score and its correlates—hypotonia, need for resuscitation, delay in first breath—indicate illness but not what kind.

pH: The relationship between low pH and neurologic symptoms, even neonatally, has not been impressive. Most acidotic babies do not develop neurologic symptoms, and most infants with these symptoms are not markedly acidotic.

Other than disasters like placental abruption, cord prolapse, or severe bradycardia, we have no reasonable means of identifying asphyxia in labor except markers with "enormously high" false-positive rates. Fetal growth retardation associates with increased risk of asphyxia, but it may be the cause of intrauterine growth retardation (IUGR) and not IUGR itself that increases risk. If so, asphyxia in labor may be irrelevant to outcome, and early delivery will not prevent bad outcomes. Asphyxia, hypoxia, and ischemia may all result from factors unrelated to labor. For example, sepsis produces many of the same signs in children and adults that are attributed to asphyxia in the neonate. The fact that certain pathologies can be produced experimentally in animals by reducing oxygen supply does not establish that this is the only or chief path to that outcome in humans.

In conclusion, the authors are unable to identify asphyxiating processes in labor without high false-positive rates. Overidentifying babies as at-risk subjects them to increased risk with no benefit because even noninvasive tests provoke a chain reaction of intervention. Clinical signs of neurologic depression indicate illness but not its cause. Their absence indicates that there was no asphyxia, but their presence does not establish the opposite.

Intrapartum Events a Rare Cause of Brain Damage (Studies)

5. Levene ML, Kornberg J, and Williams THC. The incidence and severity of post-asphyxial encephalopathy in full-term infants. *Early Hum Develop* **1985;11:21-26.** (England)

The records of birth-asphyxiated term infants born between 1980 and 1983 ($N = 126$) were graded for severity of postasphyxic encephalopathy (PAE) [neurologic symptoms believed subsequent to asphyxia]. EFM was practiced selectively [presumably in high-risk cases]. Where possible, other causes of irritability (e.g., hypoglycemia) were excluded.

Of infants with PAE, 23% had normal Apgar scores and "a proportion" of infants with low Apgars were neurologically normal. The overall incidence of PAE was 6 per 1000, of whom 25% were growth retarded [and thus suffering from a chronic problem]. This incidence rate was the same as that found in a study done in a similar hospital before EFM was available. Mild encephalopathy rarely leads to disability, and the incidence of moderate or severe PAE was only 2.1 per 1000. [Thus EFM could benefit 2.1 term babies per 1000, assuming all cases could be prevented and intervening introduced no risks of its own.]

6. Nelson KB and Ellenberg JH. Antecedents of cerebral palsy. *N Engl J Med* **1986;315(2):81-86.** (U.S.)

The authors conducted a multivariate analysis of risk factors for CP ($N = 189$) using a database of 45,559 pregnancies between 1959 and 1966 at 12 university hospitals. No intrapartum risk factor alone contributed more than 2% of the risk. Including intrapartum information did not identify many more cases than pregnancy risk factors alone. When all risk factors were considered, the 5% of babies at highest risk contributed only 37% of the CP cases. Only 2.8% of the 2177 babies in the top 5% of risk developed CP (97% false-positive rate). Only 40 of the 189 children with CP had asphyxial signs, of whom 58% (23) had at least one leading prenatal predictor. [Assuming all asphyxia-associated CP could be prevented, EFM could potentially benefit 40 of 45,559 babies (9/10,000). Assuming EFM would prevent CP only where asphyxia was the only explanation, the number drops to 17 per 45,559 babies (4/10,000).] Conclusions:

> First, if we do not know the cause or causes of most [CP] or if the causes are numerous or arise very early in development and no one cause contributes much of the outcome, then no foreseeable single intervention is likely to prevent a large proportion of [CP]. Second, information about events during labor, delivery, and the newborn period did not identify a substantially larger number of cases than information limited to major characteristices determined before labor . . . [which] suggests a relatively small role for factors of labor and delivery.

7. Blair E and Stanley FJ. Intrapartum asphyxia: a rare cause of cerebral palsy. *J Pediatr* **1988;112(4):515-519.** (Australia)

Each case of congenital CP from the western Australia CP register between 1975 and 1980 (*N* = 183) was matched with three control subjects for year of birth, birth weight, and demographics. Birth asphyxia was defined as fetal distress and 1-minute Apgar less than 7. Fetal distress was defined as meconium and/or abnormal FHR. Abnormal neurologic signs were defined as any abnormality, mild or severe. Definitions were broad to avoid missing a relationship with asphyxia. A population-attributable risk (PAR) was calculated, which is "the maximum proportion of a disease that can be attributed to a characteristic or etiologic factor (if it, in fact, were causal)." Thus a PAR is the decrease in incidence of disease that may be expected were the risk to be eliminated. Records were scored as to likelihood of asphyxial cause. In only 8.2% of cases was it thought possible or likely that birth asphyxia caused CP. The PAR was 14.1%, but this does not mean asphyxia was causal. Asphyxia may be a sign of CP, not the cause.

Measures of Asphyxia Predict Brain Damage Poorly

8. Dijxhoorn MJ et al. The relation between umbilical pH values and neonatal neurological morbidity in full term appropriate-for-dates infants. *Early Hum Develop* **1985;11(33-42.** (Holland)

Using data from the Gröningen Perinatal Project, this study ascertained the relation between blood chemistry and neurologic morbidity among 805 vaginally-born, normal-weight, singleton, term infants born between 1975 and 1978. A low-risk subgroup (*N* = 205) (no antenatal hospital admission, no meconium, no drugs in labor, second stage shorter than 60 minutes, spontaneous vaginal birth of vertex infant, no congenital malformations) was also analyzed to eliminate possible confounding factors. The study found that normal umbilical pH at birth did not guarantee normal neurology and that umbilical artery and vein pH and maternal-fetal differences in pH were all poor predictors of neonatal neurology in appropriate-for-dates infants.

9. Dijxhoorn MJ et al. Apgar score, meconium and acidaemia at birth in small-for-gestational age infants born at term, and their relation to neonatal neurological morbidity. *Br J Obstet Gynaecol* **1987;94:873-879.** (Holland)

Using the same database as the previous study, the relation between birth asphyxia and neurologic condition was evaluated for 247 small-for-gestational age (SGA) term infants (to eliminate any contribution of prematurity). Infants were grouped into moderate SGA (below tenth percentile, over 2.3 percentile) (*N* = 178) and severe SGA (below 2.3 percentile) (*N* = 46). Controls were 805 appropriate-for-gestational age (AGA) vaginally born and 82 AGA cesarean-born infants. Six infants were neurologically abnormal at ages 4 to 6. Birth asphyxia as measured by Apgar scores, blood gases, and meconium contributed only 7% of the variance in neurologic condition among moderately SGA infants and 22% among severely SGA infants. This relationship was stronger than among AGA infants but still suggests that chronic prenatal deprivation was the prime factor.

10. Ruth VJ and Raivio KO. Perinatal brain damage: predictive value of metabolic acidosis and the Apgar score. *Br Med J* **1988;297:24-27.** (Finland)

Records of infants (*N* = 982) born at a high-risk referral center were used to determine the predictive value of acidosis and/or low 5-minute Apgars for brain damage. All women had EFM. Reference values were obtained from 127 healthy, normal children whose mothers had no medical or labor complications. Abnormal was defined as ±2 standard deviations from the mean (pH 7.16 vaginal birth, 7.25 elective cesarean).

While significantly lower pH values were measured with oxytocin, epidural, vaginal delivery, labor longer than 12 hours, second stage more than 30 minutes, meconium staining, and cord compression ($p < 0.001$), the difference was clinically unimportant. Birth asphyxia could have played a role in 42 cases of death or brain damage. Sensitivities of umbilical arterial pH, lactate concentration, 5-minute Apgar, and Apgar plus pH were 21%, 12%, 12%, and 7%; specificities were: 89%, 91%, 98%, and 99%; positive predictive values were: 8%, 5%, 19%, and 27%; negative predictive values were: all 96%. Acidosis may have poor positive predictive value because abnormal outcomes do not relate to birth asphyxia or because the asphyxic insult occurred before labor. Alternatively, acidosis, the redistribution of blood flow to vital organs and the switch to anaerobic metabolism, may be a healthy adaptation to stress.

11. Dennis J et al. Acid-base status at birth and neurodevelopmental outcome at four and one-half years. Am J Obstet Gynecol 1989;161(1):213-220. (England)

The relationship between acid-base status at birth and neurodevelopmental outcomes at 4 1/2 years was determined for 192 singleton term infants. Excluded were children who suffered postnatal neurologic insults and those not speaking English. The study had an 85% chance of detecting a three-fold increase in poor outcomes in the most acidotic group (pH ≤ 7.10, base deficit > 12 mmol/l). Results showed no relationship between acid-base status and abnormal neurologic development. This was not due to an all-or-none effect (acidotic infants died or survived intact). Only three infants died, of whom none were acidotic. An acidotic shift may be a sign the fetus can adapt to stress and its absence a sign of compromise. Unimpaired infants predominated in the most acidotic group whereas non-acidotic infants with low Apgars fared worse in certain areas.

12. Low JA et al. The association of intrapartum asphyxia in the mature fetus with newborn behavior. Am J Obstet Gynecol 1990;163(4):1131-1135. (Canada)

Asphyxiated term newborns (umbilical artery buffer base value < 34.0 mmol/l) born 1987-89 ($N = 51$) were matched by gestational age and weight to the next unasphyxiated newborn. At three days old and again at two weeks babies were given the Brazelton newborn assessment test by someone blinded to whether the babies were from the study or control group. No differences were found at three days. At two weeks scores differed significantly in two of the seven areas tested, although the subgroup with severe asphyxia did no worse than the subgroup with moderate asphyxia [which means that unlike what would be expected if asphyxia caused neurologic deficit, the relationship was not dose-dependent]. Apgar scores were lower in the asphyxiated group, but only two newborns had Apgars of 0 to 3 and only four had signs of encephalopathy. Newborns with Apgars of 0 to 3 scored significantly lower in one area at three days and a different area at two weeks, a finding attributed to chance due to the numerous analyses made. As expected, newborns with encephalopathy scored lower in several areas. The results suggest that damage occurs only with severe acidosis. [Acidosis cannot even predict subtle behavioral differences, let alone major problems.]

Abnormal FHR Predicts Asphyxial Signs Poorly

13. Sykes GS et al. Fetal distress and the condition of newborn infants. *Br Med J* **1983;287:943-945.** (England)

The operative delivery rate for fetal distress among 850 infants was 8.6%, of which only 11.5% had severe acidosis at birth (umbilical artery pH < 7.12 and base deficit > 12/mmol/l), 24.1% had 1-minute Apgar less than 7, and 15.8% had both. The operative delivery rate for fetal distress among women who had EFM was 15.9% versus 2.2% among auscultated women. EFM was selective based on risk.

Comparing women who had EFM (46.5%) with auscultated women, 13.6% versus 0% of nonacidotic babies had operative deliveries for fetal distress, 2.3% versus 2.2% had operative delivery and severe acidosis, 7.8% versus 8.4% had spontaneous birth and severe acidosis, and the rest, 76.3% versus 89.4%, had neither operative delivery nor acidosis. The study confirmed that fetal distress rarely predicted severe acidosis or low Apgars. EFM did little to improve precision in predicting adverse outcome, and it is unlikely that the high operative delivery rate in the EFM population prevented higher rates of adverse outcomes since the majority of newborns with severe acidosis or low Apgars did not have fetal distress. [EFM also caused an unnecessary operative delivery rate of 13.6% because these babies were fine at birth.]

14. Curzen P et al. Reliability of cardiotocography in predicting baby's condition at birth. *Br Med J* **1984;289:1345-1347.** (England)

The relation between EFM tracing and condition at birth was examined for all babies who had continuous EFM ($N = 5962$) between 1978 and 1982. The operative delivery rate for fetal distress was 8.3%. Sensitivities of abnormal FHR for 1-minute Apgar below 7 and the subgroups that needed or did not need intermittent positive pressure ventilation (IPPV) [assistance with breathing] were 23.2% Apgar below 7, 35.2% IPPV, and 20% no IPPV. Positive predictive values were: 27.4% Apgar below 7, 8.7% IPPV, and 18.7% no IPPV. Regarding specificity, 93.4% had normal FHR and 1-minute Apgar above 7. Positive predictive values for abnormal FHR, operative delivery for fetal distress, and Apgar below 7 were: 15% forceps, and 47% cesarean. For IPPV they were 3% forceps and 18% cesarean. For no IPPV they were 12% forceps and 29% cesarean. For babies with normal EFM tracings, 5.8% of spontaneous births, 9.9% of forceps, and 38.5% of cesarean deliveries had Apgar below 7. Also for babies with normal EFM tracings, 0.6% of spontaneous births, 1.8% of forceps, and 11.7% of cesarean deliveries required IPPV. [Forceps, and especially cesareans, increased the odds of low Apgars and IPPV in infants with *normal* FHRs. This means that forceps and cesareans can themselves be asphyxiating. This also means that correlations between abnormal FHR, low Apgar, and IPPV are even poorer than values indicate because the "cure" can cause the "disease."] "[W]e should re-examine the current overdependence on fetal monitoring by cardiotocography."

15. Keegan KA, Waffarn F, and Quilligan EJ. Obstetric characteristics and fetal heart rate patterns of infants who convulse during the newborn period. *Am J Obstet Gynecol* **1985;153(7):732-737.** (U.S.)

Newborns with seizures ($N = 66$) were grouped by weight—(1) 2500 g or more or (2) less than 2500 g—and matched to normal infants for weight and gestational age. All had continuous EFM. More abnormal FHR patterns were found among study infants than controls (group 1, 85% versus 24%, $p < 0.0001$); group 2, 63% versus 31%, $p < 0.05$). Loss of FHR variability was greater only among group 1 infants (59% versus 9%, $p < 0.0001$) [which suggests variability discriminates poorly among group 2]. Confirming the prognostic importance of seizures, at six months 42% of study infants had neurologic deficits. In 11 of 14 cases of distress, infants were born less than 1 hour after onset of abnormal pattern, and although 15 group 1 infants had FHR abnormalities, none qualified as distress. If EFM enables intervention before damage occurs, why was there so much morbidity in a monitored population with prompt response to fetal distress? "Significantly, in the face of severe FHR abnormalities, poor neonatal outcome was not avoided by appropriate intervention. Equally significant was that with poor outcome and lesser degrees of FHR abnormality, nonintervention did not equate with inappropriate management."

16. Lissauer TJ and Steer PJ. The relation between the need for intubation at birth, abnormal cardiotocograms in labour and cord artery blood gas and pH values. *Br J Obstet Gynaecol* **1986;93:1060-1066.** (England)

All 56 infants beyond 32 weeks gestation and more than 1500 g requiring intubation over a six-month period were studied. Eight were delivered by *elective* cesarean, 24 had normal cardiotocograms (CTG), 17 had abnormal CTGs, and 7 could not be classified. The pH was significantly lower and the base deficit higher in the abnormal CTG group ($p < 0.01$). Mean birth weight was significantly lower ($p < 0.005$). One-minute Apgars were not related to CTG, but 5-minute scores were ($p < 0.05$). The majority (32) of infants had neither abnormal CTG nor acidosis. Of these, 8 had meconium, and 24 failed to establish breathing and had FHR less than 100 beats/min. Of the 24, 8 were elective cesareans [!], 8 were emergency cesareans, and 2 were forceps. [This suggests operative delivery is itself stressful.] Apgar scores correlated poorly with abnormal CTG or cord blood analysis. The need for ventilation also correlated poorly with acidosis, as over half were nonacidotic. "[T]he need for intubation cannot be equated directly with . . . intrapartum hypoxia, or metabolic acidosis at delivery."

17. van den Berg P et al. Fetal distress and the condition of the newborn using cardiotocography and fetal blood analysis during labour. *Br J Obstet Gynaecol* **1987;94:72-75.** (Germany)

Outcomes were analyzed for 2669 babies born at one hospital in 1984 who were alive at the onset of labor and had EFM. A scalp blood sample (22%) [usually sampling rates are about 4%] was taken for FHR decelerations or bradycardia unless the head was on the pelvic floor, in which case forceps were used. Operative delivery was performed (8% cesarean, 1% forceps) for scalp pH below 7.25 or FHR above 160 beats/min for more than 3 hours. Poor condition at birth was defined as umbilical artery pH below 7.20, Apgar less than 7 [1-minute?], or both. Sensitivities for EFM plus blood sampling were: 52.7% pH, 46.1% Apgar, and 61.5% both. Specificities were: 93.4% pH, 91.7% Apgar, and 91.5% both. False-positive rates were: 71.2% pH, 91.9% Apgar, and 95.3% both. False-negative rates were: 2.5% pH, 0.9% Apgar, and 0.3% both. That EFM plus blood sampling detected only 46% to 61% of distressed fetuses is attributed to "misinterpretation of the monitor trace and to delay between a fetal blood sample that gave a normal result and delivery." That 71% to 92% of "distressed fetuses" were fine at birth is attributed to "management that prevents acidosis." The authors find "strong justification for continuous fetal heart monitoring in labour and for fetal scalp-blood sampling." [This cannot be concluded, however, without showing that EFM and scalp blood sampling did better than auscultation.]

18. Steer PJ et al. Interrelationships among abnormal cardiotocograms in labor, meconium staining of the amniotic fluid, arterial cord blood pH and Apgar scores. *Obstet Gynecol* **1989;74(5):715-721.** (England)

This prospective study looked at all 698 women with complete labor data who gave birth during six months in 1984. Moderate acidosis was defined as between 1 and 2 standard deviations below the mean (umbilical artery pH 7.17-7.085) and severe acidosis as more than 2 standard deviations below the mean (pH < 7.085). With normal cardiotocogram (CTG), only 4% had moderate and 1% severe acidosis. Abnormal CTGs occurred during 41% of labors but acidosis in only 12.6%. Overall sensitivity of CTG for acidosis was 80% and for severe acidosis 83%. For first-stage abnormality, it was 47% for all acidosis and 67% for severe acidosis. The false-positive rate was 32% for any abnormality and 14% for first-stage abnormality. Most of the variance in pH could be explained by CTG abnormality. Adding meconium (16% incidence) did not improve the overall correlation. However, the major correlation with 1-minute Apgar was cesarean delivery and meconium and the next greatest correlation was abnormal CTG. Abnormal CTG did not correlate with 5-minute Apgar, although meconium, birth weight, mode of delivery, and gestational age did. Although CTG did best, 65% of the variability in pH, 72% of the variability in 1-minute Apgar, and 86% of the variability in 5-minute Apgar remain unexplained. "Not only do [CTG abnormality, meconium, acidosis, and low Apgar] correlate poorly with one another, but they correlate poorly with long-term neurologic outcome." [I calculated the positive predictive value for any CTG abnormality and all acidosis at 23%.]

19. Rosen MG and Dickinson JC. The paradox of electronic fetal monitoring: more data may not enable us to predict or prevent infant neurologic morbidity. *Am J Obstet Gynecol* **1993;168(3 Pt 1):745-751.** (U.S.)

A review of 10 studies failed to document that FHR patterns associated with neurologic injury (neonatal seizures, intraventricular hemorrhage, CP) or that intervening averted neurologic injury. Sensitivities of EFM for adverse outcomes ranged from 23% to 100% and specificities from 45% to 100%. Positive predictive values depended on prevalence, but in all cases this value will be low because of the rarity of these outcomes, even in high-risk populations. "It is clear from a review of these studies that a specific pattern, or group of patterns, of FHR monitoring that may predict brain damage is not available for use by the clinician today." Despite increased use of EFM, there have been no changes in incidence of CP in term infants.

The authors then analyzed FHR patterns from 55 brain-damaged infants and failed to find consistent patterns that foreshadowed the injury. This is because the majority of infant brain damage occurs outside of labor. "We do not advocate the abandonment of the use of [EFM], but we do believe that it is yet to be proved to be of value in predicting or preventing neurologic morbidity." [The are saying, in effect, that EFM is worthless, but not to abandon it.]

EFM AND FETAL DISTRESS

EFM (Review Papers and Analyses)

20. Shy KK, Larson EB, and Luthy DA. Evaluating a new technology: the effectiveness of electronic fetal monitoring. *Ann Rev Public Health* **1987;8:165-190.**

First, five of the strongest nonrandomized comparative studies of EFM were analyzed for quality. All took place in the early to mid-1970s and found improved outcomes, especially for high-risk women. Their greatest flaw was lack of definition of auscultation protocol. Without this, important differences in supervision of non-EFM labors cannot be excluded. And by their nature, comparative studies do not control for bias in assignment.

Next, eight randomized trials were analyzed. Six found no difference in outcomes; two found fewer neonatal seizures. Six found an increase in cesareans and the other two in forceps deliveries. [However, one of the two that did not find an increase in cesarean rate is MacDonald et al., Abstract 31, where the total cesarean rate was 2%.] RCTs were generally of higher quality.

> We believe that in contradistinction to the results of the comparative studies, EFM is unlikely to have a substantial impact on perinatal events. . . . Given the increasing evidence that EFM has little effect on perinatal outcomes (with the possible exception of neonatal seizure), . . . periodic auscultation should be available for all parturients who request it. This should occur in both academic and community hospitals.

21. Thacker SB. The efficacy of intrapartum electronic fetal monitoring. *Am J Obstet Gynecol* **1987;156(1):24-30.**

The quality of seven RCTs of EFM was assessed. Using a scoring system where higher than 80% is considered good, MacDonald et al. 1985 [Abstract 31] scored 86%; Kelso et al. 1978 [Abstract 30], Havercamp et al. 1979 [Abstract 29], and Neldam et al. 1986 [Abstract 34] scored over 50%; Havercamp et al. 1976 [Abstract 28] scored 45%; Wood et al. 1981 [Abstract 27] scored 32%; and Renou et al. 1976 [Abstract 26], the only RCT besides MacDonald et al. to find fewer adverse neurologic sequelae, scored only 29%.

A meta-analysis was done on pooled data from all trials except MacDonald et al. ($N = 3928$). No significant differences were found for Apgar less than 7, Apgar less than 4, perinatal death rate, or neonatal seizures, but the relative risk of cesarean section was 2.17 (CI 1.72-2.73) and operative delivery was 1.42 (CI 1.24-1.62). For high-risk pregnancy trials only, no significant differences were found for perinatal death, Apgar less than 7, neonatal intensive care admissions, or neonatal seizures. More cesareans were done (RR 2.48, CI 1.78-3.16) but not more operative deliveries. Pooling trials using fetal scalp-blood sampling showed it somewhat reduced the increased risk of cesarean (RR 1.81, CI 1.33-2.47) and the relative risk of operative delivery was unchanged (RR 1.47, CI 1.24-1.74).

Taking MacDonald et al. alone (nearly 13,000 women), neonatal seizures were reduced, but equal numbers had sequelae at one year. Seizures were associated with oxytocin and "prolonged labor." [Labors are augmented in all primiparous women progressing slower than the average 1 cm hour.] Cesareans were not significantly increased [the cesarean rate was only 2%], but instrumental deliveries were.

22. Prentice A and Lind T. Fetal heart rate monitoring during labour—too frequent intervention, too little benefit? *Lancet* **1987;2:1375-1377.**
During the 1970s comparative trials of EFM reported benefits, but these were either trials where controls came from earlier years or where some women were monitored and others were not. In the first case, other improvements were also taking place, and in the second, women selected for EFM were probably not comparable to those who were not. None of the four trials of high-risk patients (Havercamp et al. 1976 [Abstract 28], 1979 [Abstract 29]; Renou et al. 1976 [Abstract 26]; Luthy et al. 1987 [Abstract 35]) found differences in perinatal mortality. "Thus even for women with high-risk pregnancies the benefits of continous [EFM] have not been as clearly demonstrated as the practising obstetrician might suppose." Among low-risk and general population studies (Kelso et al. 1978 [Abstract 30]; Wood et al. 1981 [Abstract 27]; MacDonald et al. 1985 [Abstract 31]; Leveno et al. 1986 [Abstract 33]) although operative delivery rates were increased, no benefits were found except fewer seizures (MacDonald et al.). Even there, long-term outcomes did not differ.

> On the basis of the evidence there is no justification for a policy of routine monitoring for all women in labour. Indeed, such a policy will probably expose mothers and their babies to a higher rate of morbidity because of the increased operative intervention. . . . The ease with which the fetal heart can be monitored, the apparent sophistication of the monitors themselves, and the convenience of a paper record of the minute-by-minute changes have perhaps lulled the obstetrician into believing he knows more about the intrauterine status of the fetus than is the case.

23. Sandmire HF. Whither electronic fetal monitoring? *Obstet Gynecol* **1990;76(6):1130-1134.** (U.S.)
Based on animal data, Edward Hon, the father of EFM, and others argued that controlled studies to confirm benefits were inappropriate. "Unfortunately, the anticipated benefits . . . have not materialized," but by increasing the cesarean rate, EFM increased maternal morbidity and mortality and expense. EFM also "poses considerable legal risk"; it is no more predictive of short-term or long-term condition than auscultation but leaves a record "for hindsight interpretation by expert witnesses." The majority of Wisconsin doctors fighting allegations of brain damage said the EFM strip made their defense more difficult. EFM should be designated an "experimental procedure." Then, "because EFM increases the legal risks and insurance company payouts, without benefit to the fetus, the use of this experimental procedure should be considered in the determination of the physician's liability insurance premium."
Using the American College of Obstetricians and Gynecologists' guidelines, a protocol was developed to identify high-risk patients and provide auscultation for all women in two private community hospitals serving 3100 to 3200 laboring women annually. One nurse is provided per actively laboring woman except during peak census times. Nurses had to switch to EFM only 3% of the time.

[W]e conclude that intermittent auscultation . . . is practical and can be substituted for EFM in a high percentage of laboring patients using existing nursing staff. The routine use of EFM . . . is no longer appropriate from the standpoint of either its presumed effectiveness for improved outcome or lower nursing costs. Laboring patients should, at a minimum, receive information on both intermittent auscultation and EFM in order to make an informed choice of method

24. Grant A. Epidemiological principles for the evaluation of monitoring programs—the Dublin experience. *Clin Invest Med* **1993;16(2):149-158.**

As a young doctor enthusiastic about EFM, "it came as a shock to see the paucity of good quality evidence for the clinical use of EFM." EFM was supposed to improve identification of intrapartum asphyxia. However, most studies used Apgars or acid-base status to evaluate outcome. Low scores and acidosis may be due to factors other than asphyxia, and both measures are poor predictors of long-term disability. Intra- and interobserver variations in interpretation lead to many false positives, a problem ignored until recently. The principle that positive predictive value weakens as risk declines was disregarded as EFM went from selective to universal use. Thus, EFM went from a diagnostic to a screening test. Screening tests are almost always followed up with further tests because of high false-positive rates, but EFM is commonly used without recourse to further testing.

Studies comparing outcomes before and after introduction of EFM were confounded by other temporal changes in maternity care. Hospitals not introducing EFM showed similar improvements in outcome. When EFM was used selectively, researchers assumed that the study population was higher risk, but some control women were at very high risk (e.g., very preterm infants, anomalous infants). By 1980, four RCTs involving 2032 women had shown markedly higher cesarean rates but a possible reduction of neonatal seizures if EFM was used with fetal scalp-blood sampling. Since seizures strongly predict later disability, the Dublin trial was designed to measure the effect of EFM and scalp-blood sampling on seizure rate. The Dublin trial found that EFM reduced the risk of seizures, although outcomes for all other measures of intrapartum asphyxia were similar. However, by age four, more children had CP in the monitored group (12 versus 10). "[This] casts serious doubt on common assumptions about the extent to which obstetrically-preventable asphyxia causes childhood disability."

25. Paneth N, Bommarito M, and Stricker J. Electronic fetal monitoring and later outcome. *Clin Invest Med* **1993;16(2):159-165.**

Reliability: "The recognition that different qualified obstetricians did not always interpret monitoring strips the same way was slow to dawn on the obstetric community. . . . [L]ittle attention was paid to this essential prerequisite." Now that studies have been done, "[w]ith one exception, their results are quite dismal." Frequent lack of agreement was also found for the same person interpreting the same strip at different times.

Validity: "A remarkable omission from the fetal monitoring literature is information about the actual relationship between EFM patterns and neurodevelopmental outcome." What studies exist are far from satisfactory. In any case, almost all infants with abnormal EFM patterns will develop normally.

Is brain damage preventable? "[T]he goal of the randomized trials of EFM was to demonstrate that EFM could prevent brain damage. In fact they failed to show that EFM had any positive effect whatever." The Dublin trial showed a protective effect for neonatal seizures when accompanied by scalp pH sampling, but no difference in incidence of CP. Shy et al.'s 1990 study [Abstract 36] of very-low-birth-weight babies showed significantly higher CP rates in the monitored population. Moreover, EFM abnormalities often result from underlying brain damage or malformation. An anomaly increases the risk of c-section for fetal distress from 1-3% to 30-40%. [This means that even true positives may increase maternal risk without benefiting the baby.]

EFM (Randomized Controlled Trials and Follow-up Studies)

26. Renou P et al. Controlled trial of fetal intensive care. *Am J Obstet Gynecol* **1976;126(4):470-476.** (Australia)

High-risk women ($N = 350$) were allocated to either an intensive care unit (ICU) for internal EFM and fetal scalp-blood sampling or to usual care. Apgar scores and the incidence of resuscitation did not differ, but more control babies were admitted to intensive care, were acidotic, or had neurologic symptoms. All five "difficult forceps deliveries" were among control women. The cesarean rate was 22.3% in the ICU group versus 13.7% among controls. The difference is attributed to having all six women with previous cesareans in the ICU group, although 14 control women had a cesarean for "abnormal FHR" versus 28 ICU women (NS). All four "brain-damaged" babies were among controls, as was one stillbirth, which, without corroboration is deemed "asphyxial." More RCTs should not be necessary as "benefit is likely and techniques have little hazard for either mother or fetus."

[The usual care was not described. The ICU had extra "special staff" attached (closer supervision could affect outcome). Randomization method was not described (no assurance was actually random). One of the eight doctors withdrew because he felt EFM was effective. The explanation that the increased cesarean rate in the ICU group was due to its containing all six prior cesareans is both unconvincing and suggests randomization was indeed broken. The second study, Abstract 27, says the brain-damaged babies were midforceps deliveries, suggesting an iatrogenic component. Evaluating pediatricians were not blinded; the electrode wound would reveal the EFM group (possibility of observer bias). Only abnormal babies were followed up.]

27. Wood C et al. A controlled trial of fetal heart rate monitoring in a low-risk obstetric population. *Am J Obstet Gynecol* **1981;141(5):527-534.** (Australia)

A subsequent trial to the one above compared auscultation to a mix of external and internal EFM in 927 low-risk women. Infant outcomes were similar, but operative deliveries were increased in the EFM group (31% versus 23%, $p < 0.01$), and more babies spent time in a neonatal ICU (9% versus 6%, $p < 0.05$) or had phototherapy (3.6% versus 0.8%, $p < 0.01$). Control group women who developed abnormal FHR or meconium staining ($N = 49$) were monitored but analyzed with controls. The sole death, in the EFM group, was caused by umbilical cord prolapse during a midforceps delivery for fetal distress. "[I]t seems to be doubtful whether monitoring of low-risk patients will significantly reduce the incidence of fetal asphyxia."

[Although an attempt was made to compensate, randomization was broken at one of the two hospitals. Care in the auscultation group not described.]

28. Havercamp AD, et al. The evaluation of continuous fetal heart rate monitoring in high-risk pregnancy. *Am J Obstet Gynecol* **1976;125(3):310-320.** *(Denver)*

In this study of 483 high-risk women, *all* women had internal EFM and intrauterine pressure catheters, but EFM data were concealed in the control group. More monitored than auscultated women had abnormal FHR in early labor (16 versus 5, $p < 0.025$ and > 0.01). Among auscultated fetuses, 46 had "nonreassuring" FHR, of which 3 (7%) had either very low Apgars or prolonged neonatal problems. The authors believe access to the EFM data would not have helped. In the control group, auscultation was done every 15 minutes in first stage and every five minutes in second stage. Infant outcomes were similar, but more women in the EFM group had cesareans for fetal distress (7.4% versus 1.2%, $p < 0.01$). Maternal postpartum infection rates were higher (13.2% versus 4.6%, $p < 0.01$) and remained higher even after compensating for the increased number of cesareans. "Nursing attention to the gravida with respect to maternal comfort, emotional support, and 'laying on of hands' could have a significant [positive] impact on the [control group] fetus."

29. Havercamp AD, et al. A controlled trial of the differential effects of intrapartum fetal monitoring. *Am J Obstet Gynecol* **1979;134(4):399-412.** (Denver)

High-risk women ($N = 690$) with fetuses older than 34 weeks gestation were assigned to a mixture of external and internal EFM and intrauterine pressure catheter, EFM with pressure catheter and scalp blood sampling, or auscultation. Infant outcomes were similar, but the EFM group had significantly more cesareans (18% versus 6%, $p < 0.005$). Scalp blood sampling reduced but did not eliminate the excess cesarean rate (11%, NS). The increase was both in diagnoses of fetal distress and failure to progress. "Since no differences in outcome were found . . . among high-risk patients, it would seem very unlikely that a low-risk . . . patient . . . would benefit from monitoring if she is properly auscultated." As for the time demands of auscultation, considerable time is spent setting up machines, checking on monitor functioning, and in inservice training. The belief that monitoring reduces the cost of nursing care has not been verified.

R. Munsick, discussant, calculated that based on a cesarean mortality of 1 per 1000 operations, a doubling of an 8% cesarean rate with universal EFM, and one study's projection that EFM would save 1 in 1500 infants, "for 2,000 babies saved, we would sacrifice 240 women—one woman for eight babies. Should not this information be provided to gravidas before obtaining their informed consent for [EFM]?"

30. Kelso IM et al. An assessment of continuous fetal heart rate monitoring in labor. *Am J Obstet Gynecol* **1978;131(5):526-532.** (England)

This trial of 504 low-risk women (including inductions and meconium staining) compared internal EFM and intrauterine pressure catheter with auscultation every 15 minutes. Perinatal morbidity was similar. More EFM women had cesareans (9.5% versus 4.5%, $p < 0.05$), but fetal distress was not the source of the difference.

31. MacDonald D et al. The Dublin randomized controlled trial of intrapartum fetal heart rate monitoring. *Am J Obstet Gynecol* **1985;152(5):524-539.** (Dublin)

(This center developed active management of labor—see Chapter 5.)

All women with an apparently normal fetus older than 28 weeks gestation and without gross meconium staining ($N = 12,964$) were assigned either to internal EFM or auscultation every 15 minutes in first stage and after every contraction in second stage.

Scalp blood sampling was an option in both groups. All women had one-on-one continuous nursing care. Monitor-strip reviewers, pathologists, and neonatologists were blinded to study group (the electrode used left no mark).

The overall cesarean rate was 2% in both groups nor did the rate differ for fetal distress (0.4% versus 0.2%). Forceps delivery was more common in the EFM group (8.2% versus 6.3%, $p < 0.0001$), and more babies in the EFM group had traumatic fetal injuries (3.2/1000 versus 2.4/1000). Three babies in the EFM group (prolonged second stage) and one in the auscultation group (second twin, breech) died of a forceps injury. Neonatal seizures associated independently with labor longer than five hours and oxytocin use. Significantly fewer seizures occurred in the EFM group (12 versus 27, $p < 0.02$), but equal numbers of babies (three) had major disabilities at one year. The low cesarean rate is attributed to scalp-blood testing, "the strict audit of cesarean deliveries," and "the infrequent use of epidural anesthesia [3%], a form of pain relief . . . known to predispose to [FHR] abnormalities." [Active management restricts labor length to the average. All primiparas not progressing at 1 cm hour (40%!) are given high-dose oxytocin, and second stage may be curtailed by forceps. Infant morbidity and mortality appear to result from this supposedly benign regimen.]

32. Grant A et al. Cerebral palsy among children born during the Dublin randomised trial of intrapartum monitoring. *Lancet* **1989;2(8674):1233-1236.** (follow-up to Abstract 31)

All 30 children who suffered neonatal seizures and 125 (91%) of the remaining 138 with abnormal neurologic signs were examined at age four by a doctor blinded to both trial allocation and nature of neonatal problem. Twelve cases of CP were identified in the EFM group and 10 in the auscultation group, of which only six (22%) seemed possibly asphyxial. Of these, four were in the EFM group.

33. Leveno KJ et al. A prospective comparison of selective and universal electronic fetal monitoring in 34,995 pregnancies. *N Engl J Med* **1986;315(10):615-619.** (Dallas)

In alternate months, women were allocated to either selective or universal EFM ($N = 34,995$). During "selective months," 37% had EFM, during "universal" months, 94%. High-risk labors went to a labor ICU for more intensive nursing in both cases. Low-risk women were visited every 30 minutes for auscultation or inspection of the EFM tracing. Oxytocin, dysfunctional labor, abnormal FHR, meconium, and pregnancy complications were EFM indications in the selective months. Although abnormal FHR was diagnosed more often in the universal EFM group (7.6% versus 2.7%, $p < 0.01$) and cesarean for fetal distress was performed twice as often (0.9% versus 0.4%, $p < 0.01$), fetal outcomes were similar.

34. Neldam S et al. Intrapartum fetal heart rate monitoring in a combined low- and high-risk population: a controlled clinical trial. *Eur J Obstet Gynecol Reprod Biol* **1986;23:1-11.** (Denmark)

All women past 32 weeks gestation except those with insulin-dependent diabetes participated ($N = 969$). EFM was used after the woman no longer wished to walk; auscultation was every 30 minutes up to 5 cm dilation, every 15 minutes until second stage, then after every contraction. More epidurals were given in the EFM group (10.5% versus 6.7%), and more FHR abnormalities were diagnosed at every phase of labor in the EFM group (overall 131 versus 231) with much of the difference in brady-cardia. [Why? Is it because auscultation misses bradycardias close to normal rate? Is it the epidurals, which are known to cause bradycardia? Is it EFM itself?] Cesarean rates for fetal distress were similar (1.4% versus 1.7%), but vacuum extraction rates were increased in the EFM group (12.6% versus 6.9%, $p < 0.05$). Correcting for epidural anesthesia did not eliminate the excess vacuum extractions for distress. Fetal outcomes were similar. In the auscultated group, the sensitivity for babies with acidosis at birth or Apgars below 7 was 52%, the positive predictive value was 52%, and the specificity was 88%. For the EFM group, the numbers were 57%, 41%, and 75%. The study had 90% power to detect a 5% reduction of 1-minute Apgar below 7 and a 10% reduction in 5-minute Apgar below 7.

35. Luthy DA et al. A randomized trial of electronic fetal monitoring in preterm labor. *Obstet Gynecol* **1987;69(5):687-695.** (Seattle)

This RCT encompassed 246 women with no severe maternal illness laboring with a singleton cephalic fetus with no known congenital anomalies or placenta previa. Gestational age was 26 to 32 weeks and birth weight 700 to 1750 g. Both external and internal EFM were used, as were pressure catheters and scalp blood sampling. Auscultated women were assigned a nurse who listened every 15 minutes in the first stage and every 5 minutes in the second stage. Although more distress or ominous FHR patterns were observed in the EFM group (27% versus 18%, $p = 0.08$), cesarean rates for fetal distress were similar (8.2% versus 5.6%, NS). Fetal outcomes were similar, although if mortality is limited to deaths possibly affected by monitoring, the small difference (0.1%) favored auscultation. "[C]ompared with [EFM], any difference in the risk of perinatal mortality associated with . . . periodic auscultation at less than 33 weeks' gestation is unlikely to be clinically detectable."

36. Shy KK et al. Effects of electronic fetal-heart-rate monitoring, as compared with periodic auscultation, on the neurologic development of premature infants. *N Engl J Med* **1990;322(9):588-593.** (follow-up to Abstract 35)

Of 212 surviving infants, 189 (89%) made at least one follow-up visit, and 173 made an 18-month visit. Those making follow-up visits did not differ from those who did not, and those making the 18-month visit tended to have lower birth weight and to have had a serious intercranial hemorrhage. At 18 months, mental development scores (20% versus 9%, $p < 0.05$) and psychomotor scores (23% versus 15%) were lower in the EFM group, and more children had CP (20% versus 8%, $p < 0.25$.) The adjusted odds ratio for CP was 3.8 (CI 1.3-11.4). Among surviving infants, 26% of the EFM group had abnormal FHR compared with 16% of the auscultation group, and the time from onset of abnormal pattern to delivery was longer in the EFM group (median 104.5 min, range 15-1312 min versus median 60.5 min, range 6-351 min). The increase in CP was seen at all three study hospitals. "[C]ompared with . . . auscultation, [EFM] did not improve the neurologic development of children born prematurely."

37. Vintzileos AM et al. A randomized trial of intrapartum electronic fetal heart rate monitoring versus intermittent auscultation. *Obstet Gynecol* **1993;81(6):899-907.** (Athens)

EFM ($N = 746$) and intermittent auscultation (IA) ($N = 682$) were compared at two university hospitals. The perinatal mortality had held steady at 20.4 to 22.6 per 1000 over the previous 6 years. Women at 26 weeks or more gestation with a living fetus were included. Randomization was by coin toss.

"Nonreassuring FHR patterns" were noted in 23.4% of the EFM group versus 10.7% of the IA group ($p < 0.0001$). The cesarean rate was 5.3% versus 2.3% ($p < 0.005$). The perinatal mortality rate (PMR) was reduced to 2.6 per 1000 in the EFM group versus 13 per 1000 in the IA group and 18.5 per 1000 for non-participants during the same period. [Merely doing a study nearly halved the PMR for control women and even helped nonparticipants.] All other parameters of neonatal well-being were similar. Two neonatal deaths occurred in the EFM group, neither related to hypoxia. One of the two *died of hemorrhage from trauma to the base of the tongue during intubation for meconium.* [This procedure *killed* a baby!] In the IA arm, six deaths were attributed to hypoxia ($p = 0.03$). Routine EFM is now standard practice at one hospital, and the other is purchasing monitors to do the same.

[Randomization by coin toss is easy to subvert. It seems unlikely that PMR would differ so much but not any measure of morbidity. Of the six deaths attributed to hypoxia in the IA group, one baby had severe FHR decelerations in both first and second stage and was stillborn, which implies that staff did not respond to distress. Another was a vaginally born breech who had mild second-stage decelerations and 1- and 5-minute Apgars of 0 and 1, which suggests the baby died (or was killed) during birth. A third with mild second-stage decelerations had ruptured membranes, which suggests infection, not hypoxia, as cause of death. In fact, no causes of death are given, nor are FHR abnormalities other than decelerations reported. Monitors and financial support were provided by a monitor manufacturing company, which suggests possible bias.]

In a personal communication (November 13, 1993), M. Enkin commented on this trial:*

[T]he results are widely discrepant from those reported in all previous trials. This is a most unusual finding, and can only be caused by differences in the populations studied, the intervention carried out, or the methodology of the trial.

The method of allocation, by a coin toss, is open to enormous bias, and it is difficult to believe that all house officers involved would always be scrupulously honest. This suspicion is heightened by the discrepancies in the numbers in different strata in the two arms. For instance, of patients in spontaneous labour, there were 238 in the EFM group, 374 in the IA group, instead of the equal split that would be expected with a fair coin toss. The probabilities of such an unequal split occurring by chance would be too small to calculate. The probabilities of finding a 117 to 48 split in the 165 induced labours is too small to accept as due to chance.

Also difficult to believe is that in a hospital with a perinatal mortality of 20-22 per thousand, during the study it dropped to 2.6 per thousand in the experimental group, and [13] per thousand in the control group. The results in the EFM group could only have been obtained if the house officers in the hospitals studied were far better in interpreting the tracings and

---

*Dr. Enkin is professor emeritus of obstetrics, gynecology, clinical epidemiology, and biostatistics at McMaster University, Hamilton, Ontario. He is co-editor of *Effective Care in Pregnancy and Childbirth* (Oxford University Press).

acting on the interpretation than the investigators in all the American, Irish, British, and Australian studies reported. This still would not explain the halving of mortality in the control group.

Alternatives to Fetal Scalp Blood Sampling

38. Clark SL, Gimovsky ML, and Miller FC. The scalp stimulation test: a clinical alternative to fetal scalp blood sampling. *Am J Obstet Gynecol* **1984;148(3):274-277.**

One hundred fetuses with abnormal FHR mandating scalp blood sampling were given 15 seconds finger pressure and a 15-second pinch with a nontraumatic clamp first. FHR acceleration in response ($N = 51$) was uniformly associated with pH of 7.19 or above. Of nonresponders, 19 had a pH below 7.19 and 30 had a pH above 7.19. Magnesium sulfate, narcotics, and barbiturates diminished FHR variability but did not affect test response.

39. Edersheim TG et al. Fetal heart rate response to vibratory acoustic stimulation predicts fetal pH in labor. *Am J Obstet Gynecol* **1987;157(6):1557-1560.**

In 188 cases where scalp blood sampling was indicated, a 3-second vibratory acoustic stimulus was applied over the fetal head with an electronic artificial larynx. Specificity and positive predictive value was 100% in identifying a fetus with a pH above 7.20. Sensitivity was 63.7% and negative predictive value only 8.3%. More infants whose mothers had a narcotic failed to respond but were nonacidotic.

REFERENCES

ACOG. Intrapartum fetal heart rate monitoring. *Technical Bull* 1989;132:1-6.

Albers LL and Krulewitch CJ. Electronic fetal monitoring in the United States in the 1980s. *Obstet Gynecol* 1993;82(1):8-10.

Amato JC. Fetal heart rate monitoring. *Am J Obstet Gynecol* 1983;147(8):967-969.

Beaulieu MD et al. The reproducibility of intrapartum cardiotocogram assessments. *Can Med Assoc J* 1982;127:214-216.

Cogen J. ACOG considering new guidelines for labor monitoring. *Ob Gyn News* 1988;23(9).

Editorial. Cerebral palsy, intrapartum care, and a shot in the foot. *Lancet* 1989;2(8674):1251-1252.

Freeman R. Intrapartum fetal monitoring—a disappointing story. *New Engl J Med* 1990;322(9):624-626.

Garcia J et al. Mothers' views of continuous electronic fetal heart monitoring and intermittent auscultation in a randomized controlled trial. *Birth* 1985;12(2):79-86.

Gilfix MG. Electronic fetal monitoring: physician liability and informed consent. *Am J Law Medicine* 1984;10(1):31-90.

Hansen PK et al. Maternal attitudes to fetal monitoring. *Eur J Obstet Gynecol Reprod Biol* 1985;20:43-51.

Hodnett ED and Osborn RW. Effects of continuous intrapartum professional support on childbirth outcomes. *Res Nursing Health* 1989;12(5):289-297.

Kennell J et al. Continous emotional support during labor in a US hospital. *JAMA* 1991;265(17):2197-2201.

Klaus MH et al. Effects of social support during parturition on maternal and infant morbidity. *Br Med J* 1986;293:585-587.

Lumley J. The irresistible rise of electronic fetal monitoring. *Birth* 1982;9(3):150-152.

Murphy KW et al. Birth asphyxia and the intrapartum cardiotocograph. *Br J Obstet Gynaecol* 1990;97:470-479.

Nageotte MP. Cesarean section for fetal distress. *Clin Obstet Gynecol* 1985;28(4):770-781.

Nielsen PV et al. Intra- and inter-observer variability in the assessment of intrapartum cardiotocograms. *Acta Obstet Gynecol Scand* 1987;66:421-424.

Parer JT. The Dublin trial of fetal heart rate monitoring: the final word? *Birth* 1986;13(2):119-121.

Parer JT and Livingston EG. What is fetal distress? *Am J Obstet Gynecol* 1990;162(6):1421-1427.

Sosa R et al. The effect of a supportive companion on perinatal problems, length of labor, and mother-infant interaction. *New Engl J Med* 1980;303(11):597-600.

U.S. Department of Health and Human Services. Advance report of maternal and infant health data from the birth certificate, 1990. *MVSR* 1993;42(2 Supp):5-24.

VanTuinen I and Wolfe SM. *Unnecessary cesarean sections: halting a national epidemic.* Washington, D.C.: Public Citizen's Health Research Group, 1992.

Part II

PREGNANCY AND LABOR MANAGEMENT

My class in medical school was absorbing the idea that when it comes to tests, technology and interventions, more is better. No one ever talked about the negative aspects of intervention, and the one time a student asked about the "appropriateness" of fetal monitoring, the question was cut off with a remark that there was no time to discuss issues of "appropriateness."

Perry Klass, M.D., quoted in *Medicine and Culture,* Lynn Payer, 1988

8

Gestational Diabetes

> Myth: *You may feel fine, but we know that gestational diabetes is a serious threat to your baby.*
>
> Reality: *"[T]here is a paucity of evidence linking lesser degrees of glucose intolerance with significant disturbance of pregnancy outcome when confounding variables such as maternal age, adiposity, and parity are allowed for."*
>
> Keen 1991

In normal pregnancy, certain hormones make extra glucose available to the fetus by preventing the mother's insulin from doing its normal job of transporting glucose out of her bloodstream into her own cells. This insulin-suppressant effect increases as pregnancy advances. As a result, maternal blood glucose levels after eating rise linearly throughout pregnancy, although the pregnant woman has normal or even above-normal levels of insulin. The pancreas tries to compensate, but by the third trimester, pregnant women average higher than nonpregnant levels of blood glucose after eating (hyperglycemia). They also have lower than nonpregnant glucose levels (hypoglycemia) after an overnight fast when their bodies have had a chance to catch up (Goer 1991; Kuhl 1991; Forest et al. 1983).

In 1964 O'Sullivan and Mahan reported that pregnant women with glucose values at the upper end of the spectrum were more likely to develop diabetes later in life; the added stress of pregnancy revealed a woman's "prediabetic" status. Since diabetes was known to pose serious threats to the fetus, researchers extrapolated that subdiabetic levels of glucose intolerance during pregnancy might also do harm.

During the 1960s and 1970s doctors began studying the effects of glucose intolerance in pregnant women; however, the studies were poorly designed (Goer 1991). Sometimes they selected women for glucose testing on the basis of previous poor pregnancy outcome or risk factors in the current pregnancy and then compared outcomes with the general population. Some mixed in known prepregnant diabetics. They often failed to account for confounding factors. In short, the studies thoroughly obscured the true risk of subdiabetic glucose intolerance in pregnancy. Management protocols such as starvation diets, early elective induction, and withholding nourishment from the newborn may also have contributed to poorer outcomes among gestational diabetics. That notwithstanding, the results convinced researchers that they had discovered a serious problem, and in 1979 they convened the first of what became a series of exponentially larger international conferences (Metzger 1991a).

Opening the first conference, one of the organizers suggested that pregnancy be viewed as a "tissue culture experience." The mother becomes an "incubator" and a "supplier of medium," and "the success of the whole project depends on the extent to which optimum culture conditions have been established." The conference would seek to establish whether minimal disturbances were potentially harmful to the fetus and whether attempts at rectification were justified (Freinkel 1980).

Given the preconceived notions of the researchers, the confused state of the research, and a metaphor that reduced women to incubators supplying potentially faulty growth medium, it should come as no surprise that by the end of the second conference, gestational diabetes (GD) was established as a new disease. It was officially defined as

> carbohydrate intolerance of variable severity with onset or first recognition during the present pregnancy . . . irrespective of whether or not insulin is used for treatment or the condition persists after pregnancy. [It includes] the possibility that the glucose intolerance may have antedated the pregnancy. (Second International Workshop-Conference 1985)

Thus, women with blood glucose values in roughly the upper 3% for pregnant women have come to be defined as diabetics, although the situation is different from either type of true diabetes. In Type I diabetes, the insulin-making cells in the pancreas have been destroyed. With Type I, extremes of low and high blood sugar early in pregnancy can damage the forming embryo. On the other hand, gestationally diabetic women are usually making normal or above-normal amounts of insulin and have normal blood sugar metabolism in the first trimester (Hadden 1980). Type II diabetes, found mostly in overweight or older adults, resembles the situation in pregnancy in that the problem is insulin resistance, not insulin production. However, there are differences. In both other types, diabetes of long standing may damage the mother's blood vessels and kidneys, which may in turn jeopardize the fetus, but gestational diabetics do not have long-standing diabetes. The one problem GD shares with Type I and Type II is that chronic hyperglycemia can overfeed the fetus, resulting in macrosomia (overly large infants, usually weighing 4000 g or 8 lb 13 oz or more). Even here, though, other factors—race, age, parity, and especially maternal weight—far outweigh glucose intolerance in determining the baby's weight (Keen 1991; Phillipou 1991; Green et al. 1991; Farmer et al. 1988, all abstracted below).

The conference definition of GD confuses more than it enlightens because it jumbles together various levels of severity. This is similar to claiming that everyone with a cough and fever has pneumonia. The confusion was deliberate. The conferees considered using the term *glucose intolerance of pregnancy*, but decided on *diabetes* to make sure insurance companies would pay for high-risk management, and women themselves would take the condition seriously (Second International Workshop-Conference 1985).

The 1985 conference recommended—and the 1990 conference reaffirmed (Metzger et al. 1990b)—that all pregnant women be screened for GD between 24 and 28 weeks of pregnancy by a 50 g glucose drink and that those with values of 140 mg/dl (7.8 mmol/l) or above be given a diagnostic 100-g oral glucose tolerance test (OGTT) (Second International Workshop-Conference 1985). Women with two values meeting or exceeding O'Sullivan and Mahan's values on the follow-up OGTT should be considered to have gestational diabetes (Table 8.1). The American Diabetes Association endorsed the conference recommendations (American Diabetes Association 1987). The American College of Obstetricians and Gynecologists recommends the same screening and diagnostic values; however, it recommends selected screening only for women under age 30 (ACOG 1986). Despite ACOG's stance, many U.S. obstetricians screen everybody.

Keep in mind that O'Sullivan and Mahan chose their cutoffs for convenience in follow-up. No threshold has ever been demonstrated for onset or marked increase in fetal complications below levels diagnostic of diabetes. Instead of raising questions about the validity of GD testing, this lack of correlation with complications has led some researchers to lobby for a lowering of diagnostic thresholds, which would label even more women gestational diabetics (Ratner 1993; Kaufmann et al. 1992, abstracted below).

Articles about the diagnosis and treatment of GD almost always begin with a litany of the supposed dangers of untreated GD: perinatal death, congenital anomalies, macrosomia, neonatal hypoglycemia, hyperbilirubinemia (neonatal jaundice), other neonatal metabolic abnormalities, and maternal hypertension. Reducing the incidence of macrosomia is also supposed to reduce the number of instrumental and cesarean deliveries as well as birth injuries and asphyxia.

Accordingly, women diagnosed as gestational diabetics will find themselves plunged into anything from an unpleasant experience to a living nightmare, depending on their degree of glucose intolerance and their doctors' whim (Gillmer et al. 1986) They may have blood tests anywhere from weekly to several times a day, dietary and calorie restrictions, extra doctor visits, prenatal surveillance and weight estimate tests (all of which have high false-positive

Table 8.1: Values on the Oral Glucose Tolerance Test (OGTT)

	NDDG and ACOG 100 g glucose	Coustan* 100 g glucose	WHO* 75 g glucose
fasting	105 mg/dl (5.8 mmol/l)	95 mg/dl	140 mg/dl (7.8 mmol/l)
1 hour	190 mg/dl (10.6 mmol/l)	180 mg/dl	—
2 hour	165 mg/dl (9.2 mmol/l)	160 mg/dl	140-200 mg/dl (7.8-11.1 mmol/l)
3 hour	145 mg/dl (8.1 mmol/l)	135 mg/dl	—

- Oral glucose administered after an overnight fast.
- For the 100 g OGTT, two or more venous plasma concentrations must be met or exceeded.
- For the WHO 75 g OGTT, values are not adapted for pregnant women; both values must be met or exceeded; range represents *impaired glucose tolerance.*

Sources: Coustan and Lewis 1978; WHO Study Group 1985

rates), insulin injections, prenatal hospitalization, induction of labor, and/or repeated glucose monitoring during labor (Knopp et al. 1991; Jovanovic-Peterson and Peterson 1991; Coustan 1991; Dickinson and Palmer 1990; Chez et al. 1989; Reed 1988; Landon and Gabbe 1988; Board et al. 1986; ACOG 1986). The odds of cesarean—both scheduled and in labor—are greatly increased compared with nongestational diabetics carrying babies of the same weight (Goldman et al. 1991; Acker, Sachs, and Friedman 1985, both abstracted below). The infants of GD mothers may be subjected to repeated heel sticks to determine blood glucose, removed to nurseries for observation, or fed glucose water, which interferes with establishing breastfeeding (Hod et al. 1991).

The human and monetary cost of diagnosing and treating GD is staggering, but has it bought better perinatal outcomes? As we shall see in this chapter, for subdiabetic levels of glucose intolerance, the answer is no. A few studies have managed to reduce the incidence of large-for-gestational-age (LGA) babies (weight above the ninetieth percentile for gestational age) from 20% down to the normally expected 10%, usually by using insulin. Even so, only one study has ever shown a reduction in operative deliveries (cesarean plus instrumental deliveries) (Coustan and Imarah 1984). In that study doctors knew which women had had insulin. If they believed insulin prevented macrosomia—which Coustan's other work shows they did—this belief could well influence the decision to intervene.

In fact, GD diagnosis and treatment is doing considerable harm. As we have seen, the GD label itself buys a greatly increased cesarean rate. The price of reducing macrosomia is the manipulation of the primary growth mechanism of infants, roughly 80% of whom would not be LGA if they were left alone. And this, like GD itself, presumes without evidence that this physiologic variation in birth weight is pathological. Ironically, it may even buy higher glucose levels since one of the body's prime responses to stress and anxiety—and GD management is nothing if not stressful and worrying—is to flood the body with glucose.

Few have noticed that the diagnosis and treatment of GD is a spectacular failure. To read most studies is to fall into an Alice in Wonderland world. A review article analyzes the OGTT, finds it worthless, and recommends continuing to use it to diagnose GD (Nelson 1988, abstracted below). Researchers take note that sonography to estimate fetal weight did no better than a coin toss at predicting macrosomia and then recommend it anyway (Combs, Singh, and Khoury 1993, abstracted below). Doctors find that rigid glycemic control did not improve infant outcomes and assume that means they should try harder (Hod et al. 1991). A group reports that women with GD have one-third more cesareans compared with a matched population with normal glucose tolerance, although birth weights and complications were similar. Then they congratulate themselves on the success of their management (Goldman et al., abstracted below). After showing that current cutoffs fail to discriminate a group of women at high risk for macrosomia, obstetricians conclude they should lower the values or that insulin should be given to more women (Neiger and Coustan 1991; Weiner 1988 abstracted below; Tallarigo et al. 1986). By this logic, they could lower diagnostic cutoffs ad infinitum and still find "abnormal" women "at risk" for macrosomia.

What is going on? Robbie Davis-Floyd (1993) explains that when rituals fail to avert bad outcome, people do not abandon them as worthless. Instead, they intensify them. When Bolivian tin miners find that propitiating the gods of the underworld with flowers and fruit does not prevent mine disasters, they bring more offerings, and perhaps sacrifice a llama. Likewise, doctors engaged in rituals to ward off the supposed dangers of GD refuse to see that what they are doing is not only useless but harmful—and the juggernaut rolls on.

The fact is that only those who were true diabetics prior to pregnancy or those few whose pregnancies have tipped them into a true diabetic state benefit from special care. Beyond that, women who are overweight should try to achieve normal weight before pregnancy, because maternal weight bears the strongest relationship with infant birth weight and glucose tolerance. Women with subdiabetic glucose intolerance during pregnancy should eat a diet low in simple sugars and high in complex carbohydrates and fiber, and health permitting, they should exercise moderately and regularly. These practices improve glucose tolerance (Horton 1991; Bung et al. 1991; Fraser, Ford, and Lawrence 1988; Ney, Hollingsworth, and Cousins 1982). This, of course, is advice that would profit any pregnant woman. As for GD, after reviewing the literature, Hunter and Keirse (1989) say, "Except for research purposes, all forms of glucose tolerance testing should be stopped."

SUMMARY OF SIGNIFICANT POINTS

- GD has not been convincingly shown to increase risk—except the risk of having a big baby. Even so, most babies of GD mothers will be of normal weight and most high-weight babies will be born to women who are not gestational diabetics. (Abstracts 3-4, 6-7, 9, 11-14, 22-23)

- Even if risks exist, treatment has little effect on reducing them and introduces considerable risk, stress, and unpleasantness of its own. (Abstracts 4-5, 7, 9, 14-15, 19-23, 25-31)

- Maternal weight correlates with fetal weight (so overweight women should lose weight before pregnancy). (Abstracts 5, 10, 13-14, 20-21, 23)

- The OGTT, used to diagnose GD, does not produce reliable, repeatable values. (Abstracts 1-3, 6)

- Failure to consume adequate amounts of carbohydrate for three days prior to the OGTT, bed rest, and many medications cause false positives. (Abstract 1)

- No threshold of risk has been found short of values diagnostic of diabetes. (Abstracts 2, 5-12, 14)

- Elective inductions and cesareans for suspected macrosomia do not improve outcomes, and they increase cesarean rates. (Abstracts 21-24)

- Forceps and epidurals (probably becauses epidurals cause longer second stages and lead to instrumental deliveries) increase the probability of birth injuries, birth asphyxia, and meconium aspiration (in addition to the maternal risks of these procedures). (Abstracts 23-24, 29)

- Equally good outcomes for gestational diabetics can be achieved with far less intervention. (Abstracts 15, 23, 31-32)

ORGANIZATION OF ABSTRACTS

The Deficiencies of the OGTT

Diagosis Does Not Correlate with Risk

Research Critiques
Diagnostic Thresholds Do Not Predict Perinatal Outcomes (Review)
Diagnostic Thresholds Do not Predict Perinatal Outcomes (Studies)
Maternal Hyperglycemia Predicts Macrosomia Poorly

Treatment Does Not Improve Outcomes

Screened Versus Unscreened Populations
Treatment and Perinatal Mortality
Treatment and Macrosomic Babies
Cesareans and Macrosomic Babies

The Risks of Testing and Treatment

The Dangers of Hypoglycemia
False Positives on Prenatal Tests (see also Chapter 9, "Postdates Tests")
Intervention Introduces Risk
Intervention Is Rarely Necessary

THE DEFICIENCIES OF THE OGTT

1. Nelson RL. Oral glucose tolerance test: indications and limitations. *Mayo Clin Proc* **1988;63(3):263-269.**
Fasting plasma glucose is the most reliable and widely used test for diagnosing Type I and Type II diabetes because of its reproducibility. The OGTT leads to overdiagnosis. Subjects must have consumed at least 150 g of carbohydrate daily for three days preceding the test. Caffeine, nicotine, bed rest, and many medications impair glucose tolerance. A review of 10 studies shows that the OGTT is poorly reproducible. Nonpregnant subjects taking the OGTT on more than one occasion showed a mean difference of 26 mg/dl at one hour and 20 mg/dl at two hours for the same individual. Unless results are grossly abnormal, the OGTT should be repeated before making a diagnosis. For those with normal fasting plasma glucose values [the usual case with GD], up to 50% will retest normal. The OGTT should be discontinued as a diagnostic test for diabetes and repeated fasting hyperglycemia used instead. More harm is probably caused by overdiagnosing diabetes than by not using the glucose tolerance test. Multiple factors affect the test, and its reproducibility varies. The diagnosis of diabetes mellitus should be made with conservatism, and an oral glucose tolerance test should rarely be necessary. [Then, amazingly, Nelson reverses himself and recommends universal screening and a follow-up OGTT for pregnant women.]

2. Naylor CD. Diagnosing GD mellitus. Is the gold standard valid? *Diabetes Care* **1989 Sep;12(8):565-572.**

A test establishing a curve for normal physiologic values should be performed on a large, unselected, disease-free population representative of all subjects whose values will later be compared to the curve. The values used in the 100-g OGTT were derived in the 1950s from pregnant inner-city clinic women with a median age of 25 years, an average of 2.8 children, and a white-to-black racial mix of 60:40. These women were almost all tested in the second and third trimester. Since glucose tolerance declines as pregnancy progresses, using these values without adjustment means few abnormal tests early in pregnancy and increasing numbers of abnormal tests as pregnancy advances. Thresholds were set at two standard deviations from the mean for whole-blood glucose for each stage of the OGTT. They were not tied to any biological or prognostic differences. [This is akin to saying all people over six feet tall have a metabolic disease. Some of them may; most of them do not.] Women were tested only once, and the OGTT is poorly reproducible. Whole blood glucose was measured. Today plasma glucose is used. Simply multiplying whole blood values by a correction factor cannot be done because the ratio of red blood cells to plasma declines as pregnancy progresses. The test was not developed to predict maternal or fetal morbidity or mortality; it does not even do a particularly good job at predicting what it was developed for—future development of glucose intolerance or diabetes. The current test is a threshold test [you are either a gestational diabetic or not], but maternal-fetal risk appears to occur on a gradient with respect to glucose intolerance with the presence or absence of fasting hyperglycemia forming a significant factor. Unfortunately, these flawed criteria are so well entrenched that redoing them may be difficult.

3. Harlass FE, Brady K, Read JA. Reproducibility of the oral glucose tolerance test in pregnancy. *Am J Obstet Gynecol* **1991;164(2):564-568.**

Pregnant women ($N = 64$) who had positive 50-g oral glucose screening tests were given two OGTTs 1 to 2 weeks apart. Forty-eight women (75%) tested normal-normal; 11 (17%) tested normal-abnormal; 3 (5%) tested abnormal-normal [which agrees with Naylor, Abstract 2, who says glucose intolerance rises with gestational age]; only 2 (3%) tested abnormal-abnormal. Mean birth weights of babies born to mothers who tested abnormal were not different from babies of mothers who tested normal both times.

DIAGNOSIS DOES NOT CORRELATE WITH RISK

Research Critiques

4. Jarret RJ. Reflections on gestational diabetes mellitus. *Lancet* **1981;2(8257):1220-1222.**

The diagnostic criteria recommended by the First International Conference-Workshop and the National Diabetes Data Group were developed in an attempt to predict future development of overt diabetes, not poor outcome in the current pregnancy. Even if GD increased perinatal mortality, treatment did not help. Both treated and untreated gestational diabetics had higher perinatal mortality than normoglycemic controls.

The methodology of the studies is flawed. Most studies showing increased perinatal mortality selected women for glucose testing on the basis of factors independently associated with perinatal risk. Other studies attributed improved outcomes among gestational diabetics to treatment but lacked a control population of gestational diabetics subjected to ordinary management. Most did not examine the confounding factors of age and obesity. Increased congenital anomalies is not an issue, and the association with fetal macrosomia is questionable. Studies correcting for age and maternal weight eliminated the association. "There seems no reason to believe that haphazard screening for GD has contributed in any way to the overall reduction in perinatal mortality rates." The concept of gestational diabetes is valid only as a spur to research.

5. Ales KL and Santini DL. Should all pregnant women be screened for gestational glucose intolerance? *Lancet* 1989;1(8648):1187-1191.

No evidence is found that glucose intolerance is associated with maternal morbidity, but identification as a gestational diabetic "triggers a cascade of events, which may have their own adverse effects": dietary manipulation, insulin administration, and additional fetal surveillance. Studies showing excess perinatal mortality did not control for age, parity, or obesity, nor did they look at other medical or obstetric complications among gestational diabetics that could have affected outcomes. In any case, treatment did not improve mortality rates. Chief among perinatal complications are macrosomia and consequent birth injuries. It is impossible to determine from the evidence if gestational glucose intolerance causes macrosomia, although there appears to be a consistent association. Even if it does, birth weight-related complications become a problem only at birth weights over 4500 g [9 lb 14 oz]. Fewer than 4.4% of untreated gestational diabetics will have babies of this size. Moreover, glucose intolerance is implicated in only 5% of babies with birth weights of 4500 g or more. Even though insulin treatment has been shown to reduce birth weight, obese women, who are most likely to have a baby in this weight range, are the least likely to benefit from insulin. "Why then is there such enormous pressure to screen all pregnant women? And why is there growing pressure to treat ever-milder degrees of glucose intolerance? Until these questions can be answered scientifically, a more restrained approach than universal screening might be appropriate."

Diagnostic Thresholds Do Not Predict Perinatal Outcomes (Review)

6. Keen H. Gestational diabetes. Can epidemiology help? *Diabetes* 1991;40(Suppl 2):3-7.

Glycemic responses plot as a bell-shaped curve, as do many other biological variables. Distributions shift to the right in successive age groups, and no natural diagnostic thresholds are found at any age. When one adds the diversity of types of test and the considerable day-to-day individual variation, the difficulties of establishing diagnostic definitions for subdiabetic glucose intolerance become clear. Establishing cutoffs based on percentile or deviation from the mean is simple and exact, but diagnosis should be made on the basis of increased risk. "If the risk of lesser degrees of glucose intolerance is diminutive, nonexistent, or confined to a small subset, then many women could be submitted to the physical, emotional, social, and economic disadvantages of diagnosis and treatment for no good reason. There is relatively little evidence deriving from adequately planned controlled studies that bears on this key question." What evidence there is suggests that current diagnostic thresholds do not discriminate a population at increased risk. Confounding factors (age, obesity, and parity) may also play an important role in determining fetal outcome rather than glucose tolerance.

Diagnostic Thresholds Do Not Predict Perinatal Outcomes (Studies)

7. Li DFH et al. Is treatment needed for mild impairment of glucose tolerance in pregnancy? A randomized controlled trial. Br J Obstet Gynaecol 1987;94:851-854.
Women diagnosed as GD by the National Diabetes Data Group (NDDG) criteria ($N = 158$) were retested with the more stringent diagnostic criteria recommended by the World Health Organization (WHO) (see Table 8.1). They were then alternately allocated to treatment and control groups. Neither doctors nor women knew the results of the second test. Half the women who were abnormal by NDDG standards were normal by WHO standards. Treatment and monitoring consisted of diet, blood glucose testing three times daily, monthly ultrasound scans, weekly estriol assays starting at 32 weeks, and weekly nonstress tests from 36 weeks.

Women who were normal by WHO standards had similar outcomes, whether treated or controls. Compared with treated women who were glucose intolerant by WHO standards, untreated glucose-intolerant women had significantly heavier babies (mean of 3407 g versus 3110 g, $p < 0.01$), longer gestations (mean 39.8 wk versus 38.8 wk, $p < 0.001$) [which could account for the difference in weight], and more babies weighing over 4000 g (14% versus 0%, $p < 0.05$), but there was no perinatal morbidity in any group. Induction (13% versus 16%) and cesarean (27% versus 26%) rates were similar between treated and untreated groups. "About 52% of the women had normal glucose tolerance using the WHO criteria and treatment of these women did not offer any clinical benefit." The WHO test is recommended over the NDDG test so that "women can be spared the unnecessary anxiety of being labelled as diabetic, and they need not suffer the inconvenience and discomfort of diet control, sugar profile and fetal surveillance."

8. Farmer G et al. The influence of maternal glucose metabolism on fetal growth, development and morbidity in 917 singleton pregnancies in nondiabetic women. Diabetologia 1988;31:134-141.
Using an intravenous GTT, the relationship between maternal glucose tolerance and fetal outcome is investigated in 917 pregnant women not known to be diabetics. Age, but not parity, related to declining glucose tolerance. Birth weight gave no evidence of a "pathological" group at the diabetic end of the spectrum, although glucose intolerance associated with macrosomia. Women with fasting hyperglycemia were more likely to produce a heavier baby. Babies of glucose-intolerant mothers were more likely to have congenital anomalies, and babies born at 41 weeks gestation or later were more likely to have birth asphyxia or related problems. However, the degree of risk was graded throughout the normal range of glucose tolerance, and there was no value beyond which fetal morbidity substantially increased or below which fetal well-being was ensured. The authors conclude that the intravenous GTT "lacks predictive sensitivity in individual cases and cannot be used to identify a small pathological or high-risk group of mothers." [Consider, too, that the intravenous GTT is more reproducible than the oral GTT because the glucose does not have to be digested.]

9. Weiner CP. Effect of varying degrees of "normal" glucose metabolism on maternal and perinatal outcome. *Am J Obstet Gynecol* 1988;159(4):862-870.

The relationship between degree of hyperglycemia and outcomes is correlated among 312 women undergoing a 100-g OGTT. The 1-hour screen value and the 2-hour value of the OGTT is stratified by increments of 20 mg/dl. [Weiner does not explain why 121 women with screen values below threshold had an OGTT.] Women diagnosed as GD were controlled by diet, and insulin was given if diet did not normalize blood sugar.

Looking at screen values, birth weight correlated positively with maternal weight gain and maternal weight at time of screening. Maternal age rose linearly with screening test rank. Birth weight did not correlate with either screen or OGTT 2-hour value. No segment differed significantly from any other. Screen rank and abnormal OGTT correlated positively but without significant increase until screen value exceeded 180 mg/dl, which suggests a pathological threshold at this value rather than a gradient. There were no significant relationships between screen value and neonatal morbidity.

Looking at the 2-hour OGTT value, maternal age, nonelective operative delivery, and infants with 1-minute Apgar below 7 increased, and infants discharged simultaneously with mother correlated positively with rising glucose values, but significant differences among ranks occurred only at the highest rank (>180 mg/dl) "and was thus inconsistent with a gradient phenomenon." [The 2-hour cutoff value on the OGTT is 155 mg/dl. Thus, Weiner's data do not support the belief that mild disturbances of glucose metabolism are pathological.] Macrosomia increased but not significantly.

Among the subgroup whose OGTT was normal, birth weight and maternal weight and maternal weight gain went up with screen rank [as before]. Mean birth weight and percentage of babies weighing over 4000 g increased significantly when screen value exceeded 199 mg/dl, but weights over 4200 g and percentage above the ninetieth percentile for gestational age did not. There was no correlation between screen value and 2-hour OGTT value or between the 2-hour value and outcome. [Oral glucose testing is not very reproducible.]

Among women diagnosed as gestational diabetics [including three women who were insulin dependent], no significant relationships between screen rank, 2-hour OGTT value, and outcomes were found. As a class, they were twice as likely as nongestational diabetics to have an operative delivery (20% versus roughly 10%) and a baby with a 1-minute Apgar below 7. [The increase in operative delivery may account for this.] However, 5-minute Apgars were not significantly different. Women with GD are "perhaps inseparably at increased risk for non-elective operative delivery [although they were not at greater risk for any complication that would indicate cesarean]. . . . These findings stress the importance of screening for GD and the need for close antenatal and neonatal surveillance [despite the fact that glucose values less than 180 mg/dl do not relate to outcome]."

10. Phillipou G. Relationship between normal oral glucose tolerance test in women at risk for gestational diabetes and large for gestational age infants. *Diabetes Care* 1991;14(11):1092-1094.

If the degree of glucose intolerance is an important determinant of fetal weight, then OGTT values should predict the incidence of LGA infants. Of 2631 women, 176 had an OGTT based on a positive 50-g glucose screen or clinical factors. Of these, 18.7% tested positive for GD. The odds ratio (OR) for birth of an LGA infant for women with a positive OGTT versus all women free of GD was 5.8 (CI 2.8-12.1). The OR for women with normal OGTTs versus women not tested (negative screen) was 2.3 (CI 1.4-3.6). Other risk factors for LGA infant were multiparity (OR 2.5, CI 1.7-3.6), maternal weight 70 kg or more (OR 3.3, CI 1.9-5.7), and male infant (OR 2.0, CI 1.5-2.6). While women selected for an OGTT are at increased risk for an LGA infant, no predictive relationship could be established between OGTT values and LGA infant. Despite clinical management, women with positive OGTTs had a high incidence of LGA infants. "The results may be interpreted as either indicating a role for confounding variables, i.e., maternal weight, multiparity, and birth of a male infant, or the imprecision of the OGTT in assessing physiologically important changes in maternal hyperglycemia."

11. Kaufmann RC et al. The effect of minor degrees of glucose intolerance on the incidence of neonatal macrosomia. *Obstet Gynecol* **1992;80(1):97-101.**
The birth weights of babies of women who had one abnormal value on the OGTT were compared with normal controls ($N = 2152$) who had no maternal complications known to affect fetal size. Three different sets of values were used: group 1 ($N = 109$), Coustan's group [see Table 8.1]; group 2 ($N = 85$), Amankwah et al.: fasting 100, 1 hour 180 mg/dl, 2 hour 160 mg/dl, 3 hour 140 mg/dl; group 3 ($N = 65$) NDDG [see Table 8.1]. Infants were significantly more likely to weigh more than 4000 g in all three groups compared with controls (22.0%, 22.3%, and 20.0%, respectively, versus 12.4%). However, percentages weighing above the ninetieth (5.5%, 3.5%, 1.5%, respectively, versus 10.0%) and ninety-fifth percentiles (3.7%, 0, 0.9%, respectively, versus 5.0%) were not significantly different compared with controls. The average birth weight of infants weighing over 4000 g was no greater than controls [no drift toward higher weights among intolerant groups]. "There was no correlation between any of the GTT values and birth weight." [This study shows that no set of criteria discriminates women who will have macrosomic babies from normal controls.]

Maternal Hyperglycemia Predicts Macrosomia Poorly

12. Oats NO et al. Maternal glucose tolerance during pregnancy with excessive size infants. *Obstet Gynecol* **1980;55(2):184-186.**
Pregnancies resulting in the birth of an infant weighing 4540 g or more (roughly the upper 1% for birth weight) ($N = 137$) were compared with a control series of 5000 consecutive pregnancies. The incidence of hyperglycemia (defined as any OGTT value above the ninety-fifth percentile) was increased (20.4% versus 11.7%, $p < 0.01$). Previous studies have shown no association between maternal hyperglycemia and birth weight above the ninetieth percentile (≥ 4000 g), so association between macrosomia and hyperglycemia is evident only above the ninety-ninth percentile. Even so, 77% of mothers had normal glucose tolerance even among babies in this extreme weight category, "which indicates that hyperglycemia is not necessarily the cause of fetal overgrowth."

13. Spellacy WN et al. Macrosomia—Maternal characteristics and infant complications. *Obstet Gynecol* **1985;66(2):158-161.**
Using a computerized database involving 11 hospitals, 33,545 infants were categorized as very macrosomic (> 5000 g; N 82), mild macrosomic (4500-4999 g; $N = 492$), and controls (2500-3499 g; $N = 18,739$). The macrosomic group (> 4500 g)

represented 1.7% of the infants.

Compared with controls, women with mild macrosomic babies and very macrosomic babies were more likely to have postterm pregnancies (10.2% and 14.2% versus 2.5%), maternal weight at birth more than 90 kg [200 lbs] (33.4% and 50.2% versus 8.2%) or more than 112.5 kg [250 lb] (8.4% and 19.7% versus 1.2%), and diabetes, either gestational (4.1% and 11.0% versus 1.0%) or insulin dependent (2.8% and 3.7% versus 0.4%) (all $p < 0.0001$). Macrosomic babies were also more likely to be male (70.7% of very macrosomic babies). The probability of a macrosomic infant in a woman with a single risk factor was 5.4% postterm, 5.6% maternal weight more than 90 kg, 6.4% GD, 9.2% insulin dependent diabetes, and 10.0% maternal weight over 112.5 kg. Multiple risk factors increased the odds, but the probability of macrosomia with GD and maternal weight over 90 kg was still only 12%.

14. Green JR et al. Influence of maternal body habitus and glucose tolerance on birth weight. *Obstet Gynecol* **1991;78(2):235-240.**

The interrelations between body mass index (BMI) (weight/height^2), glucose tolerance, and race were examined for low-income black, Chinese, Latina, and white women ($N = 2069$). Pregnancies longer than 42 weeks were excluded. The majority of Latina (76%), black (66%), and white (60%) women were overweight, whereas the majority of Chinese women (63%) were at ideal weight. Maternal BMI associated significantly with increased birth weight and infant BMI. The incidence of macrosomia with respect to BMI varied by ethnic group. Whereas 7% of black or Latina macrosomic babies were born to thin mothers, 25% of white macrosomic babies were born to thin mothers, and 66% of Chinese macrosomic babies were born to thin mothers. Screening glucose values also varied by race. Black women (114.8 mg/dl) had significantly lower values than Chinese or Latina women (124.9 mg/dl), and white women were similar to Chinese and Latina women (121.5 mg/dl). Birth weights varied little for glucose values from 80 mg/dl to 200 mg/dl. Below 80 mg/dl, birth weight dropped off sharply [hypoglycemia] and at over 200 mg/dl, birth weight rose sharply [this is the diagnostic threshold for diabetes]. "The failure to find substantial effects of glucose on fetal growth throughout the range of postprandial glycemia encompassing the majority of women with [GD] suggests that glucose is not a direct mediator of fetal overgrowth and is not a reliable marker of risk." This conclusion agrees with several other studies that have continued to find macrosomia among "ostensibly 'well-controlled' gestational diabetics." [Their results argue strongly for ignoring hyperglycemia below levels diagnostic of diabetes. They also raise the issue of the effects of hypoglycemia, a potential problem with reduced-calorie diets.]

TREATMENT DOES NOT IMPROVE OUTCOMES

Screened Versus Unscreened Populations

Note: There will probably never be a randomized controlled trial assessing the impact of routine GD screening because of the large number of subjects required and the near universal belief in its value. However, the following study takes advantage of a natural experiment. In the early 1980s, some Cornell University Medical Center physicians screened routinely and others did not.

15. Santini DL and Ales KL. The impact of universal screening for gestational glucose intolerance on outcome of pregnancy. *Surg Gynecol Obstet* **1990;170 (5):427-436.**

After excluding transfers from other hospitals, multiple gestations, and known prepregnancy diabetics, there were 533 unscreened and 774 screened women. Screening should reduce macrosomia, perinatal morbidity, and cesarean section by identifying gestational diabetics for corrective therapy. However, there were no significant differences in the percentages of large babies (> 4000 g), macrosomic babies (> 4500 g), or in numbers of LGA infants as calculated by one of two different methods. Using the second method, there were significantly more LGA babies in the screened population ($p < 0.05$), the population that should have fewer because they were treated.

There were no significant differences in perinatal mortality or morbidity, including 5-minute Apgars, length of hospitalization, total perinatal mortality, perinatal mortality adjusted for nonviable infants, birth injuries, hypoglycemia (< 30 mg/dl), hypocalcemia (< 7 mg/dl), hyperbilirubinemia (> 12 mg/dl), polycythemia, respiratory complications, or intracerebral hemorrhage. Conversely, primary c-section was more likely in the screened population (19.3% versus 12.1%, $p < 0.01$), as were increased numbers of antepartum outpatient visits, supplementary tests (sonograms, nonstress tests, amniocenteses), and antepartum hospitalizations. [Not only does identifying and treating gestational diabetics not improve outcomes, it introduces risks.]

Treatment and Perinatal Mortality

16. O'Sullivan JB et al. The potential diabetic and her treatment in pregnancy. *Obstet Gynecol* **1966;27(5):683-689.**

Between 1954 and 1960 all prenatal patients at a Boston hospital were screened for glucose intolerance. All women who were above threshold on the screen; had a history of prior infant weighing over 4100 g [9 lb]; or who had a perinatal death, congenital anomaly, prematurity [defined as birth weight less than 5 lb 6 oz]; or toxemia [defined as excessive weight gain, hypertension, or proteinuria (protein in the urine)] in two or more pregnancies underwent a 100-g OGTT.

Gestational diabetics were divided into two groups: 307 positive-treated who were treated by diet and insulin and 308 positive-controls who were not treated. Outcomes were compared with 306 negative controls for which the only criterion was normal glucose tolerance. There were significantly more perinatal losses of a fetus older than 28 weeks (2.6% versus 4.3%, $p < 0.01$) among gestational diabetics compared with negative controls but *no* significant difference between treated and untreated gestational diabetics (4.3% versus 4.9%).

Treatment and Macrosomic Babies

17. Kalkhoff RK. Therapeutic results of insulin therapy in gestational diabetes mellitus. *Diabetes* **1985;34(Suppl 2):97-100.**

In two of the six studies reviewed, insulin reduced the number of macrosomic babies.

In one study insulin reduced macrosomia in women with fasting hyperglycemia, a rarer and more serious glucose metabolism disturbance, when compared with women with fasting hyperglycemia on diet alone. In one study, insulin helped gestational diabetics with normal fasting plasma glucose. In one study, insulin did not make a difference. [The sixth study is covered in Abstract 18.]

18. Metzger BE. Treatment of mild gestational diabetes mellitus. Is it time for a controlled clinical trial? *Diabetes Care* **1988;11(10):813-816.**

Of seven studies reviewed, four [two studies were by Coustan's group] found insulin-treated mothers had fewer macrosomic babies than mothers treated by diet alone; one group found that insulin reduced the numbers of macrosomic babies in normal weight but not obese gestational diabetics; and two found no difference between insulin and diet-alone mothers. However, only one of the seven studies reduced the numbers of operative deliveries by using insulin. [This was Coustan and Imarah (1984). Women were given insulin prophylactically in a study hypothesizing that it would reduce birth weight. The doctors attending the births knew which women were taking insulin. Their belief that insulin would reduce the risk of macrosomia could well influence the decision to intervene.]

Note: The following four papers were not covered in either review, three of them because they were published after Metzger (1988).

19. Philipson E et al. Gestational diabetes mellitus. Is further improvement necessary? *Diabetes* **198534(Suppl 2):55-60.**

Gestational diabetic women (*N* = 158) were matched to controls for age, race, weight, and private versus clinic status. Despite treatment, the incidence of macrosomia (> 4000 g) (25% versus 15%, *p* < 0.05) and LGA (> ninetieth percentile) (33% versus 22%, *p* < 0.05) were different from controls. Insulin did not significantly reduce macrosomia (20% versus 30%) or LGA (29% versus 39%) compared with diet alone. Gestational diabetics were more likely to have primary cesareans (18% versus 11%, *p* < 0.04). There were more perinatal deaths among gestational diabetics, although this did not reach significance. [These women were treated to achieve euglycemia so, as in Abstract 16, normalizing blood sugar did not prevent excess perinatal mortality.]

20. Maresh M et al. Factors predisposing to and outcome of gestational diabetes. *Obstet Gynecol* **1989;74(3 Pt 1):342-346.**

Women were diagnosed as gestational diabetics (*N* = 213) and then subdivided into those with normal fasting glucose (A1) and those with fasting hyperglycemia (A2). Normal-weight women were placed on an 1800-calorie diet, and overweight women [not defined] were placed on a 1500-calorie diet. [The recommended calorie intake in pregnancy is 35-38 kcal/kg of prepregnancy ideal body weight regardless of glycemic status. This works out to a minimum of about 2000 calories per day (Second International Workshop-Conference 1985).] "The effectiveness of treatment was judged by the absence of weight gain [!]." If diet failed to control blood sugar, insulin was used.

Outcomes were compared with controls matched for age, parity, and ethnic group. The percentage of LGA infants (> ninetieth percentile) was 19% of the A2 group, 14% of the A1 group, and 10% of controls, a trend that did not reach statistical significance.

[Note that treatment, even treatment as rigorous as this, did not reduce LGA to the statistically expected 10%.] Only overweight gestational diabetics delivered excessive numbers of LGA babies (24%). Normal-weight gestational diabetics did not. Maternal overweight but not maternal age or severity of diabetes was significantly related to birth weight ($p < 0.001$). [This suggests maternal weight has far more to do with macrosomia than blood sugar.] Differences in cesarean rates were not significant but substantially exceeded controls (30% A2, 20% A1, 14% controls). [Treatment did not normalize cesarean rates either.]

21. Thompson DJ et al. Prophylactic insulin in the management of gestational diabetes. *Obstet Gynecol* **1990;75(6):960-964.**
Gestationally diabetic women ($N = 95$) were randomly assigned to either diet or diet plus insulin. Women with a ripe cervix were induced between 40 and 42 weeks gestation, and all remaining women were induced at 42 weeks. Twenty-seven women "failed" therapy, that is, did not maintain normal glucose levels, in which case, depending on her assigned group, insulin was either added or the dosage increased. Women in the insulin group were less likely to have babies weighing over 4000 g (5.9% versus 26.5%, $p = 0.48$) but *more* likely to have a primary cesarean (17.6% versus 11.7%, NS). All macrosomic infants (> 4000 g) were born to women weighing 200 lb at delivery or more. Women who failed therapy were more likely to have a macrosomic baby (30% versus 13%, NS). Macrosomia did not correlate with OGTT values. [Once again, high maternal weight was the key factor.]

22. Goldman M et al. Obstetric complications with GDM. Effects of maternal weight. *Diabetes* **1991;40(Suppl 2):79-82.**
Women with GD ($N = 150$) were matched to controls ($N = 350$) for age, parity, and ethnicity. Labor abnormalities, birth trauma, and incidence of macrosomia (> 4200 g) were similar (6.7% GD versus 3.6% control) as was the incidence of LGA infants (> ninetieth percentile) (10% GDM versus 6.6% control). Despite this, both nonlabor cesareans (16% versus 8%) and labor cesareans (21.8% versus 15.6%) were more common among GD women. The overall cesarean rate was 35.3% versus 22% ($p = 0.002$). Women were more likely to have either a scheduled cesarean or a labor cesarean ($p < 0.05$) in all maternal weight categories except "underweight." [GD affected decision making independent of maternal weight, the major determinant of birth weight.] "We believe the low rates of fetal macrosomia and birth trauma justify our approach to intensive diet therapy. . . . [T]he explanation [for increased cesarean rates] is probably related to patterns of physician decision making."

Cesareans and Macrosomic Babies

23. Boyd ME, Usher RH, and McLean FH. Fetal macrosomia: prediction, risks, proposed management. *Obstet Gynecol* **1983;61(6):715-722.**
Outcomes for babies weighing over 4000 g were compared for two time periods: 1963-65 and 1978-80. During both periods, macrosomia was 1.5 to 2 times more frequent for women who were multiparous and over 35 years old, had a prepregnant weight greater than 70 kg, had a ponderal index (wgt/hgt^3) above the ninetieth percentile, was taller than 169 cm, gained more than 20 kg, or gave birth more than 7 days

postterm. Diabetic mothers had twice the risk. Among primiparas the cesarean rate for cephalopelvic disproportion/failure to progress rose from 8.7% to 19.0% ($p < 0.05$). No perinatal deaths were caused by birth asphyxia or trauma in either period. Despite the rise in cesarean rate, no differences were seen in asphyxia or trauma rates (brachial palsy [injury to the nerves serving the arm], facial palsy, or clavicular fracture [broken collar bone]) for either any affected infant (77/1000 in 1963-65 versus 83/1000 in 1978-80) or severely affected infants (22/1000 versus 34/1000). In fact clavicular fracture was more frequent in the latter period (4 versus 17, $p < 0.01$). Compared with spontaneous birth, c-section associated with meconium aspiration and severe asphyxia (defined as requiring more than three minutes resuscitation with positive pressure ventilation usually with 1-minute Apgar scores of 0-3) (10.8/1000 versus 1/1000). One explanation for the association is that labor or delivery with a macrosomic baby may be difficult, even with cesarean delivery, but the incidence of birth asphyxia in macrosomic and normal-weight babies born by elective repeat cesarean was similar (46/1000 versus 36/1000). [This could be an effect of general anesthesia rather than of the surgery itself.] Midforceps deliveries bore similar associations with trauma and asphyxia, although eliminating it would increase the cesarean rate even further. "[T]he authors would advise more judicious care with [midforceps] delivery and the avoidance of excessive force in rotation and traction. . . . An increase in [total cesarean] rate for macrosomic infants from 8% in the 1960s to 21% in 1978 to 1980 did not improve perinatal outcome."

24. Keller JD et al. Shoulder dystocia and birth trauma in gestational diabetes: a five-year experience. *Am J Obstet Gynecol* **1991;165(4 Pt 1)928-930.**
Of 210 women with GD and babies weighing 3500 g or more, 173 labored, 34 had elective repeat cesareans, and 3 had elective cesareans for suspected macrosomia [2 of the 3 weighed less than 4000 g]. Ultimately 120 women had vaginal births of whom 15 (13%) had shoulder dystocias [the head is born but the shoulders are stuck]. Of these, seven were in babies weighing less than 4000 g. More shoulder dystocias occurred after prolonged second stage (25% versus 10.6%, NS). Only 9.8% (11 of 112) followed spontaneous birth, but 50% (4 of 8) followed forceps delivery, a fivefold increase. "[T]o deliver by cesarean section all fetuses estimated to weigh > 4000 g would considerably increase the number of cesarean sections performed, but not eliminate the risk of shoulder dystocia."

THE RISKS OF TESTING AND TREATMENT

Note: If the OGTT is unreliable, diagnosis correlates poorly with infant outcomes, and treatment offers little or no benefit, then the risks of treatment become important.

The Dangers of Hypoglycemia

Note: In the zeal to drive down blood sugar levels, the dangers of too little blood sugar are overlooked.

25. Langer O et al. Glycemic control in gestational diabetes mellitus—how tight is tight enough: small for gestational age versus large for gestational age? *Am J Obstet Gynecol* **1989;161(3):646-653.**

This study matched 334 gestational diabetics with 334 control women for obesity, race, and gestational age at delivery. Diabetics were treated to achieve normal blood sugar. Women tested their blood glucose seven times daily on a home monitor with a memory chip to ensure accurate reporting. Blood glucose values for each subject were averaged and grouped into low (≤ 86 mg/dl), mid-range (87-104 mg/dl), and high (≥ 105 mg/dl). A woman in the low blood sugar group was 2.56 times more likely to have a small-for-gestational-age (SGA) infant compared with the other two groups. Twenty percent had SGA babies compared with 11% among controls ($p < 0.001$). These women had a 30% cesarean rate compared with 13% having normal-weight infants and 18% having LGA babies. Hypertension, a common cause of intrauterine growth retardation, was not the culprit.

26. Rizzo T et al. Correlations between antepartum maternal metabolism and intelligence of offspring. *N Engl J Med* **1991;325(13):911-916.**

The children of 89 prepregnant diabetics, 99 gestational diabetics, and 35 normoglycemic women were given mental development tests at age two and intelligence tests at ages three, four, and five. After correcting for socioeconomic status, race or ethnic origin, and "patient group [?]," scores correlated inversely with third-trimester levels of beta-hydroxybutyrate ($p < 0.02$) [a ketone produced as part of the metabolic response to insufficient calories]. The worse the mother's ketone levels were, the poorer was the child's intellectual development. No other correlations (e.g. prematurity and acidemia) were found. "The association between ketonemia in mothers . . . and lower IQ in their children speak for the need for continued efforts to avoid ketoacidosis and accelerated starvation in all pregnant women."

False Positives on Prenatal Tests

27. Mintz MC and Landon MB. Sonographic diagnosis of fetal growth disorders. *Clin Obstet Gynecol* **1988;31(1):44-52.**

This article reviews the use of sonograms to estimate fetal weight. Head measurements alone are not useful for identifying macrosomic diabetic babies because unlike overgrowth of genetic origin, only the body responds to excess blood sugar. Ultrasound screening reliably identifies normal-weight fetuses but not overly large or overly small fetuses. Multiple measurements and serial scans are required for greatest accuracy. [The decision to induce or perform an elective cesarean may depend on fetal weight estimate. Even the most meticulously performed scan may be misleading, and in clinical practice, scans may be less than meticulous. Therefore, the decision to intervene may be made on extremely shaky grounds.]

28. Golde S and Platt L. Antepartum testing in diabetes. *Clin Obstet Gynecol* **1985;28(3):516-527.**

This literature survey concludes, "Techniques of fetal surveillance serve to provide reassurance to the obstetrician that the fetus is tolerant of its in-utero environment.

They do not function well to identify true distress, having false-positive rates of 25-50%." [Since this study addressed prepregnancy diabetics, whose babies are at substantial risk, it seems likely that routine prenatal surveillance testing of gestational diabetics may frequently lead to unnecessary intervention.]

Intervention Introduces Risk

29. Levine MG et al. Birth trauma: incidence and predisposing factors. *Obstet Gynecol* **1984;63:792-795.**
This study assessed the incidence of and predisposing factors for brachial plexus injury, clavicular fracture, and facial nerve palsy. Injured infants (N = 162) were compared with 10,775 uninjured infants born during the study period. All three types of injuries associated with forceps delivery generally, midforceps delivery in particular, primiparity, and big baby. Brachial plexus and facial nerve injury associated with regional anesthesia and second stage longer than 60 min. [This suggests that the woman most likely to have a baby with a birth injury is a first-time mother, carrying a big baby, who elects an epidural since epidurals lead to prolonged second stage and forceps deliveries.]

30. Acker DB, Sachs BP, and Friedman EA. Risk factors for shoulder dystocia. *Obstet Gynecol* **1985;66(6):762-768.**
The predictability of shoulder dystocia was investigated in a population of 14,721 women having vaginal births of babies weighing over 2500 g. Diabetic women (mixed pregestational and gestational diabetics) having babies weighing 4000 g or more had a 46.3% cesarean rate, whereas nondiabetic women delivering babies in the same weight class had a 26% cesarean rate. [Thus, it appears that being labeled diabetic increases the risk of cesarean.] The strongest predictive factors for shoulder dystocia were the combination of diabetes and estimated fetal weight over 4000 g. The authors recommended elective cesarean section for these women despite a false-negative rate of 45.3%.
[This recomendation exemplifies the mentality that leads to excess cesarean sections in women labeled diabetics. There were 36 diabetic women who gave birth vaginally to a baby weighing 4000 g or more. Assuming fetal weight estimates were perfectly accurate, which they are not, if this recommendation had been followed, all 36 women would have had a cesarean. Twenty-five of them did not experience shoulder dystocia, so surgery offered no benefit. Of the 11 women whose babies had shoulder dystocia, 5 suffered complications, so assuming these all represented different infants, the mothers of the remaining 6 infants also would have had unnecessary cesareans. The authors are blithely consigning 31 of 36—86%—of these women to the risks and pain of major abdominal surgery, to no benefit. Moreover, the five complications were two clavicular fractures, two cases of brachial palsy, and one 5-minute Apgar below 7. Long-term outcomes were not given, but clavicular fractures heal rapidly, and few babies with a 5-minute Apgar below 7 suffer any long-term consequences. And, too, as we have seen, cesareans may increase the risk of meconium aspiration and birth asphyxia; they are not risk free even for the baby. Also, one wonders to what degree obstetric management—epidurals, forceps, poor maternal positioning for birth—contributed to the incidence of shoulder dystocia.]

31. Combs CA, Singh NB, and Khoury JC. Elective induction versus spontaneous labor after sonographic diagnosis of fetal macrosomia. *Obstet Gynecol* **1993;81(4):492-496.**

Outcomes were compared for women with term pregnancies and estimated fetal weight at or above the ninetieth percentile who either had elective inductions for macrosomia ($N = 44$) or began labor spontaneously ($N = 115$). Prostaglandin gel was used to ripen an unfavorable cervix before induction. The diagnosis-to-delivery interval was only 1.5 days less for induction than spontaneous labor. The hospital's cesarean rate was 22.5%. The cesarean rate with elective induction was 57% versus 31% for spontaneous labor ($p < 0.01$). After controlling for birth weight, parity, and care provider, induction still associated with a higher risk of c-section (OR 2.7 CI 1.2-5.9). The odds of having a cesarean with a private doctor versus a midwife or resident were 3.0 (CI 1.5-5.8). Shoulder dystocia occurred in 1 of 19 (5.3%) of elected inductions and 2 of 79 (2.5%) spontaneous labors. All weighed over 4000 g, two were forceps deliveries, and there was one clavicular fracture. Sonographic fetal weight estimates for birth weight 4000 g or more had a sensitivity of 61.3%, specificity of 70.3%, positive predictive value 65.0%, and negative predictive value of 66.9% (macrosomia was suspected in 5.6% of the population). Fewer than half of babies suspected of macrosomia (45%) weighed over 4000 g. "We conclude that elective induction of labor after a sonographic diagnosis of macrosomia increases the cesarean rate and does not prevent shoulder dystocia."

Intervention Is Rarely Necessary

32. O'Brien ME and Gilson G. Detection and management of gestational diabetes in an out-of-hospital birth center. *J Nurse-Midwifery* **1987 Mar/Apr;32(2):79-84.**

Women were screened if they had risk factors. Because 95% of the patients were Hispanic or of Native American descent (a population with a high incidence of diabetes) and more than half were over 30 years old, an unusually large percentage (10%) had GD. A 2000-calorie diet was prescribed, and women attended classes once every two weeks for information and support. Fetal movement counting began at 36 to 37 weeks and weekly nonstress testing at 40 weeks. An EFM strip was taken before admission to the birth center in labor. Dilute juice was allowed in labor. Newborns were checked frequently for hypoglycemia.

One-hundred nineteen women completed prenatal care with the midwives, meaning they maintained good glucose control and did not develop any other complications. Of them, 26% had a baby weighing 9 lbs [4100 g] or more, and 9.2% had a cesarean [roughly half the primary cesarean rate of obstetrician-run studies in the same or earlier time period (Landon and Gabbe 1985; Philipson et al. 1985, Abstract 19; O'Sullivan 1983; Coustan and Lewis 1978)]. When those who were transferred to obstetric care prenatally were added, the cesarean rate was still only 11%. Nine women experienced shoulder dystocia (7.6%) and three babies were injured as a result. [The article does not say which of the four babies with birth injuries had injuries that resulted from shoulder dystocia. The injuries were one each brachial palsy, fractured clavicle, fractured humerus, and cephalohematoma. Long-term outcomes for injured babies were not given.]

REFERENCES

ACOG. *Management of diabetes mellitus in pregnancy.* Technical Bulletin No. 92, 1986.

American Diabetes Association. Position statement on gestational diabetes mellitus. *Am J Obstet Gynecol* 1987;156(2):488-489.

Board PJ et al. Gestational diabetes definition, diagnosis, and treatment strategies. *Pract Diabetology* 1986;5(6):1-15.

Bung P et al. Exercise in gestational diabetes. An optional therapeutic approach? *Diabetes* 1991;40(Suppl 2):182-185.

Chez RA, moderator. Meeting the challenge of gestational diabetes (symposium). *Contemp Ob/Gyn* 1989;34(3):120-140.

Coustan DR. Management of gestational diabetes. *Clin Obstet Gynecol* 1991;34(3):558-564.

Coustan DR and Imarah J. Prophylactic insulin treatment of gestational diabetes reduces the incidence of macrosomia, operative delivery, and birth trauma. *Am J Obstet Gynecol* 1984;150(7):836-842.

Coustan DR and Lewis SB. Insulin therapy for gestational diabetes. *Obstet Gynecol* 1978;51:306-310.

Davis-Floyd R. Lecture, Oakland, CA, Oct 28, 1993.

Dickinson JE and Palmer SM. Gestational diabetes. *Sem Perinatol* 1990;14(1):2-11.

Forest JM et al. Reference values for the oral glucose tolerance test at each trimester of pregnancy. *Am J Clin Pathol* 1983;80(6):828-831.

Fraser RB, Ford FA and Lawrence GF. Insulin sensitivity in third trimester pregnancy. A randomized study of dietary effects. *Br J Obstet Gynaecol* 1988;95:223-229.

Freinkel N. Gestational diabetes 1979: philosophical and practical aspects of a major public health problem. *Diabetes Care* 1980;3(3):399-401.

Gillmer MDG et al. Low energy diets in the treatment of gestational diabetes. *Acta Endocrinol* 1986;Suppl 277:44-49.

Goer H. Gestational diabetes. *Int J Childbirth Educ* 1991;6(4):20-30.

Hadden D. Screening for abnormalities of carbohydrate metabolism in pregnancy 1966-1977: the Belfast experience. *Diabetes Care* 1980;3(3):440-446.

Hod M et al. Gestational diabetes mellitus: a survey of perinatal complications in the 1980s. *Diabetes* 1991;40(Suppl 2):74-78.

Horton ES. Exercise in the treatment of NIDDM: applications for GDM? *Diabetes* 1991;40(Suppl 2):175-178.

Hunter DJS and Keirse MJNC. Gestational diabetes. In *A guide to effective care in pregnancy and childbirth,* Enkin M, Keirse MJNC, and Chalmers I, eds. Oxford: Oxford University Press, 1989.

Jovanovic-Peterson L and Peterson CM. New strategies for the treatment of gestational diabetes. *Isr J Med Sci* 1991;27(8-9):510-515.

Knopp RH et al. Metabolic effects of hypocaloric diets in management of gestational diabetes. *Diabetes* 1991;40(Suppl 2):165-171.

Kuhl C. Insulin secretion and insulin resistance in pregnancy and GDM. Implications for diagnosis and management. *Diabetes* 1991;40(Suppl 2):18-24.

Landon MB and Gabbe SG. Diabetes and pregnancy. *Med Clin North Am* 1988;72(6):1493-1511.

Landon MB and Gabbe SG. Antepartum fetal surveillance in gestational diabetes mellitus. *Diabetes* 1985;34(Suppl 2):50-54.

Metzger BE. 1990 overview of GDM. Accomplishments of the last decade—challenges for the future. *Diabetes* 1991a;40(Suppl 2):1-2.

Metzger BE et al. Summary and recommendations of the third International Workshop-Conference on Gestational Diabetes Mellitus. *Diabetes* 1991b;40(Suppl 2):197-201.

Neiger R and Coustan DR. Are the current ACOG glucose tolerance test criteria sensitive enough? *Obstet Gynecol* 1991;78(6):1117-1120.

Ney D, Hollingsworth DR, and Cousins L. Decreased insulin requirement and improved control of diabetes in pregnant women given a high-carbohydrate, high-fiber, low-fat diet. *Diabetes Care* 1982;5(5):529-533.

O'Sullivan JB and Mahan CM. Criteria for the oral glucose tolerance test in pregnancy. *Diabetes* 1964;13(4):278-285.

O'Sullivan MJ. Non-insulin dependent gestational diabetes mellitus: diagnosis, management and outcome. *J Fla Med Assoc* 1983;70:757-760.

Ratner RE. Clinical review 47: gestational diabetes mellitus: After three international workshops do we know how to diagnose and manage it yet? *J Clin Endocrinol Metab* 1993;77(1):1-4.

Reed BD. Gestational diabetes mellitus. *Primary Care* 1988;15(2):371-387.

Second International Workshop-Conference. Summary and recommendations of the second International Workshop-Conference on Gestational Diabetes Mellitus. *Diabetes* 1985;34(Suppl 2):123-126.

Tallarigo L et al. Relation of glucose intolerance to complications of pregnancy in nondiabetic women. *New Engl J Med* 1986;315(16):989-992.

WHO Study Group. WHO Tech Rep Ser 1985 # 727.

9

Postdates Pregnancy: Induction Versus Watching and Waiting

> Myth: *To avoid problems, at two (or even one) weeks after the due date labor should be induced.*
>
> Reality: *"It is apparent that the overwhelmingly redundant message of the . . . literature . . . is that there is absolutely no study, no evidence whatsoever, that routine induction at any gestational age improves perinatal outcome."*
>
> Nichols 1985a

To obstetricians of the 1960s and 1970s, dealing with postdate pregnancy seemed cut and dried. The incidence of fetal distress, macrosomia (large baby, usually birth weight ≥ 4000 g), birth trauma, cesarean section, passing meconium (the baby's first stool) into the amniotic fluid, and meconium aspiration, cause of a life-threatening pneumonia, rose. Babies also displayed postmature syndrome, believed due to a failing placenta: dry, peeling skin, loss of subcutaneous fat, and meconium staining. And sometimes a healthy fetus died without warning, of unknown cause. The obvious solution was to induce labor at term.

However, inducing labor resulted in, what was for that era, appallingly high cesarean rates, primarily because a uterus and cervix that are not ready to labor will not respond effectively to oxytocin. The most common reason for this is an erroneous due date. Therefore, the next course of action was to search for a way to establish a reliable due date, to develop tests to indicate whether the pregnancy could be safely continued when the cervix was not "ripe," and to find a means of ripening an "unripe" cervix. (Probably because they would be difficult to measure, preparatory changes within the uterine muscle are not considered.)

Obstetricians believe they have accomplished these goals. Two main approaches have evolved: establish the due date by routine sonogram before the third trimester and then either (1) test repeatedly for fetal well-being until either the cervix becomes inducible or a positive test mandates intervention; or (2) induce at some arbitrary date, first ripening an unready cervix. Now that doctors believe they can confirm the due date and soften the cervix and that recent randomized controlled trials have shown inducing may even reduce the cesarean rate, the philosophy is becoming, "Why wait?" (Cucco, Osborne, and Cibilis 1989; Benedetti and Easterling 1988)

This policy would make sense, except that a number of underlying assumptions have been made about the causes of postdate complications, the accuracy of tests, and the efficacy and harmlessness of treatment that do not hold up. First, the whole concept of dating is based on a gestational length established by fiat in the early 1800s. Franz Carl Naegele officially declared that pregnancy lasted 10 lunar months (10 × 28 days), counting from the first day of the last menstrual period (Mittendorf et al. 1990; Nichols 1985a, both abstracted below). However, when Mittendorf et al. measured the median duration of pregnancy, they found that healthy, white, private-care, primiparous women with well-established due dates averaged 288 days and multiparas averaged 283 days, values significantly different from both Naegele's rule and each other. Others have found similar results (Nichols 1985b; Usher et al. 1988, both abstracted below). Mittendorf et al. also cite other studies showing racial differences in gestational length. For example, one showed that black women averaged 8.5 days fewer than white women of similar socioeconomic status.

Moreover, ultrasound-determined due dates are not accurate. One study used the date established by ultrasound at 16 to 18 weeks to test the validity of dating by the last normal menstrual period (LNMP) (Kramer et al. 1988). It found that as gestational age went past term, positive predictive values for the LNMP declined from 95% to 12%. The authors took this to mean the LNMP was inaccurate, but, of course, the ultrasound date is the problem. Even first trimester measurements have an error bar of ±5 days increasing to ±8 days in the second trimester and ±22 days in the third (Otto and Platt 1991).

Few practitioners appreciate the limitations of ultrasound or clinical data. Otto and Platt say the due date should not be changed unless the discrepancy is more than two weeks, yet they see doctors changing a due date by a few days, no trivial alteration if a woman will be induced when she exceeds a certain date. Shearer and Estes (1985, abstracted below) cite examples of doctors, changing due dates with each new datum. Nichols (1985b) points out that bigger fetuses may be erroneously assumed to be older and also that studies show that when ovulation dates were known from basal body temperature and coital records, 70% of women classified postdates were incorrectly dated.

The risks of postdates are not what they seem either because the postdates population is weighted toward complications. As we have seen, primiparous women average longer gestations, and first-time mothers are more likely to have difficult labors, complications, and cesarean sections. Poor women, a higher-risk group, are the women most likely to be misdated because they are least likely to know when they got pregnant or to seek early prenatal care (Sims and Walther 1989, abstracted below). Epidemiologic studies have found an excess of medical (fetal anomalies, hypertension) and social (teen mothers) risks in the postdate population (Eden et al. 1987a, 1987b, abstracted below).

Some risk does accrue in healthy postdate pregnancies (notably meconium passage and big babies), but it does not follow that we should induce all women. Studies have found that as gestational age goes from 37 to 44 weeks, perinatal mortality and morbidity distribute in a U-shaped pattern (Sachs and Friedman 1986; Nichols 1985b, both abstracted below). If we try to eliminate postdate pregnancies on grounds of increased complications, should we not equally logically try to delay labor onset in the early-term group?

As with the risks of postdates, postmature syndrome is also not what it seems. Postmature syndrome is derived from one doctor's subjective evaluation of 37 babies estimated to range from 285 to 325 (!) days gestation (Clifford 1954). Clifford described three grades of severity, but gestational ages widely overlapped each other within grades. He observed no control infants and had no evidence that the symptoms he noted were due to inadequate placental function. In fact, postmature syndrome neither associates exclusively with postdates pregnancy nor do its signs have clinical importance (Shearer and Estes 1985, abstracted below).

Tests of fetal well-being also contribute to the myths of postdates. When a test says the fetus is in jeopardy, it is likely to be wrong (Gregor, Paine, and Johnson 1991, abstracted below), but labor is induced or a cesarean is done. The baby usually turns out to be fine—it always was. But the test results, the intervention, and the good outcome confirm beliefs that postdatism is dangerous, testing valuable, and good outcome due to timely intervention.

High false-positive rates also create the illusion that the threshold of risk lies at ever younger gestational age. Devoe and Sholl (1983) found the distribution of test results did not change from 41 to 43 weeks nor were results different from a term population. But when doctors find substantial numbers of positive tests at a given age, they begin testing sooner, and because of false positives, they find fetuses who appear to be in trouble. This vicious cycle has led to lowering the start dates for testing and the definition of prolonged pregnancy from 42 weeks to 41 weeks (El-Torkey and Grant 1992; Dyson, Miller, and Armstrong 1987, both abstracted below) or even 40 weeks (Egarter et al. 1989; Arias 1987).

Recent randomized controlled trials generally have shown equivalent or even superior outcomes for routine induction, but this may not be a true difference. First, doctors know who is postdate and by how long. If they believe postdatism is risky, a blip on the fetal monitor is more likely to lead to intervention, especially if the mother is being induced after a positive surveillance test. Second, older studies found a wide gap in cesarean rates between spontaneous and induced labors. The gap has closed because the cesarean rate is now outrageously high in both expectantly managed and induced groups. Herabutya et al. (1992), admittedly an extreme example, concluded that the two approaches were equivalent because both groups had *47%* cesarean rates. Third, the protocols flatten the differences between induced and spontaneous labor. Many labors in the expectant arm are induced for fetal jeopardy or because a time limit was reached, and many in the induced arm are spontaneous because labor began in the period between randomization and induction. Finally, the expectant group undergoes testing and runs the risks of false positives; the induction group does not.

In fact, we have little evidence that modern postdates management offers benefits and considerable evidence that it does not. As we shall see, randomized trials of expectant management versus routine induction show few or no significant differences in outcome. Attempts to prevent postdate pregnancy by membrane stripping (lifting the amniotic sac off the cervix) or nipple stimulation initiate labor more frequently compared with controls, but studies present no data on delivery route. Vaginal application of prostaglandin-containing gel may ripen the cervix but has little effect on cesarean rates. Macrosomia may be of concern because of increased c-sections and birth injuries, but ultrasound predicts macrosomia poorly (95% confidence intervals of ±20% with accuracy worst at extremes of weight; Otto and Platt 1991), and we have no evidence that induction improves outcomes. We do know that performing cesareans for macrosomia does not decrease asphyxia or injury rates (Boyd, Usher, and McLean 1983).

Paradoxically, treatment works best on those who need it least: induction is most likely to succeed when the fetus is healthy and the mother on the verge of starting labor on her own. The inverse also holds: treatment does least for those who most need it. Whether the process has gone awry or the mother simply is not as far along as her doctor thinks, if her body is not ready for labor, induction will likely fail. When testing reveals a compromised fetus, doctors induce whether the cervix is ready or not. Inducing an unripe cervix leads to long, hard labors (Arulkumaran et al. 1985a, 1985b), yet a baby in trouble is least able to withstand the stress. Oligohydramnios (too little amniotic fluid), a complication of postdates pregnancy, predisposes to abnormal fetal heart rate (Leveno et al. 1984, abstracted below). When it is found, obstetricians induce. Membranes will almost surely be ruptured for one reason or another. Now the baby has no amniotic fluid.

We also have evidence that postdates management itself causes complications, and, as with surveillance tests, this ironically reinforces belief that postdatism is dangerous. Devoe and Sholl (1983) found that 30% of fetuses testing normal developed fetal distress when labor was electively induced, and the cesarean rate was 15% versus 2% for spontaneous labor. Ahlden et al. (1988) found that the most likely scenario to end in an infected baby was an overdue mother who was induced, had an amniotomy, internal electronic fetal monitoring (EFM), many vaginal exams, and whose labor ended in cesarean section. Guidetti, Divon, and Langer (1989) concluded that testing should begin at 41 weeks because 14% of women had a c-section for fetal distress between 41 and 42 weeks. That so many healthy women carrying healthy *term* fetuses had cesareans for fetal distress says more about management than the dangers of 41 week gestations. (*No* baby, by the way, had a 5-minute Apgar less than 7, which calls into question the diagnosis.) Likewise, Arias (1987) found huge jumps in complication rates (6% to > 20%) and cesarean rates (7% to > 25%) at 40 weeks, which he believed indicated risk at earlier fetal age than previously thought. This is when women were transferred to the high-risk clinic. I submit that the true risk, it seems, was care in the high-risk clinic.

Postdates pregnancy is far from cut and dried. Testing in order to induce selectively introduces risks. Routinely inducing creates more problems than it solves. Letting nature take its course is generally best, although that is not risk free either. No course of action (or inaction) guarantees good outcome. The reality is you pay your money and you take your choice.

SUMMARY OF SIGNIFICANT POINTS

- The median gestational length exceeds 280 days among healthy, white, middle-class women. Primiparas have longer pregnancies than multiparas. (Abstracts 2-3, 7, 17, 34)

- As a rule of thumb, add one day to gestational length for every day the menstrual cycle normally exceeds 28 days. (Abstract 2)

- Many postdate babies are not really postdates. (Abstracts 1-2, 5, 20, 26)

- Most postdates babies are not postmature. (Abstracts 2, 5)

- Postmature syndrome is not exclusive to postdates, has not been shown to have clinical importance, and may be a manifestation of intrauterine growth retardation (IUGR). (Abstracts 2-3, 5)

- Perinatal mortality and morbidity in postdates infants are usually associated with prenatal risk factors. (Abstracts 2, 5, 16-18)

- Healthy fetuses do not lose weight postdates. (Abstract 19)

- Sonographic and clinical weight and date estimates are often wrong. (Abstracts 1-2, 7, 14-15)

- Fetal surveillance tests have high false-positive rates. (Abstracts 2, 12-13, 28-29)

- Surveillance tests do not improve outcomes and may increase risk [because they lead to intervention]. (Abstracts 1, 28-29)

- Surveillance tests have low false-negative rates, but they can fail to predict impending demise. However, most deaths after a negative test were not preventable. (Abstracts 2-3, 13, 16, 20)

- Using breast stimulation for a contraction stress test (CST) is faster, cheaper, equally effective, and less invasive than IV oxytocin. (Abstract 2)

- Vibroacoustic stimulation causes prolonged fetal tachycardia. (Abstract 13)

- Local application of prostaglandin gel (PGE_2) improves cervical scores and increases the incidence of spontaneous labor but has little or no effect on cesarean rates, and it may cause uterine hyperstimulation and abnormal fetal heart rate (FHR). (Abstracts 4, 21-22)

- If cervical scores are 4 or less after local application of PGE_2, the odds of a cesarean with induction are 50%. (Abstract 29)

- Membrane stripping shortens pregnancy but does not affect the mode of delivery. It also has potential risks, although studies reported no problems. (Abstracts 6, 8-9)

- Unilateral breast stimulation safely and effectively ripens the cervix and shortens pregnancy. (Abstracts 10-11)

- Routine induction at any age does not improve perinatal outcome. (Abstracts 1, 2, 4, 16)

- Review and clinical practice papers and population studies find that inducing increases the risk of fetal distress and cesarean section, especially in primiparas. (Abstracts 4, 6, 17-18)

- Some randomized controlled trials find fewer complications and/or cesareans with observation (Abstracts 24-27, 30); some find fewer with induction (Abstracts 29, 31-32); and some find no difference. (Abstract 28).

- The risks of postdates labor are higher incidence of macrosomia (≥ 4000 g) (range at term 6-9%; range postdates 16-30%) and meconium passage (range at term 7-34%; range postdates, 25-47%). (Abstracts 1-3, 5, 14-17, 19, 29, 32-34)

However, macrosomia is not exclusive to postdates, and moving up the due date for large babies inflates the number of postdated macrosomic babies. (Abstracts 1, 3, 5, 19)

Also, postdates meconium passage does not indicate compromise. (Abstracts 1-2)

ORGANIZATION OF ABSTRACTS

Literature Reviews

Pregnancy Does Not Average 280 Days

Efforts to Eliminate Postdates Pregnancy

Stripping Membranes
Breast Stimulation

Postdates Tests

Fetal Surveillance Tests
Weight Estimates

Epidemiological Studies

Preinduction Local Application of Prostaglandin E_2

Studies of Postdates Management

Randomized Controlled Trials
Studies Where Surveillance Testing Not Routine

LITERATURE REVIEWS

1. Shearer MH and Estes M. A critical review of the recent literature on postterm pregnancy and a look at women's experiences. *Birth* 1985;12(2):95-111.
Reported incidences of postdate pregnancy vary from 2.9% to 25%. Nearly all authors concede that half of postdates women are really at term. Because many factors affect dating (not knowing the date of the last menstruation, irregular cycles, differences in time of ovulation), "the length of pregnancy should not be rigidly set at 40 weeks."

Certain risks associate with postdatism. The incidence of macrosomia (≥ 4000 g) ranges from 12.7% to 29.2%, but term infants can be macrosomic too. The practice of diagnosing postterm pregnancy when a larger fetus is detected inflates both the incidence of postterm pregnancy and the association with macrosomia. Oligohydramnios associates with fetal distress (probably by diminishing umbilical cord cushioning), thick meconium, and small babies. However, the amount of amniotic fluid does not correlate with outcome, and it is unclear to what extent oligohydramnios is characteristic of prolonged pregnancy or when intervention is warranted. The incidence of meconium passage rises, but reported numbers vary (11.9-44%). When the heart rate is normal, meconium does not indicate fetal compromise, nor is there evidence that it relates to cord compression or placental insufficiency. Studies have not shown a connection between placental aging changes and fetal distress. Clifford's signs of "dysmaturity" are subjective and have not been shown to have clinical importance. One study showed developmental disadvantages in postterm infants, but of the 40 babies, only 3 were probably actually postmature. "The importance of this study is its suggestion that older mothers with obstetric complications and/or a mother's simply being told she is overdue, might be associated with social and developmental deficits for at least the first eight months of life."

As for management regimens, all studies have found no benefits or increased risk for routine induction at 42 weeks. Studies disagree on what combination of test results mandates intervention. One task force found that few obstetricians are trained to do or interpret sonograms and over 70% were performed by their assistants. "Without a 'gold standard'—a well understood, definite biological endpoint—components of the bio-physical profile will continue to be measured against equally poorly validated fetal surveillance tests." Four randomized trials of high-risk populations where nonstress test (NST) or contraction stress test (CST) information was or was not made available found no differences in perinatal morbidity or mortality. A meta-analysis of them found *more* deaths when clinicians had access to test results. Since postdated populations contain about half normal-term women, NSTs and CSTs would have even less benefit.

Interviews with 32 overdue women found a woman who was induced three days after her second alarming NST and who was told her baby had a liver tumor; she gave birth to a healthy baby. A woman told she was 31 days late by the last of the three due dates assigned her had a baby Dubowitz dated at 41 weeks. "Sonograms were markedly misleading as to dates. . . . It also seems that sonograms were associated with a marked escalation in other tests, intervention in labor, and cesarean sections."

2. Nichols CW. Postdate pregnancy. Part I. A literature review. *J Nurse-Midwif* **1985a;30(4):222-239.**

Most postdates babies are not postmature. "Women have been subjected to the haz-ards and emotional hardships of an induced labor without apparent benefit." Except when done between 6 and 12 weeks menstrual age, ultrasound dating has a margin of error greater than dating by LMP. Primiparous women average longer pregnancies than multiparas, and the average gestational length is longer than 280 days. All clinical dating methods, including the LMP, have margins of error of more than 2 weeks. Com-paring the LMP to ovulation dates from basal body-temperature records, one study found that 70% of pregnancies classified as postdates were misclassified. Another found the proportion of pregnancies classified as postdates by the LMP was 15.5%, versus 4.5% by ovulation date. Only 2 of 110 babies were postmature, and one was not postdates. One day should be added for every day the cycle exceeds 28 days.

We have no accurate way to identify postdates fetuses at risk. Fetal movement counts are not sensitive enough. Neither hormonal assays nor placental grading are reliable. The incidence of meconium-stained fluid increases abruptly at 38 weeks, but this relates to maturing reflexes, not distress. Oligohydramnios associates with growth retardation, thick meconium, and fetal distress and may have value [but false-positive rates are high]. The CST appears to have a lower false-negative rate than the NST, but this is based on nonrandomized studies. Several studies have shown nipple stimulation to be as safe and reliable as an oxytocin drip for the CST as well as cheaper, easier, and faster. The biophysical profile accurately predicts fetal distress at extreme ends of its scale. [What about midrange scores?] Two studies found no increase in abnormal FHR with postdatism.

Studies of management have not found that tests accurately identify postmature babies or that routine induction improves perinatal outcome. Epidemiologic studies have found that much of the excess perinatal mortality in the postdates population is due to other factors: congenital anomalies, infection, or IUGR. The postmature infant is relatively rare. About 10% of pregnancies are postdates, of which 5% to 26% result in postmature babies.

3. Nichols CW. Postdate pregnancy. Part II. Clinical implications. *J Nurse-Midwif* 1985b;30(5):259-268. (U.S.)

Points made in this paper are that an unknown number of "postdates" pregnancies come from moving up a due date for cases of "size ahead of dates," and that one study found that most "postmature infants" (Clifford's syndrome) were growth retarded (43% versus 3% expected).

The paper then reports on outcomes for 170 women reaching 37 weeks gestation who were managed by the Yale midwifery group. [This group is *very* intervention oriented; their practices are nearly indistinguishable from those of obstetricians. See Chapter 15.] All were healthy, white, private patients. Women were divided into groups by length of pregnancy: (1) 37 to 38.4 weeks (7.4%), (2) 38.5 to 42 weeks (79.4%), or (3) over 42 weeks (10.3%). Women with gestations of 41.5 weeks or more had weekly NSTs and were induced at 43 to 44 weeks. The mean gestational age for primigravidas was 287.2 versus 280.1 for multiparas ($p < 0.05$). Operative delivery rates were 23.1% in group 1, 13% in group 2, and 27.8% in group 3. The postdates induction rate was 11% but would have been 33% had all women been induced at 41 weeks.

Comparing group 1 with group 3, premature rupture of membranes (30.7% versus 5.5%), induction (23.0% versus 11.1%), and jaundice (38.5% versus 22.2%) were more common in group 1 ($p < 0.05$). Oxytocin augmentation (0 versus 33.3%), fetal distress (0 versus 17.0%), thick meconium (0 versus 27.8%), and feeding problems (7.7% versus 33.3%) were more common in group 3 ($p < 0.05$). Meconium passage rates were similar (23.0 versus 22.2%) but higher than group 2 (15.8%). Feeding problems correlated with intubation for meconium. One baby died of neonatal asphyxia. The pregnancy was dated at 42 weeks, but Dubowitz assessment [a method of determining gestational age by physical assessment of the neonate] placed the baby at 39 to 40 weeks. An NST had been done the day labor began, which had normal results. Fetal distress and thick meconium developed in labor.

4. Steer PJ. Postmaturity—much ado about nothing? *Br J Obstet Gynaecol* 1986;93:105-108.

Postdates was the indication in half the inductions at a British hospital. Is induction justified? Since the increase (if any) in perinatal mortality is small, a randomized trial would require large numbers. Randomized trials focusing on perinatal morbidity have found no difference in outcomes, but one found a significant increase in cesarean section with induction (27% versus 9.8%). Large retrospective studies have also failed to substantiate benefits for induction, while finding increased forceps and cesarean rates for induced labors. Among primagravidas, cesarean rates of 30% are reported for inductions with a cervical score less than 4 to 6. Techniques to ripen the cervix still find two times the cesarean rates compared with a favorable cervix. "[I]n the absence of signs [of growth retardation] and in otherwise uncomplicated pregnancies, the safest management of prolonged pregnancy is to await the spontaneous onset of labour."

5. Sims ME and Walther FJ. Neonatal morbidity and mortality and long-term outcome of postdate infants. *Clin Obstet Gynecol* **1989;32(2):285-293.**
Studies report that 3.5% to 14.3% of births occur after 42 weeks, of which about 21% of babies are postmature. When early ultrasound confirms menstrual dating, the incidence of postdates drops from 7.5% to 2.6%. Earlier studies were likely to include women with irregular cycles or who did not know the date of their LMP. These are often poor women and thus at higher risk, which would then falsely be attributed to postdatism. Clifford's description is commonly used to diagnose postmaturity. However, more than 50% of the infants he studied were not postdates.

Recent studies have not shown an increase in perinatal mortality with postdates. At highest risk are postdate infants weighing less than 2500 g, and the most frequent cause of death is congenital malformation. The incidence of fetal distress is higher and the c-section rate is doubled with postdates [postdate management could contribute], but reports of neonatal asphyxia conflict. Meconium release and meconium aspiration are more common. The incidence of macrosomia doubles [no numbers], and macrosomic infants are more prone to birth injury.

Studies of long-term outcome conflict. The most recent, which included only women with confirmed due dates and followed the babies for two years, found no differences in mental development, physical milestones, or illness compared with term infants.

6. Satin AJ and Hankins GD. Induction of labor in the postdate fetus. *Clin Obstet Gynecol* **1989;32(2):269-277.**
This clinical practice paper contains the following warnings:

- "Stripping of membranes prior to Pitocin induction has not been shown to be efficacious. Risks of this procedure include potential infection, inadvertent rupture of membranes, and bleeding from an undiagnosed placenta previa."

- "Once amniotomy is performed, the patient is committed to delivery. . . . Restraint from a premature amniotomy, particularly when inducing an unfavorable cervix, may also reduce the incidence of operative deliveries and their complications. . . . In part [the] wide range of cesarean delivery rates [when postdate pregnancies are induced at 42 weeks (51.3-6.5%)] is accounted for by whether the patient is allowed sequential inductions or is committed to a same day delivery by amniotomy. . . . Risks of amniotomy include cord prolapse, adverse change in fetal presentation, and prolonged rupture of membranes."

- "Variability in maternal and fetal response to oxytocin demands their constant surveillance regardless of dose. . . . Qualified personnel . . . able to identify and treat both maternal and fetal complications must remain in attendance. . . . The fetal heart rate and pattern and uterine activity must be monitored vigilantly." The American College of Obstetricians and Gynecologists recommends beginning infusions at 0.5 to 1.0 mU/min with 1 mU/min increments at 30- to 60-minute intervals because one study with faster incremental dosages and higher infusion rates found that oxytocin had to be stopped or reduced for abnormal FHR or hypercontractility in 36% and 44% of women. With lower rates, the incidence was 19% [still one in five!]. When given in high dosages in conjunction with salt-free IV solutions, oxytocin may cause cardiovascular and fluid and electrolyte abnormalities (water intoxication). Symptoms are confusion, nausea, convulsions, and coma. Doses of 20 mU/min may induce antidiuresis, and doses over 40 mU/min can profoundly decrease urinary output.

PREGANCY DOES NOT AVERAGE 280 DAYS

7. Mittendorf R et al. The length of uncomplicated human gestation. *Obstet Gynecol* 1990;75(6):929-932.
This study used the LMP in women with regular cycles to establish gestational age because when ultrasound dating and menstrual dating in women with regular cycles were compared in in vitro fertilization pregnancies, the best ultrasound-based estimate resulted in 80% more error than the LMP plus a confirmatory pelvic exam. Ovulation was assumed to occur 14 days before the next expected menstrual period.

The population consisted of all women with uncomplicated pregnancies and reliable menstrual history who began labor spontaneously (primiparas, $N = 31$; multipara, $N = 83$). The women were white and had private doctors. The median gestational length [from time of ovulation] was 274 days for primiparas (CI 269-276 days) and 269 days in multiparas (CI 267-270 days). Naegele's rule predicts 266 days [280 - 14 = 266]. p-values for primiparas ($p = 0.0003$) and multiparas ($p = 0.019$) were different from both 266 days and each other ($p = 0.0032$). Other studies have found that black women (264 days) and Japanese women (264 days) may have yet shorter median gestational lengths.

EFFORTS TO ELIMINATE POSTDATES PREGNANCY

Stripping Membranes

8. McColgin SW et al. Stripping membranes at term: can it safely reduce the incidence of post-term pregnancies? *Obstet Gynecol* 1990;76(4):678-680.
Women with firm due dates were randomly assigned ($N = 180$, 90 per group) to weekly membrane stripping (the examiner lifted 2-3 cm of membrane off the cervix, first stretching open the cervix if it was long and closed) or the usual cervical exams beginning at 38 weeks. Treated women went into labor sooner (8.60 ± 0.74 days versus 15.14 ± 0.83 days) and were less likely to exceed 42 completed weeks (3.3% versus 15.6%, $p < 0.004$). [The study group had 54 multiparas versus 45 multiparas among controls. The authors say this did not affect outcome, but multiparas average shorter gestations.] The greatest benefits were derived for nulliparous women with unfavorable Bishop scores [no data given]. "The mode of delivery was not significantly different [no

data given]." No complications were found. The advantages were fewer office visits, less need for surveillance tests, decreased patient and physician anxiety, and fewer difficult inductions. [Note the lack of clinical benefits. If doctors were less anxious and their care less interventive, the "advantages" would vanish.]

9. El-Torkey M and Grant JM. Sweeping of the membranes is an effective method of induction. *Br J Obstet Gynaecol* 1992;99(6):455-458.

Women were randomly assigned at 41 to 42 weeks gestation to sweeping of the membranes ($N = 33$) or controls ($N = 32$). If the cervix would not admit a finger to lift the membranes off the lower segment, the cervix was massaged "to encourage prostaglandin release ($N = 6$)." Induction was scheduled for four days later. More women in the study group began labor spontaneously (76% versus 38%, $p = 0.002$). Of the 27 women who underwent sweeping, 89% went into labor versus 17% of the women who had cervical massage. [In other words, membrane sweeping did not help the women with an unripe cervix, the ones who really needed it.] No complications were found. Cesarean rates were similar (15% versus 12%).

Breast Stimulation

10. Elliott JP and Flaherty JF. The use of breast stimulation to prevent postdate pregnancy. *Am J Obstet Gynecol* 1984;149(6):628-632.

Two hundred healthy women at about 39 weeks gestation were randomly assigned to either breast stimulation or control group. Study women were asked to stimulate the nipple, areola, and distal breast manually one at a time for 15 minutes, alternating breasts, for one hour per session. They were "encouraged" to spend three hours per day on this activity. Control women were asked to abstain from coitus and breast stimulation. While initial Bishop scores were similar, 8 study women versus 21 control women reached 42 weeks without beginning labor. Of those completing 42 weeks, 5 study women versus 17 control women had Bishop scores less than 8 ($p < 0.01$). Women who stimulated their breasts for 3 hours or more daily had a mean days-to-delivery interval of 4.61 versus 8.54 for those stimulating for less time ($p < 0.0004$). However, "we found it difficult to motivate our patients to stimulate the breasts as much as 3 hours per day."

11. Salmon YM, et al. Cervical ripening by breast stimulation. *Obstet Gynecol* 1986;67(1):21-24.

One hundred healthy women past 38 weeks gestation were divided into two groups. The treatment group was told to massage alternate breasts gently especially around the nipples, for three hours daily. The control group was told to avoid intercourse and breast stimulation. Breast stimulation was first performed while being monitored. No uterine hypertonus was noted. The treatment group showed a change in Bishop score (3.96 ± 1.34 versus 1.04 ± 1.03, $p < 0.00001$). Within three days 36% of treated women began labor versus none in the control group ($p < 0.00008$). After three days, the remaining study group became controls and vice versa. Once again Bishop scores improved compared with controls (3.11 ± 1.42 versus 0.76 ± 0.97, $p < 0.0001$.) The authors contend that the studies in which uterine hypertonus and fetal bradycardia were noted used bilateral breast stimulation. Some patients found the stimulation tiresome. Perhaps a shorter period would be sufficient. "Breast stimulation was found to be an inexpensive, simple, noninvasive, and effective outpatient method of ripening the cervix. . . . Given the relative safety of breast stimulation as described [here], the next step would be to ascertain its applicability to high-risk pregnancies."

POSTDATES TESTS

Fetal Surveillance Tests

12. Leveno KJ et al. Prolonged pregnancy. I. Observations concerning the causes of fetal distress. *Am J Obstet Gynecol* **1984;150(5 Pt 1):465-473.**
Sonar evaluations of amniotic fluid volume were performed in 213 women either suspected (N = 143) or known (N = 70) to be past 42 weeks gestation, but results were not revealed. Oligohydramnios (defined as fewer than two 1-cm pockets of amniotic fluid) was found in 39%. Women with normal amniotic fluid volume were less likely to have a cesarean for fetal distress compared with women with oligohydramnios (5.4% versus 13.1%, p = 0.05). [However, my calculation shows the sensitivity of oligohydramnios for cesarean for fetal distress to be 61%, specificity 63%, false-positive rate 37%, and false-negative rate 39%. The positive predictive value was 13%, and the negative predictive value was 95% (prevalence of cesarean for fetal distress: 8.5%). Thus, normal fluid volume reassures, but low fluid volume predicts fetal distress in labor poorly—nor do we know whether inducing labor would reduce this incidence.]

13. Gregor CL, Paine LL, and Johnson TR. Antepartum fetal assessment. A nurse-midwifery perspective. *J Nurse Midwifery* **1991;36(3):153-167.**
The premise of antepartum testing is that uteroplacental insufficiency will be displayed in fetal responsiveness, activity, and FHR.

Fetal movement counts: Fetal movement counts measure deviations from the fetus's normal pattern. A cessation of fetal movements correlates highly with impending death. In such cases a follow-up test should be done.

Nonstress test: EFM is done for a 20-minute period. When FHR accelerations are absent, do not meet criteria, or adverse FHR patterns are present, the test is nonreassuring. The false-negative rate (deaths within one week after a normal test) is 5% to 10% of all deaths. Most deaths associated with a reactive NST are not preventable (malformations, cord accidents, sepsis, prematurity). The false-positive rate is 40% to 80%. Nonreactive NSTs should be followed by a CST or biophysical profile.

Vibroacoustic stimulation (VAS): An artificial larynx is pressed against the mother's belly over the fetal head. The sound and vibration startle the fetus and produce an FHR acceleration. This is supposed to decrease the time it takes for an NST, but because a common response is prolonged tachycardia (> 160 bpm), waiting for the FHR to return to normal results in equally long tests. This test has achieved rapid acceptance despite lack of research on the actual mechanism of action, deleterious effects, or the establishment of norms. VAS can be used to awaken a sleeping fetus, but "[w]e find the addition of a test that nonphysiologically startles a sleeping fetus, primarily to save time, to be unnecessary."

Contraction stress testing: The FHR is evaluated in response to contractions elicited either with IV oxytocin or nipple stimulation. The decision to deliver should be made cautiously and taking other factors into account because the false-positive rate may be as high as 30%. A nonreactive NST and a positive CST increase the likelihood of uteroplacental insufficiency.

Biophysical profile (BPP): The BPP combines a sonogram with an NST to score the baby 0 to 2 on five parameters: fetal muscle tone, fetal movements, fetal breathing movements, amniotic fluid volume, and FHR reactivity. As the score declines, the incidence of morbidity increases. At 6 it is 55%, and at 0 it is 100%. The false-positive rate is less than 1 per 1000. [The authors do not say what BPP value or for what outcome.]

Amniotic fluid evaluation: Oligohydramnios may indicate uteroplacental insuffi-ciency or may lead to cord compression. However, measurements of amniotic fluid volume "have been fraught with difficulty and inaccuracy." One study found a fluid volume less than 5 cm associated with a 48% incidence of meconium staining and a 10% incidence of 5-minute Apgars below 7.

Test validity: False-positive tests "can lead to undue psychological strain on the woman and her family, unnecessary intervention, and possible iatrogenic problems from the intervention." Not all poor outcomes can be predicted by testing because some are due to events unrelated to uteroplacental insufficiency. With tests in current use, a fetus testing negative is highly likely to be healthy (low false negative), but a fetus testing positive is unlikely to be compromised (high false positive).

Weight Estimates

14. Chervenak JL et al. Macrosomia in the postdate pregnancy: is routine ultrasonographic screening indicated? *Am J Obstet Gynecol* **1989;161(3):753-756.**

Healthy women with confirmed dates had ultrasound weight estimations after 41 weeks gestation ($N = 317$). Birth weights were compared with a control group of 100 healthy women at 38 to 40 weeks gestation. The incidence of macrosomia (> 4000 g) was 25.5% in the study group versus 6% in the control group ($p < 0.05$). The sensitivity of sonography for macrosomia was 61%, and the specificity was 91%. The positive predictive value was 70%, and the negative predictive value was 87%. [This positive predictive value means that when the true incidence of macrosomia is 25%, the odds of thinking the baby is macrosomic and being wrong is 3 out of 10. Thus, sonography will lead to unnecessary intervention, increasing risk.]

15. Pollack RN, Hauer-Pollack G, and Divon MY. Macrosomia in postdates pregnancies: the accuracy of routine ultrasonographic screening. *Am J Obstet Gynecol* **1992;167(1):7-11.**

Women pregnant 41 weeks or longer ($N = 519$) had sonographic weight estimations (measurements of abdominal circumference and femur length) within one week of birth. The incidence of birth weight or 4000 g or more was 23% and 4% weighed 4500 g or more. At birth weights over 3750 g, sensitivity for birth weight of 4000 g or more was 56%, specificity 91%, positive predictive value 64%, and negative predictive value 87%. Measurements systematically overestimated birth weight. "Routine ultrasonographic screening for macrosomia in postdates pregnancies is associated with a relatively low positive predictive value."

EPIDEMIOLOGICAL STUDIES

16. Sachs BP and Friedman EA. Results of an epidemiologic study of postdate pregnancy. *J Reprod Med* **1986;31(3):162-166.**

Outcomes were examined for all singleton infants born at a Boston teaching hospital from 1975 to 1982 who were 38 weeks or more gestation and had no major congenital anomalies ($N = 18,610$). Women had oxytocin challenge tests (OCTs) [same as CSTs] or NSTs regularly after 41 weeks.

Perinatal mortality rates were the same at 38 to 39 weeks gestation (3.8 per 1000) as at 42 to 44 weeks (3.7-3.8 per 1000), while the rate at 40-41 weeks was 2.3 per 1000. Perinatal mortality rates were six times higher in infants weighing less than 2500 g compared with heavier babies. Out of 10 deaths occurring after 41 weeks, five were associated with medical or obstetrical complications. Three had normal FHR tests within five days of demise. The study failed to demonstrate a significantly increased perinatal mortality in postdate infants probably because the population of nearly 20,000 was too small. [Therefore, inducing labor at 42 weeks has extremely limited potential benefit.] The incidence of meconium rose from 7% to 25% (relative risk (RR) at > 42 weeks compared with 38 to 41 weeks = 2.0). The RR of fetal distress in labor also doubled [possibly due to induced labors?], and while the RR of certain postpartum complications increased, the overall incidence at after 42 weeks was only 3%. The percentage of failed inductions rose from 2% at 38 to 39 weeks to 28% at 44 weeks or more. Likewise, the primary cesarean rate went from 7% to 25%. [Inducing substantially increases the risk of cesarean section.] "Elective induction of labor for all pregnancies > 42 weeks does not appear justified."

17. Eden RD et al. Perinatal characteristics of uncomplicated postdate pregnancies. *Obstet Gynecol* **1987a;69(3 Pt 1):296-299.**

Infants of uncomplicated pregnancies born at 42 weeks gestation or later ($N = 3457$) were compared with similar infants born at 40 weeks ($N = 8135$). Differences were small, but mothers of postdate infants were more likely ($p < 0.05$ in all cases) to be primagravidas (33.4% versus 37.9%) and to have higher blood pressure (diastolic 78.5 mm Hg versus 79.2 mm Hg). Infants were more likely to be macrosomic (> 4500 g 0.8% versus 2.8%), to experience shoulder dystocia (0.7% versus 1.3%), and to have congenital anomalies (2.0% versus 2.8%). They were more likely to pass meconium (19.4% versus 26.5%) and to aspirate it (0.6% versus 1.6%). Corrected perinatal mortality rates were not significantly different (2.7/1000 versus 4.2/1000). The difference in death rates did not relate to meconium passage or anomalies. Large differences were found in induction (2.8% versus 14.2%) and cesarean (8.3% versus 17.6%) rates. Induction with a ripe cervix and internal EFM during labor are recommended [despite minuscule differences in outcomes and large differences in induction and cesarean rates.].

18. Eden RD et al. Posdate pregnancies: a review of 46 perinatal deaths. *Am J Perinatol* **1987b;4(4):284-287.**

This study analyzes the 46 perinatal deaths that occurred among 6701 babies born at 42 weeks or more gestation. The death rate was 6.9 per 1000 births. Mortality associated significantly ($p < 0.05$) with Black or Hispanic race, maternal age 15 years or less, hypertension, birth weight less than 2500 g, meconium, cord accident, and congenital malformations. The perinatal mortality rate at 42 to 43 weeks was 4 per 1000, the same as at 36 to 42 weeks (N = 49,689), and jumped to 10 per 1000 at 43 weeks or more. "Only normal pregnancies should be allowed to progress postdate." [This conclusion is unwarranted. This study presents no evidence that terminating pregnancy sooner would improve outcomes.]

19. McLean FH et al. Postterm infants: too big or too small? *Am J Obstet Gynecol* **1991;164(2):619-624.**

Fetal growth was analyzed in a population of 7005 infants among whom early ultra-sonography confirmed due date. Pregnancies with conditions known to affect fetal growth (e.g. diabetes, hypertension, multiple births) were excluded. Mean birth weight increased, as did the incidence of large ($\geq$ 4000 g) babies (9% at 39 completed weeks, 15% at 40, 22% at 41, 30% at 42). The incidence of small babies (< 2500 g) decreased to zero by 42 completed weeks. "No evidence of postterm weight loss or lower weight for length could be demonstrated. . . . There is a lack of convincing evidence that the postterm fetus is at increased risk of distress or nutritional deprivation."

20. Grubb DK, Rabello YA, and Paul RH. Post-term pregnancy: fetal death rate with antepartum surveillance. *Obstet Gynecol* **1992;79(6):1024-1026.**

The study population was all women undergoing antepartum fetal surveillance be-tween 1986 and 1990 for the sole indication of "prolonged pregnancy" (defined as > 41 wks). Tests consisted of an NST and measurement of amniotic fluid volume, followed by a biophysical profile if the NST was nonreactive. Women with certain dates and favorable cervixes were induced after 43 completed weeks. "However, uncertain dating was very common in the clinic population" [which means many women were probably not postdates].

Of the 8038 women undergoing testing, nine had stillbirths (fetal mortality rate 1.12/1000), none due to anomalies. One woman had normal tests and did not return. Only two women had abnormal tests (but were not delivered). Two women had not completed 42 weeks gestation. "Our findings suggest that beginning antepartum surveillance between 287-293 days is not unreasonable." [On the contrary, considering that seven of nine babies had normal tests, this study demonstrates the failure of testing, even in a clinic population where, because problems are more likely, positive predictive values are higher. Consider, too, that outcomes do not represent the risks of postdatism because many women were not really postdates.]

PREINDUCTION LOCAL APPLICATION OF PROSTAGLANDIN E$_2$

21. Owen J et al. A randomized, double-blind trial of prostaglandin E$_2$ gel for cervical ripening and meta-analysis. *Am J Obstet Gynecol* **1991;165(4 Pt 1):991-996.**

Women with a nonemergent indication for induction, a Bishop score of 4 or less, and no contraindication to prostaglandin were randomly assigned to intracervical application of 1 ml of 0.5 mg/ml PGE$_2$ gel (N = 47) or a placebo (N = 53). Oxytocin induction was begun 12 hours later. A minimum of 12 hours was required to diagnose "failed induction," and serial induction was permitted after overnight rest.

During the waiting period, five women in the control group began labor, of whom two developed abnormal FHR requiring closer monitoring. In the study group, eight women began labor, of whom five developed abnormal FHR. Of these, two had cesareans and one responded to medical treatment for uterine hyperstimulation. The overall cesarean rate was 28% in the PGE_2 group versus 30% among controls.

A meta-analysis was performed on 18 randomized trials of local application of PGE_2 gel in dosages of at least 0.5 mg intracervically or 5 mg intravaginally. Reports included 944 treated women and 867 controls. The cesarean rate was not significantly different. "[O]ur data and a meta-analysis do not confirm that [local PGE_2 application] can improve the success of . . . induction of labor by significantly decreasing the cesarean rate. Given that the use of this . . . agent is not without side effects, we cannot recommend PGE_2 gel for cervical priming before . . .induction of labor."

22. Trofatter KF. Endocervical prostaglandin E_2 gel for preinduction cervical ripening. Clinical trial results. *J Reprod Med* 1993;38(1 Suppl):78-82.

This report reviews results of four U.S. and Canadian randomized controlled trials of intracervical application of 0.5 ml PGE_2 in a commercially prepared gel. Altogether, 277 women were treated and 261 were controls. Gel was inserted 12 hours before oxytocin induction in women with Bishop scores of 4 or below. Forty percent of the women were being induced for postdates. Bishop scores improved significantly ($p < 0.01$), and more women began labor (47.4% versus 9.6%, $p < 0.001$) in the treated group. However cesarean rates were not significantly different (28.5% versus 32.9%).

23. Keirse MJNC. Prostaglandins in preinduction cervical ripening. Meta-analysis of world wide clinical experience. *J Reprod Med* 1993;38(1 Suppl):89-100.

This study analyzes data from 44 randomized or quasi-randomized (e.g. alternate allocation) controlled studies of using prostaglandin to ripen the cervix. All but one trial found a statistically significant increase in cervical score, and every trial reported more women beginning labor in the study group. No single trial showed a significant reduction in cesarean rate, but in the aggregate, the cesarean section rate was reduced by about 15% (CI 1-30%). The odds of instrumental delivery were also reduced by 10% to 40%. Prostaglandin treatment associated with reduced use of epidural anesthesia [which may explain why more study women gave birth spontaneously]. Treatment also associated with uterine hyperstimulation and FHR abnormalities, but neither trend resulted in increased operative delivery or lower Apgar scores. More cesareans were performed during the latency period among study women compared with controls, but the reverse was true during labor. "Nevertheless, it is inappropriate to administer prostaglandins for cervical ripening for trivial reasons and without careful monitoring of maternal and fetal well-being."

STUDIES OF POSTDATES MANAGEMENT

Randomized Controlled Trials

Note: See also Table 9.1. Note the *tremendously* high cesarean and perinatal complication rates, especially since most studies *excluded* complicated pregnancies.

24. Suikkari AM et al. Prolonged pregnancy: induction or observation. *Acta Obstet Gynecol Scand* **1983;116(Suppl):58.** (Finland)

Women 10 days or more postdates were randomly assigned to induction ($N = 66$) or observation ($N = 53$). Among induced women, 29% had operative deliveries versus 15% among the observed group. The induction rate among controls was 26%. Infant outcomes were the same. Since follow-up is more "laborious" than induction, prophylactic induction is recommended in cases of prolonged pregnancy with a favorable cervix. [The authors are willing to double the number of operative deliveries, thereby exposing twice as many women and babies to their concomitant risks, in order to avoid the nuisance of awaiting labor.]

25. Katz Z et al. Non-aggressive management of post-date pregnancies. *Eur J Obstet Gynecol Reprod Biol* **1983;15:71-79.** (Israel)

Women with confirmed due dates who had reached 294 days gestation and had a pelvic score of 4 or less ($N = 156$) were evenly allotted to immediate induction (controls) or observation (study group). The study group was monitored at 3-day intervals until the pelvic score exceeded 4 or pathology developed. In the study group, 52 (66.6%) women began labor spontaneously after a mean duration of 299.8 days (range 295-316

Table 9.1: Randomized Controlled Trials of Induction Versus Expectant Management

STUDY	# OF SUBJECTS	% EXPECTANT POP ACTUALLY INDUCED	C-SEC RATE EXPECTANT POPULATION
Suikkari et al. 1983, Abstract 24	119	26.4 % [a]	15.1%
Katz et al. 1983, Abstract 25	156	21.8%	8.8%
Cardozo, Fysh, and Pearce 1986, Abstract 26	402[1]	23.5%	9%
Witter and Weitz 1987, Abstract 28	200	15.4%	27.8%
Dyson, Miller, and Armstrong 1987, Abstract 30	302[3]	20.7%	27.3%
Augenson et al. 1987, Abstract 30	409[5,6]	31%[7]	7.7%
Bergsjo et al. 1989, Abstract 31	188[8]	36.2%	41.5%
Hannah et al. 1992, Abstract 32	3407[9,10]	32.5%	24.5%

[a]attributed to postdates

[1]Sixty-four percent of the "induced" population was actually induced.

[2]This was a placental abruption at 292 days.

[3]PGE$_2$ gel was used to ripen cervix before induction.

[4]The morbidity for meconium (46.7% versus 19.1%, $p < 0.01$), meconium aspiration (4.0% versus 0, $p < 0.02$), and fetal distress (18.0% versus 2.6%, $p < 0.01$) was greater in the expectant population.

[5]Eighty-two percent of the "induced" population was actually induced.

days). Of the 26 inductions, 17 were because of an increased pelvic score. In the study group, 9% had cesareans versus 20.5% of controls. Among controls, half the cesareans were for fetal distress, "probably caused by the prolonged and difficult labor resulting from induction while the pelvic score was still low." The department cesarean rate was 8%. No differences in neonatal outcome were found. One neonatal death unrelated to malformation occurred. It followed a cesarean for fetal distress in the control group. "Conservative management . . . appears to be entirely justified."

26. Cardozo L, Fysh J, and Pearce JM. Prolonged pregnancy: the management debate. *Br Med J* **1986;293:1059-1063.** (Great Britain)

Healthy women were randomly allocated to active ($N = 195$) or conservative management ($N = 207$) at 290 days gestation. Due dates were confirmed by ultrasound. (This reduced the incidence of prolonged pregnancy from 10% to 6.6%.) In the active group, labor was induced between 292 and 294 days by local application of PGE_2 gel followed three hours later by amniotomy and, if necessary, oxytocin. In the conservative group, women were monitored by fetal movement charts, NSTs, and amniotic fluid volume measurements. Women were induced for abnormalities or on request. The sample size could detect a 17% reduction in cesarean rate. In the active group, 36% began spontaneous labor during the waiting period. In the conservative group, 19% were induced.

C-SEC RATE INDUCED POPULATION	PERINATAL MORTALITY[a] EXPECTANT POP	PERINATAL MORTALITY[a] INDUCED POP	PERINATAL MORBIDITY[a] EXPECTANT POP	PERINATAL MORBIDITY[a] INDUCED POP
28.8%	0/53	0/66	NS	NS
20.5%	0/78	1/78	NS	NS
13%	0-1/207[2]	0/195	NS	NS
29.1%	0/97	0/103	NS	NS
14.5%	1/150	0/152	4	4
6.5%	0/195	0/214	NS	NS
28.9%	1/94	0/94	NS	NS
21.2%	2/1706	1/2603	11	11

[6]Induction attempts could be repeated up to three times.

[7]The expectant population was allowed one more week (43 wk).

[8]Of the "induced" population, 91.5% was actually induced.

[9]PGE_2 gel was used to ripen the cervix in the induced arm but not in the expectantly managed arm.

[10]Of the "induced" population, 66.1% was actually induced.

[11]Morbidity for fetal distress (8.3% versus 5.7%, $p = 0.023$), c-section for fetal distress (8.3% versus 5.7%, $p = 0.003$), and meconium (28.7% versus 25.0%, $p = 0.015$) was greater in the expectant population.

When admitted to the hospital, conservatively managed women had higher mean Bishop scores ($p < 0.01$), lower fetal heads ($p < 0.001$), and more occiput anterior fetuses [the favorable position] ($p < 0.01$). Although the incidence of abnormal FHR was similar, women in the active group tended to have more intervention for fetal distress. The cesarean rates (13% versus 9%), forceps rates (20% versus 26%), and incidence of failed induction (1.7% versus 2.1%) were not significantly different for active versus conservative groups. Infant outcomes were similar, except the active group had lower cord pHs. The women in the active group who began labor spontaneously had a 4% cesarean rate, none for fetal distress. Compared with the rest of their group, women in the conservative group who were induced had more abnormal FHRs, more intervention for abnormal FHR, and more cesareans (23% versus 7%). Twenty had inductions on request, of whom nine had cesareans, four for failed induction. "Thus from our results we can find no evidence to support the view that women with normal prolonged pregnancy should undergo routine induction of labour at 42 weeks' gestation."

27. Pearce JM and Cardozo C. Prolonged pregnancy: the management debate. *BMJ* 1988;297:715-717. (A letter requested a supplemental analysis of the women remaining after the 2- to 4-day waiting period to allow a clearer comparison of induction versus conservative management because it would eliminate women in the active group who began labor spontaneously. Pearce and Cardozo complied.)

In the active group, 125 women remained, and in the conservative group 156 women. The conservative group maintained significantly higher Bishop's scores and lower fetal heads at labor onset. The incidence of FHR abnormalities in the active group reached significance (14% versus 7%, $p < 0.02$), as did the incidence of cesarean for fetal distress (6% versus 1%, $p < 0.05$).

28. Witter FR and Weitz CM. A randomized trial of induction at 42 weeks gestation versus expectant management for postdates pregnancies. *Am J Perinatol* 1987;4(3):206-211. (U.S.)

Healthy women at 41 weeks gestation were randomly assigned to expectant management ($N = 97$) or delivery at 42 weeks ($N = 103$). Expectantly managed women did fetal movement counts and had 24-hour urinary estriol determinations followed up by CSTs. The delivery group were induced with oxytocin at 42 weeks followed by amniotomy when contractions were established. Serial inductions were allowed. "Failed induction" was diagnosed 20 hours or more of regular, painful contractions. In the delivery group, 34% began labor spontaneously before 42 weeks, as did 40% of the expectant group. Eliminating these women did not change results. [No data are given on how many in the expectant group were induced.]

Cesarean rates were similar (expectant 27.8% versus delivery 29.1%), nor were the proportional indications for cesarean, except for "prolonged latent phase" [a.k.a. "failed induction"] (0% versus 23.3%). The number of inductions for fetal indications was higher in the expectant group (15.4% versus 4.6%, $p < 0.025$), but the percentage having cesareans was the same (40%), as was the incidence of fetal distress in labor. [This suggests that testing overdiagnosed compromised infants.] Infant outcomes were not different [but the fetal distress rates (34% versus 33%) and meconium passage rates—39% versus 34%—were extremely high]. Although a cost analysis found the delivery group cost $250 more per patient (extra time in the hospital outweighed prenatal visits and testing), induction at 42 completed weeks is recommended.

29. Dyson DC, Miller PD, and Armstrong MA. Management of prolonged pregnancy: induction of labor versus antepartum fetal testing. *Am J Obstet Gynecol* **1987;156(4):928-934. (U.S.)**

Healthy women with confirmed gestational age of 287 days and cervical scores less than 6 were randomized to either induction (N = 152) or testing (N = 150) management. In the induced group, local PGE_2 treatment was followed by induction 16 to 18 hours later if the cervical score was 5 or above or one more dose of PGE_2 and an additioal 4-hour wait if it was not. Half of women (6 of 12) with a final cervical score of 4 or less had cesareans versus 16% (15 of 95) of those with scores greater than 4. The testing group had pelvic exams, NSTs, and amniotic fluid evaluations weekly until 42 weeks and biweekly thereafter. Inductions were done for abnormal tests or cervical score of 6 or more. In the testing group, 20.7% were induced (14.7% for cervical score of 6 or more, 6% for abnormal tests). [Calculation shows 29.6% of the induction group began labor spontaneously.] Of the nine women induced for abnormal tests, five had fetal distress in labor. [The test correctly predicted fetal distress only 56% of the time.] The average gestational age at delivery in the testing group was 296.3 ± 4.2 days. [This means many did not reach 294 days (42 weeks).]

The cesarean rate was lower in the induction group (14.5% versus 27.3%, p < 0.01), mostly due to fewer cesareans for fetal distress (1.3% versus 14.0%, p < 0.01). Induced women had significantly lower incidence of meconium (19.1% versus 46.7% [!], p < 0.01), meconium aspiration (0 versus 4.0%, p < 0.02), and fetal distress (2.6% versus 18.0% [!], p < 0.01). Two-thirds of women with abnormal tests had cesareans. The only death occurred in the testing group. Labor onset was spontaneous, fetal distress developed, and a cesarean was done; the infant died of meconium aspiration and persistent fetal circulation. Thus, the data favor cervical ripening with prostaglandin gel and "aggressive" induction of labor before 42 weeks. [What did they do to these healthy, mostly term women to have such complications?]

30. Augensen K et al. Randomised comparison of early versus late induction of labour in post-term pregnancy. *Br Med J* **1987;294:1192-1195.** (Norway)

Healthy women of 290 to 297 days gestation with reliable menstrual dates were randomized to group 1, immediate induction (N = 214) or group 2, continuation one more week (N = 195). Induction was considered a failure if labor was not established by six to eight hours, in which case it was discontinued and repeated up to three times. The first induction attempt failed in 23% of women. Group 2 had NSTs every three to four days and were induced on day seven. Failed inductions were treated as in group 1. In group 1, 17.8% labored spontaneously, and in group 2, 28.2% were induced and 2.6% had elective cesareans.

Emergency cesarean rates did not differ (6.5% group 1 versus 7.7% group 2). [Group 1's rate would have been much higher had serial induction not been permitted.] Infant outcomes were similar, except 10 infants in group 1 needed phototherapy for jaundice versus 1 in group 2 (0.01 > p > 0.005). Paradoxically, induction succeeds best in women with ripe cervixes, but these are the women most likely to begin labor shortly. If the goal is preventing postmaturity syndrome, these women may not need induction. "[W]e now postpone the induction of labour in post-term cases, as the risk in monitoring the natural course, certainly up to day 308, seems minimal."

31. Bergsjo P et al. Comparison of induced versus non-induced labor in post-term pregnancy. A randomized prospective study. *Acta Obstet Gynecol Scand* **1989;68(8):683-687.** (China)

Women at 42 weeks gestation by reliable menstrual dating were either induced by stripping membranes and oxytocin infusion or allowed to continue another week ($N = 94$ in each group). Induction was continued "as long as there was some progress." Because of transportation difficulties, group 2 women stayed in the hospital and had fetal movement tests, ultrasound, and urinary estriols. The hospital cesarean rate was 16.0%.

In group 1, eight women began labor before induction. Of the remaining 86, 77 achieved active labor. Of the nine failed inductions, eight had cesareans. There were 19 additional cesareans for a total of 27 (28.7%). In group 2, 60 women began labor spontaneously, of whom 25 had cesareans. Thirty-four women were induced for fetal distress, all after 43 completed weeks. Of these, 14 had cesareans for a total of 39 (41.5%). Differences were not significant, but more babies had jaundice in group 1 (6.4% versus 3.2%) and more babies in group 2 had "respiratory distress syndrome" (4.3% versus 8.5%) and aspiration pneumonia (4.3% versus 8.5%). One baby in group 2 died of pneumonia. Overall, nine children (4.8%) weighed less than 2500 g.

32. Hannah ME et al. Induction of labor as compared with serial antenatal monitoring in post-term pregnancy. A randomized controlled trial. *N Engl J Med* **1992;326(24):1587-1592.** (Canada)

At 22 hospitals, healthy women of 41 weeks or more gestation and cervical dilation 3 cm or less were randomized to induction within four days ($N = 1701$) or monitoring until reaching 44 weeks ($N = 1706$). In the induction group PGE_2 was locally applied as many as three times at 6-hour intervals if the cervix was less than 50% effaced and less than 3 cm dilated. Oxytocin was started 12 hours after the last dose. The monitoring group did fetal kick counts and had NSTs and amniotic fluid volume determinations twice weekly. In the induction group, 33.9% began labor spontaneously, and in the monitoring group, 32.5% of labors were induced. Induction in the monitoring group was *not* preceded by PGE_2 cervical ripening. [Inducing for suspected compromise without first ripening the cervix would weight the monitoring group toward fetal distress and c-section.]

The cesarean rate was lower in the induced group (21.2% versus 24.5%, $p = 0.03$), and fewer cesareans were performed for fetal distress (5.7% versus 8.3%, $p = 0.003$). The incidence of fetal distress was also lower (10.3% versus 12.8%, $p = 0.023$), as was the incidence of meconium (25.0% versus 28.7%, $p = 0.015$). [Clinically these are trivial differences.] All other of the many measures of infant outcome were similar. Two babies in the monitoring group died (NS). In one case, three days after randomization, "intrauterine death was confirmed." [Since induction was up to four days after randomization, assignment to induction would probably not have prevented it.] In the second case, fetal distress developed during spontaneous labor five days after normal tests. The baby had aspirated meconium and could not be resuscitated after an emergency cesarean. To detect a 50% reduction in perinatal mortality would require 30,000 women. The authors acknowledge that physicians were not blinded to allocation group and might have been more anxious with postdates women and that lack of PGE_2 priming could contribute to a higher cesarean rate.

Studies Where Surveillance Testing Not Routine

33. Rayburn WF and Chang FE. Management of the uncomplicated postdate pregnancy. *J Reprod Med* **1981;26(2):93-95.** (U.S.)

Outcomes for pregnancies of confirmed gestational age > 294 days (N = 101) were compared with outcomes for pregnancies lasting 38 to 42 weeks (N = 322). No significant differences were found for meconium or fetal distress. More babies weighed over 4000 g in the postdates group (16% versus 7%, $p < 0.01$), but fewer babies weighed less than 2500 g (1% versus 7%, $p < 0.05$). Cesarean rates were higher in the postdate group (13% versus 3%, $p < 0.05$). Six of the 13 postdate cesareans involved a macrosomic fetus. The one small baby in the postdates group was from a hypertensive pregnancy. The only perinatal death was in the postdate group, also in a hypertensive pregnancy; the infant died of meconium aspiration. "An elective induction of labor may be done in an uncomplicated postdate pregnancy only if the patient is aware of the risks of induction, the gestational dating is certain and the cervix is . . . 'ripe.'"

34. Usher RH, et al. Assessment of fetal risk in postdate pregnancies. *Am J Obstet Gynecol* **1988;158(2):259-264.** (Canada)

Infants of mothers with ultrasound-confirmed due dates were grouped by gestational age at birth: (1) 273 to 286 days (39-40 wks, N =5915), (2) 287 to 293 days (41 wks, N =1408), and 3) 294 or more days (≥ 42 wks, N = 340). Induction rates were 17% group 1, 24% group 2, and 44% group 3.

Meconium passage rose from 15.3% of group 1 to 27% and 31.5% of groups 2 and 3. Meconium aspiration rose from 2.2% to 5.7% to 17.6%. Fetal distress increased from 15.9% to 21.9% to 29.7%. (p values for group 1 compared with groups 2 and 3 were all less than 0.001.) Fractures and palsies increased from 10.7% to 14.2% to 29.4% ($p <$ 0.01). However, rates of depression at birth (moderate: 23.4%, 31.3%, 26.5%; severe: 3.7%, 3.6%, 8.8%) were not significantly different, nor were postasphyxic encephalopathy rates (0.7%, 1.4%, 2.9%). [How much of these high perinatal complication rates were related to labor management, especially the rising induction rate?] Postterm pregnancies were more often primiparous (47% group 1, 60% group 2, 66% group 3). [First labors are more likely to be problematic.] Postterm fetuses more often weighed 4000 g or more (23% of primiparas and 40% of multiparas postterm versus 9% and 14%, respectively, at term.) Two nonanomalous babies died 7 days or more postterm: one malnourished baby died in utero at 41 weeks, and one baby was asphyxiated by shoulder dystocia at 42 weeks.

"The paucity of postterm antepartum deaths in the present study in the absence of a program of antepartum fetal monitoring is reassuring and consistent with the findings reported over the years from this institution of a relative absence of increased risk with postterm pregnancy." It is likely that the excess "postterm" fetal deaths in other studies come from women who are unsure of their dates. These are often poor women, and their increased risk is then falsely attributed to postmaturity. Nevertheless, no amount of scientific fact will change the natural response to a postterm death, which is to think the infant should have been followed more closely or delivered earlier.

REFERENCES

Ahlden S et al. Prediction of sepsis neonatorum following a full-term pregnancy. *Gynecol Obstet Invest* 1988;25(3):181-185.

Arias F. Predictability of complications associated with prolongation of pregnancy. *Obstet Gynecol* 1987;70(1):101-106.

Arulkumaran S et al. Failed induction of labour. *Aust N Z J Obstet Gynaecol* 1985a;25(3):190-193.

Arulkumaran S et al. Total uterine activity in induced labour—an index of cervical and pelvic tissue resistance. *Br J Obstet Gynaecol* 1985b;92(7):693-697.

Benedetti TJ and Easterling T. Antepartum testing in postterm pregnancy. *J Reprod Med* 1988;33(3):252-258.

Boyd ME, Usher RH, and McLean FH. Fetal macrosomia: prediction, risks, proposed management. *Obstet Gynecol* 1983;61(16):715-722. (abstracted in Chapter 8)

Clifford SH. Postmaturity—with placental dysfunction. *J Pediatrics* 1954;44(1):1-13.

Cucco C, Osborne MA, and Cibilis LA. Maternal-fetal outcomes in prolonged pregnancy. *Am J Obstet Gynecol* 1989;161(4):916-920.

Devoe LD and Sholl JS. Postdates pregnancy. Assessment of fetal risk and obstetric management. *J Reprod Med* 1983;28(9):576-580.

Egarter C et al. Is induction of labor indicated in prolonged pregnancy? Results of a prospective randomised trial. *Gynecol Obstet Invest* 1989;27(1):6-9.

Guidetti DA, Divon MY, and Langer O. Postdate fetal surveillance: Is 41 weeks too early? *Am J Obstet Gynecol* 1989;161(1):91-93.

Herabutya Y et al. Prolonged pregnancy: the management dilemma. *Int J Gynaecol Obstet* 1992;37(4):253-258.

Kramer M et al. The validity of gestational age estimation by menstrual dating in term, preterm, and postterm gestations. *JAMA* 1988;260(22):3306-3308.

Otto C and Platt LD. Fetal growth and development. *Obstet Gynecol Clin North Amer* 1991;18(4):907-931.

10

Premature Rupture of Membranes at Term

Myth: *Once membranes are ruptured, the baby must be born within 24 hours or infection sets in.*

Reality: *"By waiting 24 hours, avoiding cervical examination, and allowing a reasonable latent phase of labor [after induction (16 hours)], we believe that the increase in cesarean section rates with induction can be minimized."*

Garite 1985

In the 1960s a flurry of papers on the infectious hazards of prolonged rupture of the fetal membranes led to the 24-hour rule: once membranes rupture the baby must be delivered within 24 hours. In order to ensure time enough for labor, this meant inducing any woman who did not begin spontaneous labor within a few hours of membrane rupture, augmenting slowly progressing labors with oxytocin, and performing cesarean sections on those for whom delivery was not imminent by 24 hours postrupture. Babies born after or close to the 24-hour limit were likely to be subjected to a septic workup to determine if the neonate was infected, which included drawing blood and often a spinal tap.

This aptly named "aggressive approach" was enthusiastically embraced by obstetricians, who expressed delight at having a rationale for intervening—although, in what is surely unintentional irony, they did not like the word *aggressive*. They feared it might give a negative impression because *aggression* means "a first or unprovoked attack or an attack of hostility" (Russell and Anderson 1962). Concerns about potentially high cesarean section rates and the observation that infections were rare when no vaginal exams were performed were brushed aside (Russell and Anderson 1962), and by the early 1970s, the 24-hour rule had become the standard of practice in term pregnancies. Aggressive management did, in fact, lead to high cesarean rates for failed induction or fetal distress, but this was considered preferable to the lethal perinatal infections that would surely result from doing nothing.

In their enthusiasm, doctors overlooked the weaknesses of those 1960s studies. For example, Duff, Huff, and Gibbs (1984, abstracted below) point out that the studies were retrospective, meaning they depended on culling records, not conducting a controlled evaluation, and nonrandomized, meaning that women were not randomly assigned to treatment or nontreatment. They mixed term and preterm pregnancies, which confounds results because preterm fetuses are more vulnerable to infection and infection often precedes membrane rupture rather than vice versa (Duncan and Beckley 1992, abstracted below; Reynolds 1991; Perkins et al. 1987). Definitions of infection were neither uniform nor precise, and management protocols for premature rupture of membranes (PROM) were not specified. In addition, antibiotic therapies and neonatal intensive care have improved so materially that 1960s outcomes no longer apply (Monif, Hume, and Goodlin 1986).

The relationships between rupture of membranes, labor, and infection are more complex than the doctors of the 1960s (or for that matter, the decades since) believed. Cooperstock, England, and Wolfe (1987) studied the association between time of rupture and time of day and found that not all cases of PROM are alike. Women who began spontaneous labor within a day or so after membrane rupture were highly likely to have membranes rupture late at night. Women with infected membranes (chorioamnionitis) did not show this circadian rhythm. Neither did women who were not infected but who did not begin labor within that time frame. Observing that labor onset shows the identical circadian pattern, the authors theorized that in the first case, hormones regulating the onset of labor were probably responsible. The second case suggests that infection precipitated membrane rupture. In the third case, some as yet unknown mechanism appeared to be at work.

Their study illuminates the problems of PROM. It explains why inductions often fail: women whose uteruses are not primed for labor—that is, women in categories two and three—will not labor effectively no matter how much oxytocin is given (Steer, McCarter, and Beard 1985). It explains the seeming relationship between length of time postrupture and infection. Women in the second category (comprising very few term pregnancies) have an incipient infection. They are not ready to labor and will have a long latency period, which will allow that infection to blossom. In women of the third category, vaginal exams and internal monitoring start infective processes that, as with the second case, have time to take hold because these women, too, have a long latency period. Finally, it explains why almost all studies of PROM management at term done since the 1960s show major benefits for expectant management (watching and waiting) in women with no signs of infection: women who are not infected are not likely to develop infections—provided people keep their fingers and monitoring devices out of the vagina—and will do best if left alone.

The fact is, not only does leaving women alone do best for most women, but standard management could hardly do worse if it were intentionally designed that way. Standard management *causes* infections and fetal distress, the very things it is supposed to prevent. Vaginal exams and internal monitoring start infections. Induction leads to vaginal exams, internal monitoring, fetal distress, and c-sections, which themselves have much higher infection rates.

One might think that the deleterious effects of the 24-hour rule have been so thoroughly documented that expectant management would replace it. But doing nothing is anathema to mainstream obstetricians, so the expense and frustration of prolonged antenatal admission for observation become justification for induction (Guise, Duff, and Christian 1992; Duncan and Beckley 1992, both abstracted below), even though waiting for labor does not extend hospital stay by much (Marshall 1993), nor is it likely to cost more when all the excess cesareans generated by induction are factored in. And in any case, there is no evidence that PROM cannot be managed on an outpatient basis. So, too, local application of prostaglandin gel is rapidly gaining prominence as an alternative to waiting for labor, but as we shall see, it does no better than expectant management at minimizing cesareans; it sometimes does worse; and it introduces risks. Finally, as we shall also see, the 2% to 4% of women who do not proceed to spontaneous labor for whatever reason within a day or so (Duncan and Beckley 1992) are likely to prove problematic whatever is done. Induction is no panacea, even for this tiny minority.

SUMMARY OF SIGNIFICANT POINTS

- Expectant management for 24 hours and probably longer is safe. Few women or babies develop clinical infections. Waiting 24 hours before inducing allows 60% to 95% of women to start labor spontaneously. (Abstracts 5, 8-9, 11-21)

- Compared with expectant management or intravaginal prostaglandin, oxytocin induction or augmentation increases the incidence of fetal distress and cesarean delivery. This is partly a direct effect of oxytocin and partly because labor is more painful and women are more likely to want epidurals. Women with an unfavorable cervix who are induced for PROM face three to five times the risk of c-section; primiparas are at highest risk. (Abstracts 9, 10-12, 14-18, 20, 22-23, 26)

- Digital vaginal exams start infections, probably by inoculating the cervix with vaginal bacteria carried up on the exam glove. A sterile speculum exam is a safe substitute. (Abstracts 5-7, 14, 21)

- Provided no digital exams are done, infection rates do not relate to length of time between membrane rupture and birth. However, oxytocin use increases the risk of infection in both mother and baby, probably because women are more likely to have digital exams, internal monitoring, and cesareans. (Abstracts 5, 12-15, 17, 20, 22, 26)

- Infections of Group B *Streptococci* are rare (2-4/1000) in babies of vaginally colonized mothers, but the mortality rate is 50%. However, induction does not prevent ß-streptococcal colonization in infants. (Abstracts 12, 23)

- Intravaginal prostaglandin gel achieved cesarean rates similar to expectant management for 24 hours or more, but it had side effects. When only 12 hours of latency period was allowed, it achieved lower cesarean rates compared with a placebo or immediate induction. (Abstracts 9, 23-26)

- Epidurals cause maternal fever (which may lead doctors to suspect infection and act accordingly). (See also Chapter 13.) (Abstracts 18-19)

- Antibiotics provide effective treatment for perinatal infection. (Abstracts 11, 13, 15-16, 20)

- One study found periodic pelvic exams at the end of pregnancy increased the incidence of PROM; another did not. Neither found the practice provided useful information. (Abstracts 1-2)

- In equivocal cases, none of the common methods of confirming ruptured membranes is reliable. (Abstracts 3-4, 8, 15)

- Women desiring expectant management may want to find out the policies on septic workups in the infant. (Abstracts 21-22)

- PROM can be managed on an outpatient basis. (Abstracts 13-14)

ORGANIZATION OF ABSTRACTS

Do Prenatal Vaginal Exams Increase the Incidence of PROM?

Tests to Confirm Rupture Can Be Inaccurate

Postrupture Cervical Exams

Expectant Versus Aggressive Management (Clinical Practice Paper, Review)

Expectant Versus Aggressive Management (Studies)

Problems with Inducing with an Unripe Cervix
Expectant Management: No Time Limit
Expectant Management: Induction after a Time Limit
Expectant Management Versus Induction with an Unfavorable Cervix

Randomized Controlled Trials of Prostaglandin E_2

DO PRENATAL VAGINAL EXAMS INCREASE THE INCIDENCE OF PROM?

1. Lenihan JP. Relationship of antepartum pelvic examinations to premature rupture of the membranes. *Obstet Gynecol* **1984;63(1):33-37.**

Women with uncomplicated pregnancies were randomly assigned to one of two groups: weekly pelvic exams beginning at 37 weeks gestation ($N = 175$) or no pelvic exams before 40 weeks in multipara and 41 weeks in nullipara ($N = 174$). Eighteen percent of those having routine pelvic exams had PROM versus 6% of those having none ($p = 0.001$).

The author theorizes that the probing finger carries up and deposits on the cervix bacteria and acidic vaginal secretions capable of penetrating the mucous plug and causing sufficient low-grade inflammation to rupture membranes. "It would therefore seem prudent to recommend that no pelvic examinations be done routinely in the third trimester unless a valid medical indications exists to examine the cervix . . . especially since the information gained from these routine examinations is often of little or no benefit to either the physician or the patient."

2. McDuffie RS et al. Effect of routine weekly cervical examinations at term on premature rupture of the membranes: a randomized controlled trial. *Obstet Gynecol* **1992;79(2):219-222.**

Women with uncomplicated pregnancies were randomly assigned to have weekly pelvic exams beginning at 37 weeks ($N = 297$) or exams only for clinical indication, such as assessment for induction ($N = 290$). The mean number of examinations in the "routine exam" group was 2.9 compared with 0.6 in the "no exam" group. No effect on PROM was found. "Though we found no harm from routine cervical examinations, we could also find no benefit."

TESTS TO CONFIRM RUPTURE CAN BE INACCURATE

3. Gorodeski IG, Haimovitz L, and Bahari CM. Reevaluation of the pH, ferning, and nile blue sulphate staining methods in pregnant women with premature rupture of the fetal membranes. *J Perinat Med* **1982;10:286-291.**

Women were grouped into those known to have intact membranes ($N = 60$), those known to have ruptured membranes ($N = 176$) either because of history and confirmation by the attending physician or because membranes were deliberately ruptured to induce or augment labor, or a test group of equivocal cases ($N = 26$). The equivocal cases were classified as ruptured or intact retrospectively based on whether rupture was seen to occur before delivery.

High false positive rates for all three tests were found in the women known to have intact membranes, especially in those with copious vaginal discharge. In women with ruptured membranes, high-false negative rates were obtained for all three tests. The false-negative rate increased over time, and by 24 hours postrupture, it reached 50%, or no better than chance. Performing all three tests on multiple samples for the test group reduced the number of incorrect results, but even so, correct, unequivocal diagnosis was made in only 61.5% of cases.

4. Davidson KM. Detection of premature rupture of the membranes. *Clin Obstet Gynecol* **1991;34(4):715-721.**

"Despite significant advances in technology, no one test has been found to be completely accurate, and diagnosis still requires an integration of historic factors, physical examination, and laboratory testing." When free-flowing amniotic fluid is observed, or both nitrazine [amniotic fluid is more alkaline than vaginal secretions, and nitrazine impregnated test paper changes color in response to it] and arborization tests [amniotic fluid forms a characteristic pattern when streaked onto a microscope slide and air dried] are positive, "PROM is confirmed," but when fluid is not seen draining from the cervix and only one of the two tests is positive, diagnosis is equivocal. [This means the tests are least reliable when they are most needed.] If diagnosis is questionable, dye can be injected transabdominally. Then, either a speculum exam can be done or a tampon placed and removed a few hours later to check for dye staining. [This invasive, potentially risky procedure would not be needed if the mother was not going to be induced for PROM. Moreover, inserting a tampon increases the risk of infection. Once again, doctors are causing the very thing they say they are trying to prevent.]

POSTRUPTURE CERVICAL EXAMS

5. Schutte MF et al. Management of premature rupture of membranes: the risk of vaginal examination to the infant. *Am J Obstet Gynecol* **1983;146(4):395-400.**

In a study of 321 pregnant women who had spontaneously ruptured membranes for more than 24 hours before delivery, two factors were found to have independent correlation with clinical symptoms of perinatal infection and mortality: duration of gestation ($p < 0.0001$) and interval between vaginal exam and delivery more than 24 hours ($p < 0.0001$). If no vaginal exams were performed, the relationship between infection and interval from rupture to delivery disappeared. "In our opinion, vaginal examination performed after rupture of membranes winds the clock of infection."

6. Munson LA et al. Is there a need for digital examination in patients with spontaneous rupture of the membranes? *Am J Obstet Gynecol* **1985;153(5):562-563.**

Cervical dilation and effacement in 133 women were assessed by both digital exam and visualization using a sterile speculum. The correlation was measured. There was less than 20% variance, "a difference that is not clinically significant."

7. Brown CL et al. Cervical dilation: accuracy of visual and digital examinations. *Obstet Gynecol* **1993;81(2):215-216.**

Both a speculum exam and a digital exam were performed by the same person on 64 pregnant women with ruptured membranes. For determining whether the mother was less than 4 cm dilated or dilated 4 cm or more, the speculum exam had a sensitivity of 100% and a specificity of 63.2%. Positive and negative predictive values were 86.5% and 100% (19% of women were dilated 4 cm or more).

EXPECTANT VERSUS AGGRESSIVE MANAGEMENT (Clinical Practice Paper, Review)

8. Garite TJ. Premature rupture of the membranes: the enigma of the obstetrician. *Am J Obstet Gynecol* 1985;151(8):1001-1005.

A protocol is proposed for diagnosing and managing PROM. History of a large gush of fluid followed by persistent leakage diagnoses PROM in 90% of cases. When diagnosis is uncertain, other tests should be used, although cervical secretions, blood, or vaginal infection can cause false positives with nitrazine paper. For managing PROM at term, recommendations are as follows:

- Speculum exam to document diagnosis and rule out cord prolapse.
- Rule out fetal distress with EFM and infection by monitoring for maternal fever.
- No digital exams unless immediate delivery is planned or anticipated.
- Continuous external EFM. [In 1988 the American College of Obstetricians and Gynecologists declared that auscultation [frequent listening] was equivalent to EFM even in high-risk cases, which this is not.]
- Induce 24 hours postrupture, which allows 80% to 90% of women to start labor spontaneously.
- Induce immediately if infection develops.
- Allow at least 16 hours for active-phase labor to develop before diagnosing a failed induction.

Waiting longer than 24 hours before inducing is not recommended because of insufficient data on the safety of ruptured membranes beyond 48 hours.

9. Duncan SLB and Beckley S. Prelabour rupture of the membranes—why hurry? *Br J Obstet Gynecol* 1992;99:543-545.

Fear of maternal or neonatal sepsis is the justification for inducing or augmenting labor when PROM occurs, but waiting "a while" seems to reduce the odds of cesarean, and "the policy appears to be safe." About 2% to 4% of term births will involve PROM with no labor within 24 hours. Older studies found an inexorable rise in infection rates as time passed after PROM, but they often mixed term and preterm pregnancies. Preterm pregnancies have longer latent periods and higher perinatal mortality. Infection often causes PROM in preterm pregnancies, and some perinatal deaths were due to other factors, such as cord prolapse. Oxytocin associates with increased cesarean rates, and the earlier it is used, the higher the rate is. Vaginal prostaglandins shorten the latent period, but a randomized controlled trial [Mahmood et al. 1992, Abstract 25] found it did not affect the cesarean rate. In term or near-term pregnancies with PROM and no evidence of obstetric hazard, a delay of 12 hours will allow many women to achieve active labor spontaneously and will improve the chances of spontaneous delivery.

"Open-ended antenatal admission is not popular with women," so beyond 12 hours, the woman's wishes and the resources for surveillance should determine whether to induce. [The decision to intervene is predicated on the unsupported belief that PROM cannot be managed on an outpatient basis.]

EXPECTANT VERSUS AGGRESSIVE MANAGEMENT (Studies)

Problems with Inducing with an Unripe Cervix

10. Rydstrom H et al. **Premature rupture of the membranes at term.** *Acta Obstet Gynecol Scand* 1986;65(6):587-591.

Outcomes were measured for 303 women with uncomplicated term pregnancies who were being induced for PROM with no contractions during a 2-hour observation period. Women were grouped based on favorable ($\geq$ 2 cm dilation) versus unfavorable (< 2 cm dilation, cervix not fully effaced, station -2 or higher) cervix. All women had internal electronic fetal monitoring (EFM). "Failed induction" was defined as failure to reach 4 cm dilation after 12 hours of stimulation.

The cesarean rate among nulliparas with a favorable cervix was 3.6% versus 19.4% with an unfavorable cervix. Among multiparas, the cesarean rate was 4.2% with a favorable cervix versus 11.1% with an unfavorable cervix. Nulliparas with an unfavorable cervix were more prone to "ominous" fetal heart rate (FHR) decelerations compared with an unselected population (28.3% versus 4.5%). Nulliparas with a favorable cervix and all multiparas had FHR findings similar to an unselected population. "These decelerations have previously been found to be associated with [oxytocin] induced abnormal activity." Newborns of nulliparas with unfavorable cervix were more likely to be transferred to neonatal care units compared with nulliparas with a favorable cervix or multiparas (14.3% versus 4.8% and 1.6%). "[Nulliparas with an unfavorable cervix] may benefit from an expectant . . . attitude to treatment" [yet the authors do not recommend expectant management for for multiparas with an unfavorable cervix even though they nearly tripled their cesarean rate].

Expectant Management: No Time Limit

11. Kappy KA et al. **Premature rupture of the membranes at term.** *J Reprod Med* 1982;27(1):29-33.

Women who had ruptured membranes, no signs of infection, no labor, and an unfavorable cervix were followed ($N = 150$). Sixty percent of those managed expectantly began labor by 24 hours postrupture—88% within 48 hours. No digital vaginal exams were performed. Since not all attending physicians agreed with expectant management, 38 women were induced, four for possible infection.

Of the induced population, 39% had cesareans either for lack of progress or fetal distress compared with only 10% of the 112 women who labored spontaneously ($p < 0.01$). Lack of progress was defined as "lack of cervical effacement and dilation despite good labor for at least 1.5 hours." Nineteen infants (13%) were placed on antibiotics either prophylactically or for treatment. There were no infant deaths or cases of sepsis in mothers or infants. "We feel that a conservative approach in patients at term with PROM and an uninducible cervix is warranted. . . . This approach decreases the incidence of cesarean sections in these patients without increasing infectious morbidity."

12. Morales WJ and Lazar AJ. Expectant management of rupture of membranes at term. *South Med J* **1986;79(8):955-958.**

Women with term uncomplicated pregnancies (including women with previous cesarean) and PROM who were not in labor were randomly assigned to expectant management (monitoring for infection or fetal distress) ($N = 167$) or induction ($N = 150$). No digital exams were done until active labor. Most (85%) began labor within 48 hours. Women randomized to induction had internal EFM and pressure catheter. "Failed induction" was defined as failure to enter active-phase labor after 12 hours of regular contractions.

The cesarean rate was 7% for women managed expectantly compared with 21% for induced women. No cesarean was done for failure to progress in expectantly managed multiparas versus a 15% cesarean rate for this cause in induced multiparas. Infection rates after cesarean section (24% versus 5% [no p value]) reflected the "well documented significant increase in postpartum endometritis after abdominal delivery." Intrapartum infection and endometritis rates after vaginal birth were increased in the induced population (12% versus 4%, $p < 0.01$). [Why? Did the internal monitor lead and catheter provide a route for ascending infection? Does induction predispose to infection?] No infant in either group was infected. Group B *Streptococcus* was isolated in 20% of cervical cultures. [I do not know if this prevalence is typical.] This resulted in 20 colonized infants because standard culturing takes two days, longer than the latency period of most women with PROM. No cases of neonatal infection occurred, but group B *Streptococcus* is still a danger because although the infection rate is low (2-4/1000), the mortality rate is 50%. A "rapid latex particle agglutination test" is recommended to detect Group B *Streptoccocus* antigen. If the test is positive, labor should be induced and prophylactic antibiotics given. "These findings . . . support the observation that contrary to previously accepted belief, prolonged interval between rupture of membranes and delivery does not increase the maternal and neonatal infection rate. Rather, with PROM the interval from digital examination to delivery is the critical parameter in the incidence of infection."

13. Gilson GJ et al. Expectant management of premature rupture of membranes at term in a birthing center setting. *J Nurse Midwifery* **1988;33(3):134-139.**

In order to minimize hospitalization for freestanding birth center patients, 59 women with uncomplicated pregnancies, PROM, and no labor for longer than 24 hours were followed as outpatients. All women were free of infection, including Group B *Streptococcus* colonization, and had had either no or one digital cervical exam. Women made daily visits to the clinic for white blood cell count, temperature, and nonstress test. Once labor began, oral castor oil and breast stimulation were used to stimulate slow labors. Half of the women reaching 24 hours without labor gave birth within the next 24 hours and 80% by 72 hours postrupture.

The cesarean rate was 20.3% versus 7.5% for non-PROM birth center clients. Of the 12 cesareans, six were for cephalopelvic disproportion (arrest of progress after 5 cm dilation despite augmentation and good labor), three for failure to progress (inability to get past 5 cm dilation despite augmentation for 12 hours), and three for fetal distress. The authors believe cesarean rates for failure to progress would have been much higher with standard management because the majority in the study still had an unripe cervix at 24 hours postrupture.

Only two women (7.4%) were transferred to hospital care for suspected infection. Length of rupture did not seem to relate to infection. Of women giving birth vaginally, only one (2.1%) developed true endometritis (fever, uterine tenderness and/or foul-smelling discharge, elevated white cell count), the same incidence as among non-PROM birth center clients. Chorioamnionitis was diagnosed in five patients (8.5%) during labor, of whom three had a cesarean. Three babies had suspected sepsis and were treated with antibiotics, but none had positive blood or cerebrospinal cultures. One mother (2.1%) had a positive culture for Group B *Streptococcus*. [This conflict with the study's entry criteria is not explained.] The baby was fine.

14. Marshall VA. Management of premature rupture membranes at or near term. *J Nurse Midwifery* 1993;38(3):140-145.

Outcomes for women with term PROM and no labor for 1 hour or more were compared between two New York hospitals, both serving indigent women. At Metropolitan Hospital (MH) labor ($N = 347$) was managed by obstetricians, and women were induced 12 hours postrupture. At North Central Bronx (NCB) midwives cared for women ($N = 562$), monitoring them for signs of infection and setting no time limits on latency period. The incidence of PROM at term was 6% at both hospitals.

Mean length of latency was shorter at MH (15.2 hr versus 34.2 hr, $p = 0$), and mean labor length (either spontaneous or induced) was shorter (9.9 hr versus 11.7, $p = 0.0015$). Women at MH had more vaginal exams (mean, 4.3 versus 3.7, $p = 0.0001$), internal EFM (71% versus 34%, $p = 0.0001$), Pitocin (58% versus 44%, $p = 0.0001$), and analgesia (60% versus 25%, $p = 0$). Few epidurals were done (10% versus 16%). The cesarean rate was higher at MH (17.5% versus 5.9%, $p < 0.0001$). (Department cesarean rates were 21.7% versus 12.1%.) No differences in uterine infection rates were found (8.3% versus 9.3%). Birth route and number of vaginal exams were strong predictors of uterine infection. Length of latency "barely achieved significance." Incidence of 5-minute Apgar score less than 7 was similar. Babies born at MH were frequently admitted to the neonatal ICU for observation, so admission rates were "startlingly" higher (60.4% versus 9.3%, $p < 0.0001$). Despite more use of neonatal antibiotics, the neonatal sepsis rate was higher at MH (4.1% versus 2.5%, NS). Although women were admitted to NCB to await labor onset, average total maternal stay was only a half-day longer (3.9 ± 2.1 versus 4.4 ± 4.0, $p = 0.0048$), and infant stay was longer at MH (5.7 ± 6.4 versus 4.2 ± 2.8, $p < 0.0001$). [One argument for induction is that the cost of antenatal admission for observation makes induction more economical.] NCB clients often have no safe place to live, are substance abusers, or cannot care for themselves. For other clients, outpatient care during the latent period "may be a sensible alternative." Conservative management resulted in one-third the number of cesareans with no increase in infection rates. "[C]onservative management can be safe for both mother and infant, and . . . [if] inefficient use of neonatal intensive care units [is avoided], it can be cost effective."

Expectant Management: Induction after a Time Limit

15. Conway DI et al. Management of spontaneous rupture of the membranes in the

absence of labor in primigravid women at term. *Am J Obstet Gynecol* **1984;150(8):947-951.**

This prospective trial of management assigned 135 healthy, term primigravid women with confirmed PROM for less than 24 hours, no fever, and no contractions to be induced the morning following hospital admission. Nitrazine swabs were not used because of their high false-positive rate. Labor began spontaneously for 105 women (78%), 95% of them within 24 hours, although 60% of those were subsequently augmented. The remaining 30 women (22%) were induced, all but two within 18 hours postrupture.

Six percent of those starting labor spontaneously had cesareans versus 27% of those induced ($p < 0.01$). The cesarean rate among augmented women was 10% compared to 0% among women with completely spontaneous labors. Women who had oxytocin were also more likely to have forceps deliveries (39% versus 10%) and epidural anesthesia (65% versus 19%) compared with spontaneous labors. Eight of the 26 forceps deliveries in the augmented population were to rotate posterior babies. "[Perhaps] the high forceps rate in the augmented group (41%) reflects inefficient uterine action or perhaps our management of these patients was not aggressive enough." [The authors link epidurals to forceps, but they do not connect that induced and augmented labors are more painful and lead to epidurals and that epidurals lead to forceps and persistent posterior babies—see Chapter 13.] Although 26 women gave birth beyond 24 hours postrupture, and several vaginal and placental swabs cultured positive, only one baby cultured positive for ß-Hemolytic *Streptococcus* [same as Group B *Streptococcus*]. Penicillin was administered and no clinical infection developed. "We . . . recommend allowing up to 24 hours to elapse after spontaneous rupture of the membranes before considering induction."

16. Egan D and O'Herlihy C. Expectant management of spontaneous rupture of membranes at term. *J Obstet Gynaecol* **1988;8:243-247.**

Women with uncomplicated pregnancies and PROM at term ($N = 1285$) were managed in the following manner:

- No vaginal digital or speculum exams were done.

- Maternal and fetal heart rates and maternal temperature were monitored every four hours.

- On the morning following admission, if more than 24 hours had elapsed since rupture, induction was attempted.

- EFM and/or fetal scalp sampling were used only with symptoms of fetal distress.

- If labor was not established within six to eight hours, and there was no evidence of sepsis or distress, induction was stopped for 24 to 48 hours before trying again.

- Labor was managed according to the principles of active management [see Chapter 5].

- If unexplained fever or fetal distress developed, a cesarean section was performed unless vaginal delivery was imminent.

- Antibiotics were given to the infant only for clinical maternal or neonatal signs of infection or positive blood cultures in the baby.

Of the 88 (6.8%) women going past 24 hours, 47 began labor before the deadline, so only 41 (2.9% overall) were induced. In addition, 15 labors were augmented, two-thirds of them primiparas. Membrane rupture-to-delivery time exceeded 48 hours in 15 patients. In two of these, both primiparas, the first induction attempt failed, but the second was successful. Of the 88, four women (4.5%) had cesarean sections—two for fever during induction, two for poor progress in labor.

Vaginal cultures grew pathogens in 59 mothers (67%). Three were of Group B *Streptococcus*. Only seven women had significant fever before, during, or after labor. None had spontaneous births. Five babies had positive blood cultures and were given antibiotics. None developed clinical signs of infection. "In the absence of any obstetric intervention, spontaneous labor ensued within 24 hours in over 90 percent of patients without serious associated infectious morbidity. Expectant management for 24 to 48 hours was associated with a high rate of spontaneous delivery with oxytocin induction required in only 3 per cent of cases."

17. Cammu H, Verlaenen H, and Perde MP. Premature rupture of membranes at term in nulliparous women: a hazard? *Obstet Gynecol* **1990;76(4):671-674.**

Healthy nulliparous women with ruptured membranes for less than 24 hours, no labor, no fever, and clear amniotic fluid ($N = 105$) were matched to two controls each ($N = 210$) with respect to spontaneous, induced, or augmented labor. The controls had had membranes ruptured artificially. Induced control women had inductions either for postdates longer than 10 days or "patient comfort." PROM women had a single sterile speculum exam, nonstress test, and EFM every six hours. Labor was induced with oxytocin 24 hours after rupture or the following morning if the 24-hour interval ended at night. Internal EFM was done in conjunction with induction. Labor was augmented if 1 cm/hr progress in dilation was not made. Control group women with unfavorable cervixes who were being induced had a single dose of prostaglandin gel the night before to ripen the cervix. Labor was managed identically in both groups. Among study women, 72% began labor within 24 hours, of whom half were augmented. Assuming a 5% prevalence of perinatal infection, this study had a power of 80% for detecting a threefold increase.

No differences were found between study group and controls with respect to cervical ripeness on admission, mean number of vaginal exams (5.2 versus 5.5), cesarean rate (5.7% versus 5.2%), or epidural rate (53% versus 48%). [This would be expected because the groups were matched for oxytocin use, the key variable affecting these outcomes.] Ninety percent of cases of neonatal asphyxia and subsequent intubation were seen after oxytocin use. Asphyxia also associated with abnormal pushing phase. "Perhaps the higher incidence of epidural analgesia in the oxytocin groups played a role." Infectious morbidity correlated with oxytocin use but not prolonged rupture of membranes. All seven clinical infections occurred among induced or augmented women in the study group. Nine of the ten infections in the control group were in oxytocin-induced or augmented labors. "This study shows that expectant management of PROM at term . . . does not cause additional morbidity."

18. Grant JM et al. Management of prelabour rupture of the membranes in term primigravidae: a report of a randomized prospective trial. *Br J Obstet Gynaecol* **1992;99(7):557-562.**

This randomized trial of term primigravidas compared active (induction with oxytocin on hospital admission) (*N* = 219) versus conservative (induction the next morning, range 9-33 hr) management (*N* = 225) of PROM. Induction was not delayed longer because of the fear of infection and the belief that women would object to longer antenatal admissions. This study had the power to detect a halving of cesarean rate. All women in the conservative group were managed according to protocol, as were 93.2% of the active group. In the conservative group, 24% were induced, and a further 35% were augmented.

The cesarean rate for conservatively managed versus actively managed women was 11.1% versus 17.4% (*p* = 0.06). Estimates were made of cesarean rate when the latency period was less than 12 hours versus 12 hours or more. When less than 12 hours, cesarean rates were 14.2% in the conservative group versus 18.4% in the active group; when 12 hours or more, they were 8.0% in the conservative group versus 10.3% in the active group. Women were more likely to have epidurals in the active group (70.3% versus 57.3%, *p* < 0.005) [which suggests induced labors were more painful and which could affect cesarean rate]. There were no differences in maternal or infant indicators of infection. Maternal fever associated with epidural use but did not signal infection [but doctors might want to rule out the possibility with septic workups]. One infant in the conservative group became septic, but recovered. The optimum latent period is longer than 12 hours, but this trial cannot provide a more precise number.

19. Rydhstrom H and Ingemarsson I. No benefit from conservative management in nulliparous women with premature rupture of the membranes (PROM) at term. A randomized study. *Acta Obstet Gynecol Scand* 1991;70(7-8): 543-547.

Healthy nulliparous women with term singleton pregnancy, confirmed PROM, dilation less than 4 cm, and no contractions during a 2-hour observation period were randomly assigned to immediate induction (*N* = 139) or conservative management (in-hospital observation and monitoring, induction on the morning of the third day, range 56-80 hr; *N* = 138). Induced women were to be delivered within 24 hours. In the conservative group, 76% gave birth within 40 hours, 15% during the next 40 hours, and 9.4% remained for induction. Epidural rates were similar (35% induced versus 37% conservative). Cesarean rates were similar (2.9% induced versus 3.6% conservative). The department cesarean rate is 7% to 8%. The incidence of fever was not more likely in the conservative group. Fever in labor associated with epidural use (*p* < 0.01). Similar numbers of mothers were treated with antibiotics (four versus five women), and more induced mothers had retained placenta (7.1% versus 0.7%, *p* < 0.05). Infants were slightly more likely to be infected (clinical signs) in the conservative group (0.7% versus 4.3%, *p* < 0.05). [True, immediate induction did not increase cesareans in this population, but look how low the rates were—especially considering that these were nulliparous women. Their findings cannot be extrapolated to U.S. populations.]

Expectant Management Versus Induction with an Unfavorable Cervix

20. Duff P, Huff RW, and Gibbs RS. Management of premature rupture of membranes and unfavorable cervix in term pregnancy. *Obstet Gynecol* 1984;63(5):697-701.

Women with an unfavorable cervix (defined as effacement ≤ 80%, dilation ≤ 2 cm) were randomly assigned to expectant management (latency range 3.5-161.5 hr, *N* = 75) or induction 12 hours after rupture (*N* = 59). Failed induction was defined as failure to enter active phase after 12 hours of regular contractions. One digital vaginal exam was performed on all patients. Most of those (75%) expectantly managed entered labor within 24 hours postrupture. By 48 hours, that number had risen to 88%. Among those assigned to induction, 8.5% started labor before 12 hours. Ten percent of each group had an epidural.

The induced population had higher incidences of both intra-amniotic infection (17% versus 4%, $p < 0.05$) and cesarean section (approximately 20% versus 7%, $p < 0.05$). Seven of the 12 cesareans were for failed induction and the other five for arrest of dilation in active phase. The authors attribute the increased infection rate to the use of internal EFM, pressure catheters, and vaginal exams. The only infant with a positive blood culture was in the induction group. The mother had a cesarean for failed induction and had no intra-amniotic infection before surgery. The baby was successfully treated. One infant in the expectant management group had a scalp abcess at the internal EFM electrode attachment site. The authors critique several older articles that concluded prolonged PROM led to infections and conclude that healthy women with an unfavorable cervix may safely be managed expectantly.

21. Wagner MV et al. A comparison of early and delayed induction of labor with spontaneous rupture of membranes at term. *Obstet Gynecol* **1989;74(1):93-97.**

Women with uncomplicated pregnancies, an unfavorable cervix, PROM, and no labor were randomly assigned to either induction at six hours postrupture ($N = 86$) or 24 hours postrupture (mean time to induction 26.2 ± 4.0 hr; $N = 96$). Randomization was not blinded. Possibly as a result of selection bias, women in the delayed group were more likely to be younger and nulliparous (77% versus 64%). Some of the women had one digital vaginal exam. Of the delayed group, 38% were induced. If the interval from membrane rupture to delivery was less than 24 hours, diagnostic evaluation for sepsis in the infant was based on clinical condition. After 24 hours, blood and gastric aspirate were evaluated and [IV] antibiotics given, depending on certain findings. After 48 hours, a full septic workup including blood, urine, spinal fluid, and gastric aspirate was done, and antibiotics were given prophylactically until cultures came back negative.

Ninety percent of the early induction group gave birth within 24 hours versus 60% of the delayed group ($p < 0.001$). There were no significant differences in cesarean rates (14% early induction, 15.6% delayed induction). Since this contradicts other studies, the authors speculate that having more nulliparas in the delayed group tilted that group toward longer labors and more cesareans. However, analyzing nulliparas separately did not alter findings.

Postpartum endometritis rates were not significantly different (2.3% early induction, 8.3% delayed induction). Three mothers and three infants cultured positive for ß-Hemolytic *Streptococcus*. In one case, both mother and baby cultured positive. More infants in the delayed induction group (48% versus 8%, $p < 0.001$) had a septic workup and antibiotic therapy (15.6% versus 3.5%, $p < 0.006$). [Septic workup and antibiotic therapy were triggered by time limits, and delaying induction meant more women giving birth beyond 24 hours postrupture.] Five infants in the delayed group had infections versus none in the early group ($p < 0.06$). All five infected infants' mothers had digital vaginal exams, "a finding that must be interpreted with care because these digital examinations were not randomized." Arguing that expectant management puts infants at risk for septic evaluations and antibiotic therapy along with the pain, anxiety, and cost that entails, the authors advise against expectant management [a circular argument since their time-triggered septic workup protocol and vaginal exams caused the problems in the first place].

22. Guise JM, Duff P, and Christian JS. Management of term patients with premature rupture of membranes and an unfavorable cervix. *Am J Perinatol* 1992;9(1):56-60.

Term women with confirmed PROM and Bishop score of 4 or less were observed 2 to 36 hours before induction. (Women were not allowed a longer period because "a more extended period of observation and hospitalization is difficult to justify to third-party payers.") This protocol is a modification of Duff, Huff, and Gibbs 1984 (see Abstract 20). Outcomes were compared among spontaneous ($N = 44$), augmented ($N = 29$), and induced ($N = 39$) labors. A single digital exam was done on admission. Women having oxytocin had internal EFM.

Induced women were more likely to have epidurals: 33% versus 17% augmented and 16% spontaneous (NS). Women laboring spontaneously were less likely to have cesareans (7% versus 21% augmented and 20% induced, $p < 0.05$) or chorioamnionitis (7% versus 14% augmented and 33% induced, $p < 0.01$ for induced versus spontaneous). Septic workups were performed on fewer babies after spontaneous labor (25% versus 34.5% and 53.8%, $p < 0.05$ for induced versus spontaneous). In the induced group 5.1% had proven sepsis versus none in the other groups (NS). Optimal management of women with an unfavorable cervix remains to be defined because women who required oxytocin after an extended period with ruptured membranes were more likely to become infected and to have cesareans. [All women had a digital exam, which "starts the clock" on infection. Women having oxytocin had internal EFM but not women laboring spontaneously. Oxytocin use increased the likelihood of cesarean. Both internal monitoring and cesarean greatly increase the likelihood of infection. Note that the authors imply that waiting is the problem rather than their interventions.]

RANDOMIZED CONTROLLED TRIALS OF PROSTAGLANDIN E₂

23. Van der Walt D and Venter PF. Management of term pregnancy with premature rupture of the membranes and unripe cervix. *S Afr Med J* 1989;75(2):54-56.

Sixty women with uncomplicated pregnancies, PROM, unfavorable cervix, and no labor were randomly and evenly assigned to one of three groups: (A) expectant management, (B) oxytocin induction, and (C) intravaginal prostaglandin E₂. In group A, 75% began labor within 24 hours postrupture and 90% began labor by 48 hours.

The mean duration of labor was about six hours in both the expectant management and prostaglandin groups, whereas it was 12 hours in the oxytocin group. The epidural rate was 5% in all three groups. All six cesarean sections occurred in the oxytocin group, as did the sole case of sepsis, an infant with a positive blood culture for ß-Hemolytic *Streptococcus*. While outcomes were similar, the authors preferred prostaglandin gel to expectant management because hospitalization time is shorter. [But PROM can be managed on an outpatient basis.]

24. Chung T et al. Prelabour rupture of the membranes at term and unfavourable cervix; a randomized placebo-controlled trial on early intervention with intravaginal prostaglandin E2 gel. *Aust N Z J Obstet Gynaecol* 1992;32(1):25-27.

Women with confirmed term PROM and Bishop score of 4 or below were randomly assigned to receive either 3 mg PGE₂ (N = 30) or K-Y Jelly (N = 29) intravaginally. Expectant management was followed for the next 24 hours. Women who received PGE₂ went into labor sooner and had shorter labors, but there were no significant differences in use of oxytocin (36.7% versus 44.8%) or cesarean rate (23.3% versus 24.1%). Women were more likely to have fever in the PGE₂ group (43.3% versus 13.8% [p value not given for peripartum fever]). There was no evidence of maternal infection, and fever is a "known side-effect of prostaglandins" [which could lead doctors to suspect infection and treat mother and baby accordingly]. One case of uterine rupture occurred in a woman who was laboring with her second child in the PGE₂ group. She required a hysterectomy. No baby was infected, and other outcomes were similar. "We conclude that early intervention with . . . PGE₂ intravaginally confers no advantage compared with conservative management except for earlier confinement."

25. Mahmood TA et al. Role of prostaglandin in the management of prelabour rupture of the membranes at term. *Br J Obstet Gynaecol* 1992;99(2):112-117.

Primigravidas with confirmed term PROM were randomly assigned to either conservative management (hospital observation for 24 hours) or treatment with prostaglandin (2 mg PGE₂ followed by another 1 mg six hours later if no labor; N = 110 in each group). A single digital exam was done. All were less than 3 cm dilated on trial entry. In both groups oxytocin was given after 24 hours if labor had not begun. The study had 80% power to detect a halving of cesarean rate.

PGE₂ reduced the PROM-to-delivery interval and the need for oxytocin augmentation (31% versus 51%, $p < 0.0001$). However, the groups were similar with respect to epidural use (30% versus 29%), cesarean rate (12% versus 11%), and infant outcomes. Even among the subgroup with unfavorable cervix (score ≤ 5), cesarean rates were similar (11% versus 12%). Two women in the PGE₂ group had cesareans for fetal distress within four hours of PGE₂ insertion. Women in the conservative group were more likely to have postpartum pyrexia (4% versus 14%, $p < 0.05$) but not more likely to require antibiotics (13% versus 15%). Three babies in the conservative group and two in the PGE₂ group had positive bacteriological screens. None stayed in the neonatal ICU because of infection.

26. Ray DA and Garite TJ. Prostaglandin E₂ for induction of labor in patients with premature rupture of membranes at term. *Am J Obstet Gynecol* 1992;166(3):836-843.

Women with confirmed PROM were randomized to immediate induction (N = 55), intravaginal insertion of 3 mg PGE₂ with a second dose if necessary six hours later (N = 40), or insertion of a placebo gel (N = 45). At the end of 12 hours oxytocin was given to induce or augment labor if necessary. No digital exams were done until labor began or oxytocin was given. Internal EFM and pressure catheters were used to evaluate fetal distress or contraction strength. Infection was diagnosed by the presence of fever and/or uterine tenderness.

Women were less likely to have oxytocin with PGE₂ than placebo (37.5% versus 64.4%, $p < 0.05$). They were less likely to have cesareans (14.3% PGE₂ versus 20.7% oxytocin versus 19.0% placebo, NS) or infections (9.5% PGE₂ versus 34.5% versus 33.3%, $p < 0.05$). [Keep in mind that diagnosis was based solely on fever and tenderness. Still, these numbers are extremely high for only a 12-hour latency, which suggests that the use of internal EFM and pressure catheters played a role.] No infant became septic, although two each from the PGE$_2$ and oxytocin groups and three from the placebo group were admitted to the neonatal ICU for septic workups. "We were unable to document any improvement in outcome with 12 hours of expectant management" [probably because 12 hours is not long enough].

REFERENCES

Cooperstock M, England JE, and Wolfe RA. Circadian incidence of premature rupture of the membranes in term and preterm births. *Obstet Gynecol* 1987;69(6):936-941.

Monif GRG, Hume R, and Goodlin RC. Neonatal considerations in the management of premature rupture of the fetal membranes. *Obstet Gynecol Surv* 1986;41(9):531-537.

Perkins RP et al. Histologic chorioamnionitis in pregnancies of various gestational ages: implications in preterm rupture of membranes. *Obstet Gynecol* 1987;70(6):856-860.

Reynolds HD. Bacterial vaginosis and its implication in preterm labor and premature rupture of membranes: a review of the literature. *J Nurse Midwifery* 1991;36(5):289-296.

Russell KP and Anderson GV. The aggressive management of ruptured membranes. *Am J Obstet Gynecol* 1962;83(7):930-937.

Steer PJ, Carter MC, and Beard RW. The effect of oxytocin infusion on uterine activity level in slow labour. *Br J Obstet Gynaecol* 1985;92:1120-1126.

11

IVs Versus Eating
and Drinking in Labor

> Myth: *An IV is necessary in labor because eating and drinking are dangerous—you never know when general anesthesia might be required.*
>
> Reality: *"From the sparse data available, we conclude that [eating and drinking in labor] is generally a safe, healthy, and natural practice. . . . It would seem prudent, given the gaps in scientific information, to offer this option primarily to healthy, unmedicated women, and to restrict high-risk women to clear fluids and perhaps intravenous fluids later in labor."*
>
> McKay and Mahan 1988

The policy of forbidding food and drink in labor because general anesthesia may unexpectedly be necessary depends on these assumptions: that aspiration (vomiting and inhaling the vomitus into the lungs) is a common problem, that a policy of nothing by mouth (non per os or NPO) prevents aspiration, and that intravenous fluids are a harmless way to replace oral intake. However, none of these assumptions is correct.

The policy of forbidding food to surgery patients began in the 1940s when doctors realized that vomiting under general anesthesia and inhaling food particles into the lungs was a grave and often fatal complication of surgery. The policy was extended to laboring women, many of whom were heavily drugged during labor and had general anesthesia even for vaginal birth. On no grounds whatsoever, and despite knowing that liquids emptied rapidly from the stomach, the ban included drinking too. NPO before surgery and during labor thus became standard practice (Maltby et al. 1986, abstracted below).

Doctors devised this dictum in the days when anesthesia was given by mask. With modern practices such as intubation (putting a tube down the throat) and better training, aspiration has become a vanishingly rare event. The maternal death rate from all anesthesia causes is 5 to 6 per 1 million births (Kaunitz et al. 1985; JAMA 1986) and from aspiration alone 2.6 per 1 million births (Renfroe and Halfhill 1984; Morgan 1986). The incidence of failed intubation during cesarean section, a necessary precursor to aspiration, was 1 in 300 (0.3%) at a teaching hospital (Lyons 1985). If we assume that 16% of pregnant women will have an unplanned cesarean and 25% of those cesareans will require general anesthesia, then 4% of laboring women will have a cesarean under general anesthesia. Of this 4% of laboring women, 0.3%, or 1 in 10,000 laboring women will be difficult to intubate—which is not to say they will then aspirate. For this we are denying all laboring women food and drink.

But this is not all. The two main factors that make aspiration dangerous are volume of stomach contents of 25 ml or more and acidity (pH) of 2.5 or less. (Quantities below and pH above these levels are not generally considered to cause severe problems.) Fasting does not empty the stomach: "No time interval between the last meal and the onset of labour guarantees a stomach volume of less than 100 ml" (Johnson et al. 1989), and the residue, pure stomach juice, is highly acidic: "It is only since we began to starve our labouring patients . . . that we have experienced the epidemic of acid-aspiration syndrome" (Crawford 1984). Doctors have tried to reduce acidity with antacids, but fasting women who have had antacids have aspirated and died.

In fact, measures taken to reduce risks may actually increase them. Particulate antacids are dangerous if inhaled, and liquid antacids increase the amount of stomach contents. Glucose IVs, the replacement for oral intake, inhibit stomach emptying (Sieber et al. 1987). IVs in general, by disturbing normal fluid balance, can cause swelling that makes intubation more difficult (MacLennan 1986). Drugs to reduce stomach acid secretion are known to affect adult liver and kidney function adversely (Moir 1983, abstracted below), so clearly they could harm the far more sensitive fetus. One randomized controlled study of a "potent" antiemetic in healthy women at term undergoing elective cesarean concluded the drug did not affect the baby, yet 3 of 23 babies were excluded because they developed respiratory distress. The study did not say, but apparently all came from the medicated group (Bylsma-Howell et al. 1983).

Doris Haire (1993), a writer and commentator on maternity care issues, says, "I have searched back through 20 years of the medical literature and there is not a single documented case of aspiration in an individual [not just pregnant women] who was properly anesthetized by today's standards of anesthesia whether that person had eaten or not." Full stomachs are not the problem; the problem is the occasional incompetent anesthesiologist.

Interestingly, in Michigan from 1978 to 1984, five women died of regional anesthesia (Endler et al. 1988), but no one is suggesting limiting the number of epidurals. Narcotics slow gastric emptying and cause vomiting (Hazle 1986, abstracted below), but no one is recommending withholding them either for fear general anesthesia should be needed.

The best way to reduce the risk of aspiration is not to forbid oral intake. A much more practical and fruitful approach is to reduce the number of cesareans, minimize the number done under general anesthesia, and ensure that all anesthesiologists are properly trained and use up-to-date equipment.

Doctors are complacent about an NPO policy in labor because they mistakenly believe IV fluids to be a risk-free replacement. This ignores the misery that IVs inflict (Simkin 1986), but this issue aside, IVs are a perfect illustration of the dangers of trying to fix what is not broken. Hunger and thirst and our natural responses invoke complex feedback loops that maintain delicate chemical balances in both mother and fetus. These balances are disrupted when they are bypassed by dumping huge amounts of fluids, often over a short period of time [bolus], directly into the bloodstream. Indeed, pregnancy renders women particularly vulnerable because the physiologic changes (increased amounts of fluids in the tissues, for example) cut down on the margin for error (Lind 1983). As we shall see, complications believed to be "just one of those things" or intrinsic to pregnant women, difficult labor, or cesarean surgery can be linked to IVs.

Moreover, while the clinical symptoms that studies found were few and relatively mild, the women and babies in the studies were usually healthy and the babies mature. What might results be when that is not true? Ironically, a bolus of IV dextrose, the worst offender, has long been prescribed to remedy fetal distress (Blomstrand et al. 1984, abstracted below) or preoperatively to combat blood loss and surgical stress, but far from being a cure, it causes problems of its own. I am not suggesting that IVs are never indicated, only that they should be used carefully.

Some doctors, acknowledging that IVs cause problems, have responded by declaring that depriving women of food and drink for up to 12 hours will not do any harm. They claim ketosis, the body's metabolic response to starvation, is a "normal" occurrence in labor and no cause for alarm (Dumoulin and Foulkes 1984). A statement as illogical and unfeeling as this one can come only from someone who thinks of every laboring woman as a presurgical patient. Only a person wedded to the medical model of childbirth would be willing to dismiss the potential problems of starvation and dehydration—and the laboring woman's sufferings possibly of hunger and certainly of thirst (Simkin 1986)—rather than admit that laboring women need calories and water.

Try thinking of laboring women as athletes (Hazle 1986, abstracted below). A sports medicine physician would be horrified at the suggestion that an athlete engage in a prolonged athletic contest with no food beforehand and no nourishing drinks or even water during the event (O'Shea 1993). Yet while reams of studies have looked at nutritional requirements during heavy physical exercise, I could not find a single study on nutrition in labor. Until we require NPO and IVs for downhill skiers, boxers, basketball and football players, and drivers entering the freeway, all potentially dangerous activities where surgery might suddenly become necessary, we should not require it of laboring women. And while it may be prudent to deny high-risk women solid food, there is no rationale for denying them and likely benefit in prescribing them small, frequent sips of clear, calorie-containing liquids.

Notes: Hartmann's solution is the same as Ringer's lactate. They are electrolyte replacements.

We do not know what the normal biochemistry of laboring women and newborns is because almost universally, all control groups were kept NPO or as near to it as makes no difference, and usually they had an IV too. Exceptions are one study where fluid intake was as desired (Abstract 19) and another where amount of oral intake was unspecified (Abstract 25).

The standard recommendation of 8 glasses of water a day is 2 liters per 24-hour period. Thus, giving one liter of IV fluid in an hour or less is grossly unphysiological—even over two to three hours is excessive.

SUMMARY OF SIGNIFICANT POINTS

- Aspiration is an extremely rare event, almost always associated with substandard anesthesia practices. (Abstracts 4, 6-7, 10-11)

- Fasting does not guarantee an empty stomach. (Abstracts 1, 4-5, 12-15)

- Clear fluids are rapidly absorbed. (Abstracts 13,15)

- Drugs to control stomach acidity have risks. (Abstracts 5, 16)

- Unlike those given IVs, women allowed oral liquids maintain normal blood chemistry. (Abstracts 19, 25)

- Labor (e.g. NPO, narcotics, IVs) and surgical (e.g. IVs, positioning, fundal pressure) management increase the risk of vomiting and aspiration. (Abstracts 1, 4-7, 12-13)

- Although narcotics delay gastric emptying, water absorption may be unaffected. (Abstract 15)

- Starvation in labor causes ketosis, which associates with longer labor, oxytocin use, forceps delivery, and fetal acidosis (in animal studies). (Abstracts 1, 4, 7-9)

- Any IV can:

Cause pain and inflammation. (Abstracts 2, 17)

Cause fluid overload, which can cause pulmonary or cerebral edema. (Abstracts 1-3, 8, 18-19, 23)

Add water weight to the baby's birth weight, causing larger weight loss in the days after birth. (Since the infant is supposed to regain its birth weight by two weeks of age, this artifactual weight loss could potentially lead a doctor or mother to conclude mistakenly that breastfeeding was inadequate.) (Abstracts 1, 3, 25-26)

- Glucose/dextrose IVs cause:

  Maternal hyperglycemia (high blood sugar) at diabetic levels. (Abstracts 1-2, 20, 23-24)

  Fetal hyperglycemia, neonatal hypoglycemia (low blood sugar). (Abstracts 1-3, 5, 8, 20-21, 24)

  Maternal and fetal hyponatremia (low sodium). (Abstracts 1, 3, 5, 8, 21, 24-26, 28)

  Lactate formation, leading to lowered maternal and fetal pH and raised pCO_2 (fetal acidosis), one of the definitions of fetal distress. (Abstracts 1, 5, 8, 21, 23-24)

- Glucose/dextrose IVs may:

  Increase cases of maternal hypotension when given as a bolus before epidural anesthesia, precisely what the bolus is supposed to prevent. (Abstract 24)

  Reduce the ability of the fetal brain to withstand hypoxia (animal studies). (Abstracts 2-3, 8, 22)

- Ringer's lactate or Hartmann's solution increases lactate levels, which may be equated with fetal acidosis. (Abstracts 23-24)

- NPO plus sugar-free IVs causes maternal hypoglycemia and ketosis. (Abstracts 21, 23-24)

- Fluid overload and hyponatremia cause transient neonatal tachypnea (wet lung syndrome) and neonatal jaundice. (Abstracts 1, 3, 5, 8, 24, 27-28)

- Problems caused by IVs are amplified when large amounts of solution are given rapidly. (Abstracts 2, 8, 23-24, 28)

- Maternal complications (hypertension, cardiopulmonary problems) and medications such as those used to stop preterm labor magnify the problems of fluid overload. (Abstracts 8, 18)

ORGANIZATION OF ABSTRACTS

Literature Reviews

Risk of NPO: Ketosis

Risk of Aspiration

Fasting Does Not Guarantee an Empty Stomach
Drugs to Raise pH and Reduce Stomach Contents Have Risks

Risks of IVs

Pain and Inflammation
Fluid Overload (IVs in General)
Hyper- and Hypoglycemia (Dextrose IVs)
Hyponatremia (Salt-Free IVs)

LITERATURE REVIEWS

1. Hazle NR. Hydration in labor: is routine intravenous hydration necessary? *J Nurse Midwifery* **1986;31(4):171-176.**

We do not know whether ketosis causes problems, although ketonuria [ketones in the urine] associates with prolonged labor. However, curing it with IV-dextrose causes maternal and fetal hyperglycemia, followed by rebound neonatal hypoglycemia. IV-dextrose also causes neonatal hyponatremia and jaundice and increases neonatal weight loss. Metabolizing glucose lowers fetal blood pH, which may cause or worsen fetal acidosis, a symptom of fetal distress. Fluid overload also causes pulmonary edema.

As for the risk of aspirating oral fluids, prolonged fasting does not guarantee small stomach volumes, and the residue is highly acidic. Delayed gastric emptying, believed intrinsic to labor, actually results from narcotic use. Moreover, both narcotics and starvation before heavy physical effort may cause vomiting.

"For years women in labor have been treated, monitored, and studied as if their unique condition were comparable with a passive surgical patient. Perhaps a laboring woman more closely resembles an athlete." Marking the many physiologic similarities, it is noted that for long athletic competitions, "optimum performance . . . depends on good nutrition, good hydration, and periodic carbohydrate intake." Therefore, women should be encouraged to load carbohydrates in early labor and to drink at least 4 oz of fluid that contains calories and electrolytes per hour—more if diarrhea is present [or she is leaking amniotic fluid]. If an IV is required, care should be taken with the amount of fluid and the use of dextrose.

2. Newton N, Newton M, and Broach J. Psychologic, physical, nutritional, and technologic aspects of intravenous infusion during labor. *Birth* **1988;15(2):67-72.**
The following points are made:

- IVs increase pain in labor. The insertion is painful, pain at the site may develop, and a glucose infusion has been shown to lower pain threshold.

- IVs adversely affect how staff see laboring women. They signal that she is "sick," and make it all too easy to give medications without "thinking twice."

- The amount of extra stress from partial immobility is unknown but clearly exists. Inhibiting mobility affects labor length. IVs also make holding and breast-feeding the newborn awkward.

- Phlebitis [vein inflammation] frequently occurs.

- IVs can be a means of fluid overdose. Double or more the ordered amounts are commonly given. Also, boluses are given prior to an epidural or as a way of "doing something" for fetal heart rate abnormalities.

- Little is known about nutritional requirements in labor, but IVs are inadequate.

- Typical IV glucose solutions cause diabetic levels of hyperglycemia, which triggers feelings of being tired and ill and may slow labor. It also causes neonatal hypoglycemia. Hyperglycemia may be dangerous. Unfed monkeys survived anoxia without brain injury; those fed or given glucose infusions were damaged or died.

3. Keppler AB. The uses of intravenous fluids during labor. *Birth* **1988;15(2):75-79.**
A healthy woman at term has at least two extra liters of water stored in her tissues. Infusing large volumes of IV fluids to combat dehydration, especially when salt free, may cause hyponatremia (water intoxication) leading to weight gain, vomiting, convulsions, pulmonary edema, oligouria [deficient urine output], and transient neonatal tachypnea [rapid breathing]. "Women who have uncomplicated labor and who have quenched their thirst with clear fluids and ice chips probably do not need intravenous fluids."

Ketosis is common in pregnancy, and mild ketonuria in labor may be normal. Giving IV glucose to cure it reduces the brain's tolerance for asphyxia and causes neonatal hypoglycemia. Giving salt-free fluids causes hyponatremia, resulting in a transfer of water weight to the fetus. This artifactual weight increase may be important because infants are expected to regain their birth weight by two weeks. Because of its antidiuretic effect, giving oxytocin may worsen these problems, especially when infusion amount exceeds one liter. "[T]he administration of intravenous fluids to laboring women in an effort to treat ketosis or dehydration is a questionable practice. . . . Inappropriate use of intravenous fluids results in some undesirable outcomes for both mother and infant."

4. Broach J and Newton N. Food and beverages in labor. Part II: the effects of cessation of oral intake during labor. *Birth* **1988;15(2):89-92.**
Problems with data collection make it hard to get a clear picture of aspiration-related maternal death, but aspiration causes only about 0.35% to 2.75% of all maternal deaths. Eating and drinking in labor are not always factors, but faulty anesthesia administration

almost always is. The belief that gastric emptying is prolonged in labor is pivotal to NPO policies, but in the absence of narcotic use, gastric emptying is not delayed. Moreover, gastric volume increases after 16 to 20 hours of fasting.

The physiologic effects of fasting in labor are unknown, but ketonuria is common and associates with long labor and forceps delivery. Blood studies done during a 24-hour religious fast concluded that the changes could impair blood supply to vital organs in cases of vascular insufficiency, which has implications for pregnant women with placental insufficiency. Moreover, hunger, thirst, and IVs are stressful. Eating and drinking would allow the woman to retain control of her routine, possibly reduce anxiety, and avoid discomfort. "Regarding all laboring women as surgical patients reinforces the tendency to view birth as pathologic. It might be beneficial to regard the birth process otherwise."

5. McKay S and Mahan C. Modifying the stomach contents of laboring women: why and how; success and risks. *Birth* **1988;15(4):213-221.**
The following points are made:

- Gastric emptying is not delayed in labor.

- Analgesics delay gastric emptying.

- Aspiration is virtually nonexistent in Holland and Japan, where eating and drinking in labor are normal, but analgesia is rare.

- Other drugs, especially when combined with large IV fluid loads, may provoke aspiration or aggravate its effects by contributing to pulmonary edema. These include oxytocin, opiates, ergometrine, and drugs used to stop preterm labor.

- Fasting does not empty the stomach and leaves a highly acidic residue. "For laboring women (or anyone else), an empty stomach does not seem in accord with nature's plan; regardless of the kind of intervention attempted or NPO status."

- Stomach pumping and emetics do not guarantee safe volumes, nor does an antiemetic (metoclopramide). Metoclopramide crosses the placenta.

- Antacids and H_2 receptor antagonists (H_2 receptor antagonists reduce stomach acid secretion) have not proved effective at reducing aspiration risks and may introduce problems. With oral antacids, particulate antacids can be aspirated; antacids increase gastric volume; acid rebound may occur. H_2 receptor antagonists do not affect acid already present, have adverse side effects, and cross the placenta. The literature has ignored the neutralizing effect of food and drink and the contradiction between NPO and antacids, which increase stomach volume.

- IV fluids cause iatrogenic problems, including fetal and neonatal hyperglycemia and neonatal hypoglycemia, hyponatremia, and jaundice; falls in fetal blood pH and rises in lactate [fetal acidosis]; maternal hyponatremia; adverse behavioral changes; and slowing of labor.

- Moderate ketosis appears to be harmless. "What is infrequently acknowledged is that ketosis may develop because of the practice of starving women. . . . It is remarkable that studies of the nutritional needs of laboring women are virtually nonexistent, although such research has been done in exercise physiology to understand optimal human nutrition patterns under conditions of hard work."

6. McKay S and Mahan C. How can aspiration of vomitus in obstetrics best be prevented? *Birth* 1988;15(4):223-229.

The authors surveyed institutional policies on eating and drinking in labor ($N = 217$) and found that 47% of hospitals limited women to NPO or ice chips only. Many of the others placed restrictions on oral intake. Statements such as, "It is better to want food than to inhale it" or "You're caving in to consumerism and courting disaster," were made. Others cited the need to placate anesthesiologists. "[I]t is poor science to base practice on anecdotal reports and threats to withdraw anesthesiology services."

Aspiration-related deaths are rare. Factors contributing to pregnant women's aspirating are supine or Trendelenburg [delivery table tilted head down] position, fundal pressure, certain drugs, the rising cesarean rate, general anesthesia for cesareans, difficult or failed intubation, and lack of availability of obstetric anesthesiologists.

> [W]e question whether parturients should be kept from eating and drinking or on restricted liquid intake to protect them from what appears to be . . . inadequate anesthesia practices. Implementing NPO policies based on inadequate scientific rationale . . . may not only contribute to maternal discomfort and physiologic imbalance, but distract clinicians from . . . addressing other more important antecedents of aspiration.

7. Elkington KW. At the water's edge: where obstetrics and anesthesia meet. *Obstet Gynecol* 1991;77(2):304-308.

Although often stated as being a major cause of maternal mortality, aspiration is actually a rare cause of death. No data demonstrate that risk-reduction methods work and a large study of freestanding birth centers reported no aspiration-related morbidity despite unrestrictive policies. "[Restrictive] policies may persist on the basis of anecdotal experience, institutional inertia to change policies begun in the 1940s, compromise with anesthesia department policy to ensure adequate coverage, exaggerated notions of risk, or fears of litigation." Preoperative fasting does not ensure low gastric volume. Factors predisposing to aspiration include increased acidity due to dehydration and ketosis, narcotics, lithotomy position, fundal pressure, and upper airway edema. [I selected iatrogenic factors from Elkington's list.] Improperly administered anesthesia, especially difficult intubation, causes most morbidity and mortality. Risks can be minimized by using regional anesthesia, having well-trained personnel, reducing cesarean rates, and giving antacids before surgery. "Restrictive oral intake policies cannot substitute for any of these. . . . At the very least, institutions favoring restrictions should allow parturients some choice after fairly representing the extremely low risk involved and the lack of data implicating oral intake as a risk factor."

8. Wasserstrum N. Issues in fluid management during labor: general considerations. *Clin Obstet Gynecol* 1992;35(3):505-513.

"[E]ven for the normal term fetus of an uncomplicated pregnancy, with its tolerance for our misadventures, we must try to optimize physiologic conditions. Appropriate fluid management contributes to this optimization." Osmotic effects depend on the type of dissolved particles. Particles that can be metabolized (dextrose) exert no effect ("free water"), while those containing ions or crystalloids (saline [also Ringer's lactate]) do. The effects of saline versus dextrose IVs are compared: saline increases extracellular volume, thereby increasing plasma volume and causing a fall in hematocrit [could this cause problems with clotting?] and an increase in pulmonary capillary hydrostatic pressure, which causes pulmonary edema. Saline contains sodium, so sodium levels are unaffected. Free water distributes both extra- and intracellularly. Therefore, dextrose IVs cause neither pulmonary edema nor a fall in hematocrit. However, because they are sodium free, they cause hyponatremia complicated by tachypnea and jaundice in the child. Bolus administration and oxytocin induction with dextrose IVs increase the risk. Both saline and dextrose IVs swell total fluid volume. This can cause a rise in intracranial pressure "with potentially disastrous consequences" because the adult cranium cannot expand. The risks of free water increase "markedly" with complications such as hypertension.

Because oral intake is commonly proscribed during labor, glucose must be prescribed or ketonemia will "inevitably" develop. Animal studies show that fetal hyperketonemia causes fetal acidosis and that maternal ketones cross the placenta, causing fetal acidosis. However, infusing glucose increases acidosis and increases fetal brain injury when there is hypoxia. Glucose infusions also associate with neonatal hypoglycemia and jaundice. Therefore, glucose should be infused, although it is difficult to recommend rates because of the many variables, and bolus administration should be avoided. [The biases of the medical model blind him to seeing that the obvious solution to the drawbacks of IVs is oral intake.]

RISK OF NPO: KETOSIS

9. Foulkes J and Dumoulin JG. The effects of ketonuria in labour. *Br J Clin Pract* 1985;39:59-62.

When glycogen stores are depleted, the liver metabolizes fat, giving rise to ketone bodies, which are normally oxidized by peripheral tissues. Under more severe conditions (e.g. diabetes mellitus, starvation [!], and excessive exercise [!]), peripheral metabolisis cannot cope, and ketosis occurs. Ketones cross the placenta. Pregnant women are "extremely" susceptible to ketosis.

In this study of 3511 laboring women (kept NPO), the overall incidence of ketosis was 40%, with incidence doubling and trebling as labor lengthened. Ketosis associated with primiparity, augmentation of labor, forceps delivery, and high postpartum blood loss. Examining interrelationships, ketosis associated independently with labor length, induced labors, augmented labors, and forceps. [But does ketosis cause long labors, or do long labors cause ketosis?] Since large quantities of IV-glucose can cause complications, care must be taken to provide physiologic quantities of IV fluids, alternating Hartmann's and 5% dextrose. [As in Abstract 8, the authors do not suggest abandoning NPO.]

RISK OF ASPIRATION

10. Olsson GL, Hallen B, and Hambraeus-Jonzon K. Aspiration during anaesthesia: a computer-aided study of 185,358 anaesthetics. *Acta Anaesth Scand* 1986;30:84-92.

An examination of the records found 87 cases of aspiration among 185,358 surgeries (4.7/10,000). In 15 cases there were no predisposing factors. Four patients died

(0.2/10,000). Four aspirations occurred during c-sections (15/10,000), of which none was fatal. These rates are of the same magnitude generally reported in the literature. The greatest risk was among emergency cases anesthetized late at night by an inexperienced anesthetist. Prognosis after aspiration was not "excessively poor" if the patient was in good general health.

11. Stephens ID. ICU admissions from an obstetrical hospital. *Can J Anaesth* **1991;38(5):677-681.**
All obstetric admissions to the intensive care unit (ICU) from 1979 to 1989 were identified. Of the 118 patients admitted, 16 were for complications of anesthesia, of which 12 were of general anesthesia and four of regional anesthesia. Only one was for suspected aspiration, but this turned out not to be the case. The number of general anesthetics given was 7452. The proportion of general to regional anesthesias for cesarean decreased from 85% in 1979 to 44% in 1989.

Fasting Does Not Guarantee An Empty Stomach

12. Miller M, Wishart HY, and Nimmo WS. Gastric contents at induction of anaesthesia. Is a 4-hour fast necessary? *Br J Anaesth* **1983;55:1185-1187.**
[Nonpregnant] women having gynecological surgery were randomly allocated to fasting overnight ($N = 22$) or having one slice of buttered toast and one cup of tea or coffee with milk between 5 A.M. and 7 A.M. ($N = 23$). Some were given narcotic and some nonnarcotic premedication. Stomach volumes were similar among all groups. Two women each in the fed and unfed groups had volumes over 40 ml. No significant differences were found for pH below 3. The shortest interval between feeding and anesthesia induction was 105 minutes, after which 5 ml of fluid was found. In only one patient was breakfast residue found. Two patients yielded bits of undigested premedication tablets.

13. Maltby JR et al. Preoperative oral fluids: is a five-hour fast justified prior to elective surgery? *Anesth Analg* **1986;65:1112-1116.**
Women having first trimester abortions fasted overnight. [In addition to water versus no water, this study also tested a stomach acid antagonist versus placebo. I report only the placebo groups.] Two to three hours before surgery all were given a dye in 10 ml of water, and half, 35 per group, were randomly assigned to receive 150 ml of water. No preoperative sedatives or narcotics were given.

Women who had water had significantly less gastric volume than those having no water (17.6 ± 14.5 ml versus 26.7 ± 18.9 ml, $p < 0.02$). The pH was similar (1.75 ± 0.94 versus 1.92 ± 1.27). No dye could be found, which means all preoperative oral fluid had passed through. The severity of thirst, but not hunger, was reduced in those given water.

The scientific basis for withholding clear fluids before surgery is unclear. Both saline and glucose water empty rapidly unless very concentrated. Opiates are "potent antagonists of gastric emptying," and their role in premedication should be evaluated. "We conclude that prolonged withholding of oral fluid does not improve the gastric volume and pH and may indeed worsen them." Giving water also increases patient comfort.

14. Lewis M and Crawford JS. Can one risk fasting the obstetric patient for less than 4 hours? *Br J Anaesth* **1987;59:312-314.**

Forty women having an elective cesarean fasted overnight. Half were offered a breakfast of tea and toast; all drank the tea, and 11 ate the toast. All were given an oral antacid. The interval between ingestion and anesthesia induction was 216 ± 21 min for those having tea only and 159 ± 53 min for those having toast too. The fasted group had an aspiration volume of 33.2 ± 22.0 ml versus 64.5 ± 21.5 ml in those having tea only and 73.4 ± 52.7 ml in those having toast too. The pH was high [less acidic] in all groups. Two women had "recognizable particles of toast." "Despite the fact that no harm came to any of these patients, the normal overnight fast was resumed at this hospital." [Note that most of the women, fed or not, had aspirate volumes exceeding the 25-ml danger point.]

15. Agarwal A, Chari P, and Singh H. Fluid deprivation before operation: the effect of a small drink. *Anaesthesia* **1989;44:632-634.**

Elective surgical patients (excluding pregnant women) were divided into three groups ($N = 50$ in each group): (1) continued overnight fast, (2) had 150 ml water 152 minutes before surgery, and (3) had 150 ml water plus preoperative injection of narcotic. Those having water had significantly less gastric volume than those fasting (29.9 ± 18.2 ml versus 20.6 ± 14.1 ml and 22.3 ± 10.5 ml, $p < 0.05$). Amounts were similar whether or not morphine was given. [Narcotics do not affect water absorption.] More people had gastric volumes above 25 ml in the fasted group. The pHs were slightly higher [less acidic] among those given water, but the difference was insignificant (1.85 ± 1.26 versus 2.05 ± 1.41 and 2.06 ± 1.34). Significantly more people who had a drink felt less thirsty and hungry ($p < 0.05$).

Drugs to Raise pH and Reduce Stomach Contents Have Risks

16. Moir DD. Cimetidine, antacids, and pulmonary aspiration. *Anesthesiol* **1983;59(2):81-83.**

Oral antacids, usually magnesium trisilicate, had been given to 12 of 18 women who died of aspiration. Some possible reasons for death are narcotic analgesia, which promotes high stomach volume by delaying emptying, and inhalation of particulate antacid. Alkali can be as damaging to the lungs as acid. Clear antacids (sodium citrate) are probably safer, but studies indicate that 20 to 30 ml are needed to be effective [thus raising volume past the 25 ml danger point]. Antacids are needed because 43% of laboring women have a pH less than 2.5 [probably because they have been kept NPO].

H_2 receptor antagonists (cimetidine and ranitidine) inhibit gastric acid secretion but have no effect on acid already present. Biochemical disturbances and adverse effects on liver and kidney function have been reported with cimetidine. Cimetidine crosses the placenta freely, although studies have not found an adverse effect on Apgars or neurobehavioral tests [but they did not test for biochemical, hepatic, and renal effects]. Intravenous injections may cause mild to severe cardiac problems.

The author recommends oral and intramuscular injection of cimetidine before planned cesarean and sodium citrate before emergency cesarean despite stating: "There is, as yet, no hard evidence that the use of antacids or cimetidine reduces maternal anesthetic mortality from pulmonary aspiration."

RISKS OF IVs

Pain and Inflammation

17. Jones JJ and Koldjeski D. Clinical indicators of a developmental process in phlebitis. *NITA* 1984;7:279-285.

The infusion of intravenous fluids . . . tends to be viewed as a commonplace routine by nurses; however, it is not considered to be routine by patients who experience both psychological and physiological effects of I.V. therapy and some of these may linger long after discharge from the hospital.

Phlebitis is an inflammatory response in the vein walls to the injury of being pierced by a needle. Patients ($N = 23$) were observed at 8-hour intervals. Within the first eight hours, 14% of subjects had clinical signs of phlebitis, increasing to 57% by the sixteenth hour. Overall, 61% of subjects developed phlebitis. Of those who did, 14% had tenderness at the site by eight hours, about 42% by 16 hours, and over 50% by 24 hours. Induration [hardening of the surrounding tissue from infiltration of IV fluid] developed in 35% of those who developed phlebitis. [Induration causes a painful, long-lasting bruise.]

Fluid Overload (IVs in General)

Note: Colloid osmotic pressure is a measure of the factors keeping fluid from leaking out of capillaries into tissues.

18. Cotton DB et al. Intrapartum to postpartum changes in colloid osmotic pressure. *Am J Obstet Gynecol* 1984;149(2):174-177.

Healthy women at term ($N = 72$) were ordered to receive IV crystalloids at 125 to 150 ml/hr. [Crystalloids are any nonprotein solutes including glucose, salt, or those found in Ringer's lactate.] Half had vaginal births and half cesarean deliveries. Overall, the mean colloid pressure declined from 21.0 ± 2.1 mm Hg in labor to 15.4 ± 1.9 mm Hg after birth. Although the mean value for those having cesareans was similar to those having vaginal births, of the 15 women who had a postpartum value of 13.6 or less (21%), 10 had cesareans. Five women (6.9%), two with cesareans, had values below 12.5 mm Hg. No women had clinical symptoms, but pulmonary edema occurs at pressures below 16.0 mm Hg and deaths have occurred among gravely ill patients at values below 12.6 mm Hg.

Despite orders, women received fluid at rates averaging more than twice that ordered, with those having cesareans receiving two and a half to more than three times as much. "Aggressive crystalloid therapy" may explain why 50% of chest X rays in postpartum women show pulmonary effusions. Care should be taken especially with women already at risk: those with known cardiopulmonary complications or hypertension or those taking drugs to stop preterm labor.

19. Gonik B and Cotton DB. Peripartum colloid osmotic pressure changes: influence of intravenous hydration. *Am J Obstet Gynecol* 1984;150(1):99-100.

Sixteen women with routine vaginal deliveries with orders for IV fluids at a rate of 125 to 150 ml/hr were compared with 12 similar women in the birthing suite who had no IV and were allowed to drink clear liquids. Mean intrapartum colloid pressures were similar (21.8 ± 2.0 mm Hg versus 21.9 ± 2.3 mm Hg), but postpartum values were higher among birthing suite women (16.4 ± 2.2 mm Hg versus 19.2 ± 2.1 mm Hg, $p < 0.001$) No birth room woman had values below 15.6 mm Hg versus five in the IV group. [Where drinking was allowed, pressure values remained normal, and the drop in postpartum colloid pressure, believed intrinsic to labor, did not occur.]

The IV group received fluids at more than twice the rate ordered. Women with colloid pressures < 15.6 mm Hg are "dangerously close" to levels causing pulmonary edema, which calls into question "aggressive hydration" for fetal distress. "The data presented here do not negate the routine use of intravenous fluids in the laboring patient. Conversely, they point out the resilience of the pregnant women's cardiovascular and renal systems when confronted with iatrogenic stresses." [To this Hazle, Abstract 1, trenchantly responds, "'The resilience' of the pregnant woman does not justify the risk of fluid overload."]

Hyper- and Hypoglycemia (Dextrose IVs)

Note: Maternal glucose values over 180 mg/dl are *highly* abnormal; 200 mg/dl is the cutoff for insulin-dependent diabetes. Babies become hypoglycemic because they respond to high glucose level by pouring out insulin. After birth the excess insulin causes their glucose levels to fall precipitously.

20. Mendiola J, Grylack LJ, and Scanlon JW. Effects of intrapartum maternal glucose infusion on the normal fetus and newborn. *Anesth Analg* 1982;61(1):32-35.

Healthy term women ($N = 56$) were studied, of whom 14 had elective cesareans. All mothers received IV glucose in accordance with standard practice. Newborns fed before four hours (except for low blood glucose) were excluded. A Dextrostix reading below 45 mg/100 ml was considered abnormal.

Maternal blood glucose at delivery had a median of 110 mg/dl (range 68-230 mg/dl). Six babies (11%) were hypoglycemic at one hour old, and low blood glucose correlated ($p < 0.05$) with maternal blood glucose of 120 mg/dl or above and glucose infusion of 20 g/hr or above. Maternal glucose load should be monitored, and babies whose mothers received excess glucose should be monitored for hypoglycemia for the first two hours. [This means the baby will have one or more painful heel sticks and possibly be fed sugar water or formula from a bottle, which can interfere with establishing breastfeeding.]

21. Grylack LJ, Chu SS, and Scanlon JW. Use of intravenous fluids before cesarean section: effects on perinatal glucose, insulin and sodium homeostasis. *Obstet Gynecol* 1984;63(5):654-658.

Healthy term women undergoing elective cesarean were randomly allocated to three groups, all receiving 1 liter IV fluid before surgery: (A) Ringer's lactate ($N = 20$) in one hour, (B) 5% dextrose ($N = 20$) in one hour, and (C) 5% dextrose ($N = 19$) in 2½ hours.

Neonatal hypoglycemia was defined as 30 mg/dl or less of glucose and hyponatremia as 130 mEq/l or less of sodium.

Mean maternal serum glucose at delivery differed among all three groups (A): 70.3 ± 13.7 mg/dl, (B): 234.4 ± 74.6 mg/dl, (C): 154.4 ± 59.4 mg/dl ($p < 0.001$). Umbilical cord blood glucose and insulin values corresponded with maternal glucose. No infants were hypoglycemic in group A versus three in group B and four in group C (A compared with B and C, $p < 0.05$). Maternal hyponatremia at delivery was found in none of 19 women in group A versus 2 of 17 in group B and 1 of 17 in group C. Neonatal hyponatremia was found in 1 of 19 babies in group A versus 9 of 17 in group B and 7 of 17 in group C ($p < 0.05$). Since hyperglycemia increases the production of lactic acid, fetal hyperglycemia could exacerbate fetal acidosis. While hyperglycemia and hyponatremia are hazardous, so is maternal hypoglycemia. Four women in group A had glucose levels of 40 to 60 mg/dl. [This has implications for laboring women too.]

22. Blomstrand S et al. Does glucose administration affect the cerebral response to fetal asphyxia? *Acta Obstet Gynecol Scand* **1984;63:345-353.**

This study of ewes and their fetuses showed that high fetal blood glucose decreased the ability of the fetal brain to withstand hypoxia. Administering extra glucose to an asphyxiated fetus, far from being beneficial, did harm by aggravating lactacidosis [acidosis due to lactic acid formation]. These results agree with other studies in monkeys and rats. Both showed that hyperglycemic, hypoxic animals produced more lactic acid in the brain than controls.

23. Morton KE, Jackson MC, and Gillmer MDG. A comparison of the effects of four intravenous solutions for the treatment of ketonuria during labor. *Br J Obstet Gynaecol* **1985;92:473-479.**

This study randomly allocated 40 healthy, term laboring women to receive one liter in one hour of normal saline, Hartmann's, 5% dextrose, or 10% dextrose ($N = 10$ per group). Blood samples were taken at 30, 60, and 90 minutes.

Both 5% and 10% dextrose produced a rapid fall in ketones compared with the nonglucose groups ($p < 0.0001$), but IV dextrose produced rises in glucose concentration to 16.2 mmol/l and 24.3 mmol/l respectively, at 60 min. [The authors dismiss concerns about ketosis in the introduction. If you have decided you cannot cure the problem, simply deny it is a problem.] Lactate concentration also rose, with levels continuing to rise after completion of the infusion. Hartmann's also produced a significant rise, although not as high as dextrose. [Hartmann's contains lactate.] Serum osmolality [osmotic pressure] was within normal range for all subjects at the beginning but rose significantly ($p < 0.001$) with 10% dextrose and fell in all other cases. With Hartmann's, values continued to decline after infusion had stopped. "It is concluded that rapid infusions of dextrose or Hartmann's should not be administered during labour."

24. Philipson EH et al. Effects of maternal glucose infusion on fetal acid-base status in human pregnancy. *Am J Obstet Gynecol* **1987;157(4 Pt 1):866-873.**

Healthy term women having elective cesareans under epidural anesthesia were randomly allocated to receive one liter given over 20 to 30 minutes of 5% dextrose (group 1, $N = 12$), Ringer's lactate (group 2, $N = 11$), or saline (group 3, $N = 9$). After this, normal saline was given at 125 ml/hr.

Dextrose caused a rapid rise in maternal serum glucose, reaching a peak of 225 ± 66 mg/dl at 20 minutes and slowly declining thereafter. [Ignored are hypoglycemic levels in women not receiving dextrose.] Glucose levels were elevated in umbilical cord blood in group 1 ($p < 0.001$), and by two hours after birth, neonatal glucose was significantly lower ($p < 0.01$). Four babies in group 1 developed hypoglycemia (defined as < 25 mg/dl), as did two in group 2 versus none in group 3. One infant in group 1 had meconium below the vocal cords, and another, with a glucose level of 18 mg/dl, developed tachypnea. Maternal and cord blood insulin levels were elevated in group 1. Maternal lactate levels rose in groups 1 and 2 compared with group 3 ($p < 0.01$). Lactate levels continued to increase after the infusion ended in group 1 but declined rapidly to normal in group 2. Lactate was elevated in group 1 infants at 30 minutes after birth compared with groups 2 and 3 ($p < 0.004$). [Not discussed is that lactate in group 2 was elevated in cord blood, although not as high as in group 1 babies.] Umbilical artery pH was lower in group 1 (7.21 ± 0.06) and pCO_2 was higher ($p < 0.05$). [Other studies (see Chapter 7) have called pHs this low "acidotic."] Maternal serum sodium was lower in group 1 compared with groups 2 and 3 ($p < 0.01$). Six women developed hypotension [a side effect of epidurals that the IV bolus is supposed to prevent] in group 1 versus two in group 2 and one in group 3. Hypotensive women had lower pH ($p < 0.05$). Umbilical artery pHs were also lower in their babies ($p < 0.02$). [IV-dextrose appears to be counterproductive.] At delivery there were fewer ketones in both maternal ($p < 0.001$) and umbilical arterial ($p < 0.04$) blood. Ketones rose over time in groups 2 and 3. "In summary, short-term maternal administration of glucose before delivery is associated with fetal hyperglycemia, hyperinsulinemia, an increase in lactic acid, and a significant decrease in pH." [And Ringer's is not problem-free either.]

Hyponatremia (Salt-Free IVs)

25. Dahlenburg GW, Burnell RH, and Braybrook R. The relation between cord serum sodium levels in newborn infants and maternal intravenous therapy during labour. *Br J Obstet Gynaecol* 1980;87:519-522.

This study used data from a survey determining normal ranges of serum electrolytes in umbilical cord venous blood taken from term infants of uncomplicated pregnancies. The correlations between electrolyte values and IV fluids in labor were examined. Of the 203 mothers, 106 had IV fluids (5% dextrose) and 97 had oral fluids. Sodium (Na) levels were lower in the IV group (133 ± 4.2 mmol/l versus 138 ± 4.3 mmol/l, $p < 0.001$), and 29 babies had cord serum values of 130 mmol or less [hyponatremia], of whom 26 were in the IV group. Neonatal weight loss was greater in the IV group (6.17 ± 3.36% versus 4.07 ± 2.20%, $p < 0.01$). Six infants (6.7%), all with cord sodium values of 129 mmol/l, had symptoms possibly attributable to hyponatremia: poor feeding (six); pale, floppy, poor suck (one), bradycardia, or seizure of unknown cause (one). "When hyponatremia is induced in the mother there must be a net transfer of water to the fetus and/or Na to the mother (probably both) and this can occur in a very short time."

26. Tarnow-Mordi WO et al. Iatrogenic hyponatraemia of the newborn due to maternal fluid overload: a prospective study. *Br Med J* 1981;283:639-642.

The study was undertaken after observing unexplained large weight losses in healthy, term newborns. All laboring women were eligible. IVs were 5% and/or 10% glucose or glucose plus Hartmann's. There were five groups: (1) oral fluids only (14 ± 4 ml/hr [effectively NPO], $N = 41$), (2) IV only ($N = 19$), (3) IV plus oxytocin ($N = 24$), (4) IV plus epidural ($N = 15$), and (5) IV plus oxytocin plus epidural ($N = 37$).

In the oral group, 24 of 41 infants had cord plasma sodium values from 136 to 145 mmol/l. Only 14 of the 95 in the IV group had sodium values in this range, 16 were 130 mmol/l or less, and six were 125 mmol/l or less. Sodium levels bore an inverse relation with rate of maternal IV fluid administration ($p < 0.001$). The mean infusion rate for women in group 4 was 195 ml/hr, or a daily amount of 4.7 liters. The maximum neonatal weight loss in group 1 was 3.6 ± 0.2% versus 5.5 ± 0.4% in group 2, 5.4 ± 0.4% in group 3, and 6.4 ± 0.5% in group 4.

27. Singhi S, Choo Kang E, and Hall J. Hazards of maternal hydration with 5% dextrose. *Lancet* 1982;2:335-336.

Forty-three mothers given 5% or 10% dextrose were compared with 51 who had no IV. After excluding premature babies, known blood group incompatibility, congenital malformations, septicemia, and growth retardation, jaundice (serum bilirubin ≥ 85 µmol/l) was more common in babies in the IV group (33% versus 11%, $p < 0.05$) as was hyperbilirubinemia (serum bilirubin ≥ 170 µmol/l) (15% versus 4%, $p < 0.05$). Mean cord serum sodium was lower among jaundiced babies in both study and control groups ($p < 0.01$). Hypo-osmolal plasma causes an inflow of water across the red cell membrane, with consequent swelling and increased fragility. The increased breakdown rate leads to higher bilirubin levels.

28. Singhi SC and Chookang E. Maternal fluid overload during labour; transplacental hyponatraemia and risk of transient neonatal tachypnoea in term infants. *Arch Dis Child* 1984;59:1155-1158.

In this nonrandomized study, the study group ($N = 186$) had glucose IVs and the control group ($N = 107$) was allowed "sips of water." Transient neonatal tachypnea (wet lung syndrome) was defined as respiration 60 breaths per minute or more for more than 3 hrs, minimal grunting and retraction, need for oxygen, spontaneous improvement within 24 hours, and suggestive X-ray findings. [Aside from concerns about the baby's health, treatment would interfere with bonding and breastfeeding.] Exclusions were sepsis, congenital heart disease, pneumonia, meconium aspiration, preterm birth, or low birth weight.

Hyponatremia (cord serum sodium ≤ 130 mmol/l) was seen in 39% of study infants versus 6% of controls ($p < 0.01$). Transient tachypnea was seen in 15% of hyponatremic infants versus 3% of normonatremic study infants and 3% of the control group ($p < 0.005$). Serum sodium values and amount of IV fluid given were negatively correlated ($p < 0.0001$), as was amount given and cord serum osmolality ($p < 0.025$). Normally fluid rapidly reabsorbs from the lungs after birth. Lowered plasma osmotic pressure would delay in this process and is the probable cause of transient neonatal tachypnea. In addition, adrenalin-induced reabsorption uses a sodium pump, and hyponatremia could impair this mechanism. Giving a preoperative bolus of IV fluid may be one reason why more cesarean-born babies develop neonatal tachypnea.

REFERENCES

Bylsma-Howell M. et al. Placental transport of metoclopramide: assessment of maternal and neonatal effects. *Can Anaesth Soc J* 1983;30(5):487-492.

Crawford JS. The pre-anaesthesia fasting period. *Br J Anaesth* 1984;56:925-926.

Dumoulin JG and Foulkes JEB. Ketonuria during labour. *Br J Obstet Gynaecol* 1984;91:97-98.

Endler GC et al. Anesthesia-related maternal mortality in Michigan, 1972 to 1984. *Am J Obstet Gynecol* 1988;159(1):187-193.

Haire D. Personal communication, Feb 18, 1993.

JAMA. Maternal mortality: pilot surveillance in seven states. *JAMA* 1986;255(2):184-185.

Johnson C et al. Nutrition and position in labour. In *A guide to effective care in pregnancy and chilbirth*. Enkin M, Keirse MJNC, and Chalmers I, eds. Oxford: Oxford University Press, 1989.

Kaunitz AM et al. Causes of maternal mortality in the United States. *Obstet Gynecol* 1985;65(5):605-612.

Lind T. Fluid balance during labour: a review. *J Royal Soc Med* 1983;76:870-875.

Lyons G. Failed intubation. *Anaesth* 1985;40:759-762.

MacLennan FM. Maternal mortality from Mendelson's syndrome: an explanation? *Lancet* 1986;1(8481):587-589.

Morgan M. Editorial: the confidential enquiry into maternal deaths. *Anaesth* 1986;41:689-691.

O'Shea M. Better fitness. *Parade Magazine* Mar 28, 1993.

Renfroe SL and Halfhill D. Maternal deaths in Florida, 1977-1982. *J Fla Med Assoc* 1984;71(9):721-723.

Sieber FE et al. Glucose: a reevaluation of its intraoperative use. *Anesthesiol* 1987;67(1):72-81.

Simkin P. Stress, pain, and catecholamines in labor: Part 2. Stress associated with childbirth events: a pilot survey of new mothers. *Birth* 1986;13(4):234-240.

12

Amniotomy

Myth: *We'll rupture membranes and get this show on the road.*

Reality: *"[T]he status of the membranes has but a small effect on the length of labor. . . . We conclude that a routine clinical practice of rupturing membranes in the presence of normal labor progress adds little to labor management and should be questioned."*

Rosen and Peisner 1987

[I]n an unscientific poll, we asked a group of clinicians in our community whether they thought amniotomy had an effect on the length of labor. The majority answered affirmatively; this has been a widely held obstetric concept. (Rosen and Peisner 1987, abstracted below)

Although most obstetricians believe that amniotomy, also called artificial rupture of membranes (ARM), is a harmless intervention that speeds up labor, this has never been established in the medical literature. Some studies support this belief; others have found amniotomy neither effective nor harmless. One recent review of routine interventions in low-risk labors concluded, "The available literature on early elective amniotomy does not support its routine use in the low risk obstetrical patient. . . . [A]mniotomy should not be done to merely 'hurry things up a bit' or to satisfy a need to 'do something'" (Davis and Riedmann 1991). Another analysis of the literature states, "Artificial rupture of the membranes has been used to augment labor for decades, but whether the procedure confers more benefit than harm is still undetermined" (Crowther et al. 1989).

Some of the earliest evidence against amniotomy comes from the Latin American Collaborative Study (Caldeyro-Barcia et al. 1974). Healthy, unmedicated term women who labored and gave birth spontaneously were randomly assigned to amniotomy or control groups. Amniotomy associated with significantly greater head molding and higher incidences of caput succedaneum (a pressure-caused swelling on the fetal head) and early heart rate decelerations, a symptom of fetal distress. The effect on the fetal heart rate (FHR) was particularly pronounced when the fetus had a loop of umbilical cord around the neck, which occurred 25% of the time. The authors explained that by equalizing hydrostatic pressure, intact membranes protected fetal-placental circulation and distributed pressure more evenly on the descending fetal head. The authors believed that amniotomy-caused complications were likely to be more frequent and severe in situations where, unlike the population they studied, the fetus is already compromised.

Subsequent research confirms that oligohydramnios (too little amniotic fluid) increases the incidence of variable and prolonged FHR decelerations, a pattern emblematic of umbilical cord compression (blood flow through the umbilical cord is impeded or stopped by uterine contraction pressure) (Leveno et al. 1984), and in this chapter we shall see an association between abnormal FHR and amniotomy. Nor is abnormal FHR the only danger. Amniotomy can cause umbilical cord prolapse (the umbilical cord comes down ahead of the baby, creating a life-threatening situation usually requiring an emergency cesarean) (Levy et al. 1984, abstracted below).

The only reason for rupturing membranes is to shorten labor, although if the procedure works—and sometimes it does not—it curtails labor only by an hour or two. That shortening labor is advantageous seems to be taken as a given; however, the only apparent benefit derives from a circular argument: Crowther et al. list amniotomy under treatments "that appear promising, but require further evaluation" because amniotomy may "possibly" reduce oxytocin use and instrumental delivery. In other words, because obstetricians will intervene if progress is not as rapid as they think it should be, amniotomy avoids yet more invasive and riskier procedures. In fact, one randomized controlled trial did find that oxytocin augmentation was more frequent in the "no amniotomy" group (Garite et al 1993, abstracted below), but no trial has found that amniotomy reduced operative delivery rates. Caldeyro-Barcia et al. state, "It should be emphasized that acceleration of labor is not necessarily beneficial for the fetus and newborn, and that it may be associated with a poor outcome of the offspring."

Ironically, while proponents of amniotomy deny that amniotomy can be hazardous, other researchers, convinced that insufficient amniotic fluid in labor can lead to fetal distress in a compromised fetus, are experimenting with putting it back (Grant et al. 1989). This procedure, called amnioinfusion, involves inserting a uterine catheter through the vagina and adding physiologic saline.

Adding to the doctrinal confusion, even those who are not in favor of routine amniotomy believe that this procedure should be done in order to set a scalp electrode for internal electronic fetal monitoring (EFM) or to check for the presence of meconium (the baby's first bowel movement) in the amniotic fluid when fetal distress is suspected. One can imagine a labor ward where in one room an obstetrician is rupturing membranes to verify fetal distress while next door another doctor is putting fluid back in hopes of alleviating it.

Does amniotomy ever make sense? Clearly, rupturing membranes at the threshold of active labor disrupts the natural timing of this event. Left alone, two-thirds of women who begin labor with intact membranes reach full dilation with membranes intact (Caldeyro-Barcia et al. 1974). Moreover, Caldeyro-Barcia et al. found that the severity and frequency of related complications correlated with length of time since membrane rupture. On the other hand, amniotomy may sometimes make sense as a treatment for slow progress if it is done late in labor. Amniotomy at this time would not violate the normal timing, and it might help by bringing the head against the cervix where it could act as a more effective dilating wedge.

However, as a routine procedure, early amniotomy appears to have little value and potential risks: What if *this* baby has a hidden problem or cannot tolerate labor with ruptured membranes? Turning the tables on those who defend intervening on a "just in case" basis, shouldn't we refrain from routine amniotomy—just in case?

SUMMARY OF SIGNIFICANT POINTS

- Routine amniotomy may shorten labor by an hour or two, but: (Abstracts 1-3, 11)

    Amniotomy is a minor variable with respect to labor length, and the large standard deviation means it varies widely in individual effect. (Abstracts 1-2, 5)

    Amniotomy does not reduce cesarean rates, even among nulliparas, the subgroup most likely to experience dystocia. (Abstracts 3, 6, 10-11)

    The only advantage to speeding up labor is reducing the use of oxytocin (which is an advantage only because doctors are timetable driven). (Abstracts 1, 11)

- Amniotomy may have little or no effect on labor length or have effect only in some subgroup. (Abstracts 3-6, 10)

- Early amniotomy may inhibit progress in women dilating slowly. (Abstract 4)

- Some studies found that amniotomy increased the incidence of FHR abnormalities in healthy, term fetuses, although it did not affect neonatal outcomes. If the fetus's ability to cope with stress is already compromised, adverse effects on FHR are likely to be more common and severe. (Given this probability, the wisdom of amniotomy to ascertain meconium staining, confirm fetal distress, or insert an internal electrode becomes questionable.) (Abstracts 3, 8, 10-11)

- Other studies found that amniotomy had no adverse effect on FHR. However, the lack of problems in healthy term babies does not mean higher-risk fetuses would be equally tolerant. (Abstracts 1, 6-7)

- Amniotomy may cause umbilical cord prolapse. (Abstract 9)

ORGANIZATION OF ABSTRACTS

Amniotomy Speeds Up Labor

Amniotomy Has No or Minimal Effect on Rate of Progress

Amniotomy Has No Adverse Effects

Amniotomy Has Adverse Effects

AMNIOTOMY SPEEDS UP LABOR

1. Stewart P, Kennedy JH, and Calder AA. Spontaneous labour: when should the membranes be ruptured? *Br J Obstet Gynaecol* **1982;89:39-43.**
Women in spontaneous labor who were 4 cm or more dilated were randomly allocated to amniotomy or not. Four women who had cesareans were excluded, leaving 34 in the amniotomy group (17 each primiparas and multiparas) and 30 in the control group (15 each primiparas and multiparas). In the control group, 70% reached full dilation with membranes intact. Three had spontaneous ruptures, and six had amniotomy for lack of progress or suspected fetal distress.

The only significant difference between groups was that the amniotomy group had a shorter first stage (4.9 ± 2.6 hr versus 7.0 ± 3.7 hr, $p < 0.002$). Other (nonsignificant) differences were that the amniotomy group had less oxytocin (23.5% versus 46.7%), fewer epidurals (47.1% versus 60%), and fewer (principally rotational) forceps (26.5% versus 43.3%). The incidence of abnormal FHR patterns was similar, as were other parameters of fetal well-being.

Without offering evidence, the authors state that there is "a slow inevitable development of acidosis in the fetus throughout labor" [although their own results would seem to contradict this] so that labor becomes "a race between progressive fetal acidosis and dilatation of the cervix." On this basis and because amniotomy facilitates EFM, the authors "see no reason at present to strive to maintain the integrity of fetal membranes." [If the problem they describe is real, it could be iatrogenic since many women have amniotomies. Removing the hydrostatic protection of the fluid may well slowly deplete fetal abilities to compensate over time for the stress of contractions.]

[This study had the following problems: small study size, mixed parity, lack of definition of "poor progress," large overlap in range of length of labors, and the possibility of oxtyocin and epidurals being confounding factors.]

2. Franks P. A randomized trial of amniotomy in active labor. *J Fam Pract* 1990;30(1):49-52.

Criteria for study admission were term spontaneous, uncomplicated labor with intact membranes, dilation 6 cm or less, and no epidural anesthesia. The average dilation at time of randomization in the amniotomy group ($N = 26$) was 4.8 cm versus 4.5 cm among controls ($N = 27$). In the amniotomy group 58% were nulliparous versus 48% among controls. In the control group 59% had an amniotomy before full dilation. Time from labor onset to randomization averaged 3.67 hours in the amniotomy group versus 4.4 hours in the control group. After adjustment for confounding variables, amniotomy shortened the time from randomization to delivery by 155 minutes (CI 9-301 min, $p < 0.05$).

[The problems with the study are small size of study, huge confidence interval, mixed parity, and no information on the time of spontaneous rupture in no amniotomy group. Considering that the control group was stacked in favor of shorter labor (fewer nulliparas, women labored longer before randomization, 59% of them had an amniotomy), a 2.6 hour difference in length of labor from 4.5 cm dilation to birth seems highly unlikely.]

3. Fraser WD et al. Effect of early amniotomy on the risk of dystocia in nulliparous women. *N Engl J Med* 1993;22;328(16):1145-1149.

Nulliparous women in spontaneous labor with healthy fetuses were stratified by degree of cervical dilation and randomly assigned to have membranes ruptured or not. The groups were: less than 3 cm, amniotomy ($N = 72$); less than 3 cm, no amniotomy ($N = 80$); 3 cm or more, amniotomy ($N = 390$); 3 cm or more, no amniotomy ($N = 383$). Half (51%) the no amniotomy group had amniotomies for failure to progress or fetal distress. Equal numbers in the amniotomy and no amniotomy groups had epidurals (73%), and similar numbers had oxytocin in the absence of dystocia (19% versus 16%). Dystocia was defined as 4 hours or more after achieving 3 cm dilation where the average rate of progress was less than 0.5 cm per hour.

Median labor length was shorter in the amniotomy group (136 min, $p < 0.001$), and dystocia was less frequent (34% versus 45%, RR 0.8 CI 0.6-0.9). However, amniotomy had less effect on labor length for women less than 3 cm dilated (66 min versus 125 min), and reduction in dystocia occurred only among women in the group with 3 cm or more dilation (33% versus 48%, RR 0.7 CI 0.6-0.8; compared with 36% versus 30%, RR 1.2 CI 0.8-1.9). Despite this, oxytocin use was similar (36% versus 41%) as were cesarean rates (12% amniotomy versus 11% no amniotomy). Fetal distress played a role in 28 of 56 (50%) of cesareans in the amniotomy group versus 15 of 50 (30%) in the no amniotomy group. Infant outcomes were similar.

[Note that one-third of women were diagnosed as having dystocia even *with* amniotomy, more than one-third of the total population were deemed to require oxytocin, and amniotomy did not reduce cesarean rates. Interestingly, the authors neither analyze nor comment on the sizeable difference in cesareans involving fetal distress. The relative risk calculates to be 1.8.]

AMNIOTOMY HAS NO OR MINIMAL EFFECT ON RATE OF PROGRESS

4. Seitchik J, Holden AE, and Castillo M. Amniotomy and the use of oxytocin in labor in nulliparous women. *Am J Obstet Gynecol* **1985;153(8):848-854.**

Labor progress and oxytocin use in relation to amniotomy were explored in a group of term nulliparous women who began labor spontaneously and gave birth vaginally ($N = 452$). Of them, 242 underwent amniotomy during first-stage labor, 29% of whom were augmented with oxytocin.

Although the large standard deviation implies that individual variation was great, amniotomy enhanced the mean rate of dilation from 1.6 ± 1.9 to 2.8 ± 3.8 cm per hour in women not destined to receive oxytocin ($p < 0.01$) and slowed the dilation rate from 0.8 ± 0.9 to 0.3 ± 0.8 cm hour ($p < 0.01$) in women destined to be augmented. Women dilating less than 1 cm per hour before amniotomy continued to dilate at the same rate after amniotomy whereas labor speeded up in 45% of women dilating 1 cm per hour or more before amniotomy. The greater the dilation at time of amniotomy, the faster the rate of dilation from amniotomy to complete dilation, but the large standard deviations mean that some women experienced rapid dilation after amniotomy and others did not. "Our data generate the ironic but realistic attitude that amniotomy works best to enhance the speed of labor when it is needed least" and that because amniotomy adversely affects progress in some cases, "[A]mniotomy should not be performed during labor without significant indications."

5. Rosen MG and Peisner DB. Effect of amniotic membrane rupture on length of labor. *Obstet Gynecol* **1987;70(4):604-607.**

In order to determine the effect of membrane rupture on labor progress, records were reviewed of 2564 complication-free women who began labor spontaneously with intact membranes. Women could have labor augmented or pain medication, and amniotomy was at physician discretion.

When women were grouped according to dilation at time of rupture, the rate of dilation was fastest for those with spontaneous rupture, next fastest for artificial rupture, and slowest for intact membranes. A stepwise regression determined the influence of parity, membrane rupture (artificial, spontaneous, or none), dilation, and station of the fetal head on dilation rate after membrane rupture and time from rupture to birth. Rupture of membranes had a "small positive effect." However, all of these factors together explained only 25.9% of the variance in the two outcomes. "This is another way of stating that despite all the scientific analyses, we still know but a few of the factors that affect labor."

6. Fraser WD et al. A randomized controlled trial of early amniotomy. *Br J Obstet Gynaecol* **1991;98(1):84-91.**

Term nulliparous women in complication-free spontaneous labor with dilation less than 5 cm and intact membranes were randomly assigned to early amniotomy ($N = 47$)

or a control group ($N = 50$). The power to detect a 20% reduction in labor length was only 55%. In the treatment group, if dilation was less than 3 cm, amniotomy was performed on further dilation and when the fetal head fixed in the pelvis. After 3 cm dilation, amniotomy was performed when the fetal head fixed in the pelvis. Among control women, amniotomy was permitted before full dilation for suspected fetal distress or lack of progress for two hours or more. Doctors were "requested" not to use oxytocin unless progress had stopped for two hours or more. EFM tracings were analyzed by observers blinded to allocation. Tracings were graded "normal" or "abnormal" based on definitions for abnormalities that would have significance for making labor management decisions. Sixty percent of controls achieved 8 cm dilation before membrane rupture versus 2% (one subject) in the amniotomy group. Among control women, 38% had an amniotomy for either labor augmentation or suspected fetal distress.

Similar percentages in both groups were augmented (32% amniotomy, 30% control) and had assisted vaginal deliveries (23% amniotomy, 28% control). The cesarean rate was 17% in the amniotomy group versus 8% among control women (no significance calculation). Times from randomization to delivery were not significantly different nor were times from randomization to full dilation. Maternal morbidity was not different nor were EFM variables, Apgar scores, or umbilical artery pH values.

Next, vaginal deliveries were analyzed separately. Maternal weight and birth weights were higher and mean dilation on admission was lower in the treatment group, but a linear regression found that these differences did not affect outcomes. When survival curves for continuance in labor were constructed, amniotomy did not predict earlier delivery after adjustment for birth weight, dilation at admission, and maternal weight.

The strengths of this study were as follows: careful blinding of the randomization process, clearly defined classifications of fetal heart rate tracings based on findings that could affect decision-making, and keeping participants in their group regardless of what happened to membranes after randomization. "The results of the study fail to support the long held belief that early amniotomy is an effective method in reducing labor duration." Since no trends in the data were found, a larger trial would be unlikely to demonstrate differences between treatment and controls.

AMNIOTOMY HAS NO ADVERSE EFFECTS

7. Bruner JP and Gabbe SG. Effect of amniotomy on uteroplacental and fetoplacental flow velocity waveforms. *Am J Perinatol* 1989;6(4):421-423.

In order to determine the effect of amniotomy, the authors used ultrasound to analyze the blood flow in the uterine and umbilical arteries in 15 healthy women in normally progressing spontaneous labor. With amniotomy, small changes in blood flow velocity were seen in both positive and negative directions. Changes among the three smokers were not different from those of the nonsmokers. In this study, the head was well applied to the cervix, and only minimal amounts of amniotic fluid were released. One cannot assume changes would be equally benign if large amounts of amniotic fluid were released. "[W]e conclude that early elective amniotomy exerts no demonstrable effect on impedance to uteroplacental or fetoplacental blood flow *in healthy women at term* [emphasis mine]."

AMNIOTOMY HAS ADVERSE EFFECTS

8. Kariniemi V. Effects of amniotomy on fetal heart rate variability during labor. *Am J Obstet Gynecol* 1983;147(8):975-976.

This study measured the effect of amniotomy on FHR variability among 32 women with term pregnancies, no pain medication [because narcotics affect FHR variability], and normal FHR. All women had completed cervical effacement, and the mean dilation was 4 cm (range 2-8 cm). Early decelerations occurred in two fetuses for 10 and 20 minutes postamniotomy. Late decelerations occurred for 20 minutes in another fetus. Variability decreased for approximately 30 minutes before recovering, which the authors attribute to decreased uterine perfusion and placental blood flow. (A decrease in variability in the absence of analgesia "reflect[s] fetal hypoxia.") [A healthy fetus is likely to withstand the stress of amniotomy, but what if the fetus were already compromised?]

[The problem with the study was lack of a control group.]

9. Levy H et al. Umbilical cord prolapse. *Obstet Gynecol* 1984;64(4):499-502.

All cases of umbilical cord prolapse between 1969 and 1982 were reviewed ($N = 79$). The incidence was 0.26%, of which 38% involved preterm infants and 50.6% involved abnormal presentation. In the 68 cases where the woman was in labor, 68.4% had cesareans. In 10 cases, prolapse followed amniotomy (12.7%). Eight babies of 26 weeks or more gestation died; one of them was a term vertex infant who died of cord prolapse after an amniotomy.

10. Barrett JF et al. Randomized trial of amniotomy in labour versus the intention to leave membranes intact until the second stage. *Br J Obstet Gynaecol* 1992;99(1):5-9.

Low-risk term women were randomly assigned to have artificial rupture of membrane (ARM) ($N = 183$) or not ($N = 179$. Of those allocated to ARM, 97% had ARM. Of those allocated to no ARM, 46% had ARM. Mean dilation at rupture was 5.0 cm in the ARM group versus 7.9 cm in the no ARM group. The trial had the power to detect a doubling of FHR decelerations from 12% to 24% and an increase in epidural rate from 30% to 50%, but not a rise in cesarean rate from 5% to 10%.

ARM did not shorten labor except for a modest decrease in length of first stage in nulliparas (8.3 ± 4.1 versus 9.7 ± 4.8, $p < 0.05$). Women in the ARM group were more likely to have epidurals (34% versus 22%, $p < 0.01$) and to have oxytocin (15% versus 9%, NS). [Epidural use may increase oxytocin use.] FHR decelerations were more likely in the ARM group (10% versus 4%, $p = 0.04$). However, other indicators of infant well-being (meconium staining, cord blood pH, Apgar scores) were unaffected, as were cesarean rates (2.7% versus 1.1%). The study may have been too small [and cesarean rates too low] to show "a small but important increase in this end point."

11. Garite TJ et al. The influence of elective amniotomy on fetal heart rate patterns and the course of labor in term patients: a randomized study. *Am J Obstet Gynecol* 1993;168(6 Pt 1):1827-1832.

Healthy women in term, spontaneous, active labor (defined as dilation 4-6 cm) were randomly allocated to amniotomy ($N = 235$) or intact ($N = 224$) groups. Mean dilation at time of rupture was 5.5 cm in the amniotomy group versus 8.1 cm in the intact group

($p < 0.01$). In the intact group 26% had amniotomy [presumably in first stage] for indication; in 6%, timing and reason were not documented.

Amniotomy reduced the mean length of first stage in all women by 82 minutes (276 ± 202 versus 358 ± 236), in nulliparas by 110 minutes (347 ± 206 versus 457 ± 233), and in multiparas by 54 minutes (230 ± 186 versus 284 ± 209) (p for all three comparisons < 0.05). However, the amniotomy group was less likely to have totally normal tracings (24% versus 36%, $p < 0.003$) during the first stage and more likely to have mild and moderate variable FHR decelerations (66% versus 49%, $p < 0.0003$) and prolonged decelerations (8% versus 4%, NS). Women in the intact group were more likely to have oxytocin (16% versus 34%, $p < 0.000005$). Cesarean rates (4.2% versus 2.0%) and neonatal outcomes were similar. [In the discussion following, Garite says that epidural use was similar. He gives no numbers.]

[Women in the intact group were twice as likely to have oxytocin. Oxytocin causes fetal distress and may have contributed to abnormal FHR in the intact group, so differences in incidence of abnormal FHR may be more pronounced than it appears. Moreover, these were low-risk fetuses. Higher-risk fetuses may be less tolerant.]

REFERENCES

Caldeyro-Barcia R, et al. Adverse perinatal effects of early amniotomy during labor. In *Modern perinatal medicine.* Gluck L, ed. Chicago: Yearbook Medical Publishers, 1974.

Crowther C, et al. Prolonged labour. In *A guide to effective care in pregnancy and childbirth.* Enkin M, Keirse MJNC, and Chalmers I, eds. Oxford: Oxford University Press, 1989.

Davis L and Riedmann G. Recommendations for the management of low risk obstetric patients. *Int J Gynaecol Obstet* 1991;35(2):107-115. (abstracted in Chapter 15)

Grant A et al. Monitoring the fetus during labour. In *A guide to effective care in pregnancy and childbirth.* Enkin M, Keirse MJNC, and Chalmers I, eds. Oxford: Oxford University Press, 1989.

Leveno KJ et al. Prolonged pregnancy. I. Observations concerning the causes of fetal distress. *Am J Obstet Gynecol* 1984;150(5 Pt 1):465-473.

13

Epidural Anesthesia

Myth: *Natural childbirth makes about as much sense as natural dentistry, and epidurals are the Cadillac of anesthesia.*

Reality: *"Reported maternal complications of epidural analgesia . . . include: dural puncture; hypotension; . . . increased use of operative delivery; neurological complications; bladder dysfunction; headache; backache; toxic drug reactions; respiratory insufficiency; and even maternal death. The fetus may also suffer complications as a result of maternal effects (for example, hypotension) or direct drug toxicity."*

Simkin and Dickersin 1989

"Planning Your Childbirth," a brochure put out by the American Society of Anesthesiologists (ASA), encapsulates the mainstream medical viewpoint on epidural anesthesia. Equating it with "pleasant, safe, and comfortable," the brochure begins by inverting the meaning of natural childbirth:

> Today's mothers are reconsidering the idea that childbirth is "natural" only without medication, and they are choosing to have pain relief . . . to help them experience a more comfortable birth.

It misrepresents the effect on labor:

> Will it slow down my labor? Some may have a brief period of decreased uterine contractions. Many . . . are pleasantly surprised to learn that after the epidural . . . [has] made them more comfortable and relaxed, their labor may actually progress faster.

> Can I "push" when needed? Epidural analgesia allows you to rest during the most strenuous part of labor. . . . [W]hen it is time to push . . . [t]he epidural block can reduce your pain while allowing you to push when needed.

It glosses over the risks of epidurals:

> Will the epidural block affect my baby? Considerable research has proven that epidural . . . anesthesia can be safe for both mother or baby. . . . However, special skills, precautions, judgements and treatments are required.

> What are the risks . . . ? [C]omplications or side effects can occur even though you are monitored carefully and your anesthesiologist takes special precautions to avoid them. To help prevent a decrease in blood pressure . . . [etc.]. By holding as still as possible during the needle placement, you help to decrease the likelihood of a headache [so it is her fault!]. The discomfort, sometimes lasting a few days, often can be reduced or eliminated by simple measures. [T]he anesthetic . . . may . . . affect the chest muscles and make it seem harder to breathe. Sometimes oxygen might be given to relieve this feeling and help the breathing. . . . To help avoid unusual reactions [stemming from injecting the medication into a vein], your anesthesiologist will administer a test dose.

They tell no lies, but they sure skate around the truth.

If an epidural is a Cadillac, it is a used one with concealed defects. The risks of epidurals convert normal labor to a high-tech event. An IV must be started to help counteract the tendency of epidurals to cause hypotension. Electronic fetal monitoring (EFM) is necessary because epidurals can cause fetal distress, and the mother's vital signs must be closely monitored to warn of maternal adverse reactions. If the needle or catheter pierces a blood vessel, which is easy to do in pregnancy because blood vessels are enlarged (Corke and Spielman 1985, abstracted below), or the needle goes deeper than the epidural space, convulsions, respiratory paralysis, and/or cardiac arrest can occur. Tests are done to confirm proper placement before giving the full dosage, but these are not completely preventative. Trained personnel, resuscitation equipment, and medication must be immediately available.

In labor, epidurals increase the need for oxytocin, instrumental delivery, episiotomy, and bladder catheterization. The first-time mother is more likely to have a cesarean. Temporary postpartum complications include urinary incontinence, nerve injury causing muscle weakness or abnormal sensation, and headache, which can last for days and is excruciatingly painful. Instrumental delivery and episiotomy increase the probability of deep perineal tears, which can have long-term effects on sexual satisfaction and fecal continence (see Chapter 14). Backache and headache may become chronic. In the newborn, epidurals may cause jaundice, and there may be adverse behavioral effects. Finally, no one is collecting figures, but having an epidural must add considerably to the cost of the birth.

Recent innovations have not helped. Even when the dosage was so small that many women could walk despite the epidural, cesarean rates were not reduced (Oriol 1992).

Within the past decade, epidurals went from being reserved for particularly prolonged or difficult labors or cesarean sections—when they are, indeed, a godsend—to the norm at American deliveries. An overwhelming number of doctors and an increasing number of nurses think epidurals should be routine. Why should any woman suffer in this day and age? they ask. Their patients have bought this, making epidurals all but universal at many hospitals.

To reach this point, doctors swept the dark side of epidurals under the rug (Brownridge 1991; Reynolds 1989; Richardson 1988; Cheek and Gutsche 1987, abstracted below; Clark 1985). They attributed life-threatening complications to poor technique. And if nobody made any errors, well, complications occurred rarely, and if handled right, mother and baby were almost always fine. They denied that epidurals lead to other interventions and that these interventions introduce risks. Or if they did not deny it, they did not see intervention rates as a problem. They also dismissed adverse effects on the baby as either nonexistent or too insignificant to worry about.

Labor pain became not only something to be blotted out, but in a stunning reversal, the pain, not epidurals became the danger. The mother's stress hormones are accused of causing fetal distress. Women who do not want an epidural are portrayed as masochistic, misguided, or misinformed, even, by virtue of this last twist, uncaring of their baby's welfare (Brownridge 1991; Reynolds 1989).

Does it make sense to tell women to avoid even a single glass of wine during pregnancy and then push drugs during labor? This contradiction is one tipoff that attitudes toward epidurals are culturally determined beliefs masquerading as objective truths. Inversions of this kind are rife in the popular press on epidurals, as well as in the medical literature. As examples, in a newspaper article, a psychologist and an anesthesiologist denounce childbirth educators for leading women to think they can cope with labor pain unaided by drugs and for telling them epidurals have risks (*San Jose Mercury News* 1993). These same experts describe the guilt, anger, and sense of failure (even to feeling suicidal) women experience after they ultimately "require" an epidural. Epidurals are safe, they contend, but labor pain and attempting natural childbirth are hazardous to psychological health. The ASA brochure warns in oversized uppercase letters not to eat or drink after labor begins. Epidurals are safe, even part of natural childbirth, but quenching thirst and eating during hours of strenuous activity are dangerous.

The need to make reality match belief leads to considerable distortion of the facts and prevents a rational evaluation of the risks and benefits. For example, Cheek and Gutsche (1987), as do others, recommend epidural block to protect high-risk fetuses from the dangers of maternal stress response to labor pain, shortly after they say a maternal drop in blood pressure is "the most common side effect" of epidurals and warn that a compromised fetus may not tolerate even a 15% to 20% fall in maternal pressure.

Another tipoff is the attitude toward those who do not conform. Cultural norms are traditionally enforced by exerting pressure through ridicule or scorn, Most women with mainstream medical care who make an effort to resist epidurals will find this out for themselves.

In fact, the pain and stress of normal labor have value. The stress hormones produced in response to labor, adrenaline and noradrenaline, trigger the final preparation of the fetal lungs to breathe air, mobilize fuel for energy, and, by shunting fetal blood away from the extremities and to the brain and heart (exactly opposite of the effect in adults), protect the fetus against hypoxia (oxygen lack) during labor (Lagercrantz and Slotkin 1986).

Nerves in the cervix, and later the pelvic floor muscles and vagina, transmit stretching sensations as well as pain. These stretch receptors signal the pituitary to produce more oxytocin, which increases the tempo of the labor, causing further cervical dilation. Once the cervix is completely open and the head distends the pelvic floor and vagina, surges of oxytocin are produced, creating the urge to push. Numb the nerves with an epidural, and you also wipe out the positive feedback mechanism (Johnson and Everitt 1988; Bates et al. 1985; Goodfellow et al. 1983).

Pain guides the mother. Commonly, the positions and activities she chooses for comfort are also those that promote good labor progress or help shift the baby into the right position for birth. Remove the pain, and you kill that feedback mechanism too.

The pro-epiduralists see the mother as needing rescue, but in reality her body prepares her to meet labor's challenge. Stress hormones give her stamina. By the time of the birth, endorphins, the body's natural painkillers, are found at levels 30 times higher than in nonpregnant women, and levels can be 20 times higher in women with prolonged or difficult labors as in uncomplicated labors (Jimenez 1988). Endorphins, produced in response to pain and stress, are also mood elevators. They are responsible, for example, for "runner's high." Oxytocin has mood-elevating and amnesiac properties too (Fuchs 1990).

Unlike epidurals, natural childbirth strategies facilitate labor both physiologically and psychologically. They raise endorphin levels, whereas epidurals reduce them (Jimenez 1988). They give the mother knowledge, skills, and confidence. Studies show that the key to a positive labor experience is mastery—a sense of control over events. With an epidural, control is completely given over to medical staff (Simkin 1991; Humenick 1981; Humenick and Bugen 1981).

While the normal stress of labor is beneficial, extreme anxiety or fear may have adverse effects (Simkin 1986). However, this type of stress may be extrinsic to labor. The animal studies that reported that stress in labor caused hypoxia in a compromised fetus—and which are quoted as an argument for epidurals—took laboring monkeys, pinched their toes, shined bright lights in their eyes, or jumped up and down in front of their cages (Simkin 1986). The monkeys did fine—*until doctors hurt or frightened them.*

Moreover, although epidurals relieve pain, one study found they did nothing to relieve stress. Wuitchik, Bakal, and Lipshitz (1990) asked laboring women what they were thinking at various points in labor and rated their reponses on a scale measuring coping versus distress. No differences were found between women who had epidurals and those who did not. The solution to undue stress in labor seems to be not an epidural, but supportive care and a relaxed, peaceful environment. As Simkin says, "Much of the stress of labor is preventable because many of the stressors . . . are imposed in the form of thoughtless routines, unfamiliar personnel, and technological interventions."

Meanwhile, one report on serious nonfatal epidural complications in 500,000 women yielded an incidence rate of life-threatening complications of roughly 1 in 14,000 cases and a serious complications rate overall of 1 in 5000 (Scott and Hibbard 1990, abstracted below). Another study reported a 1 in 3000 life-threatening complication rate (Crawford 1985, abstracted below). Women have died of epidural anesthesia but never of the pain of labor.

Drugs have been withdrawn from the market or forced into restricted use because of serious adverse reactions in the range of 1 in 1000 to 1 in 30,000 (Cohn 1989), yet epidurals are enthusiastically promoted to healthy women undergoing a normal process who are told the advantages are overwhelming and the risks are nil. I am not suggesting banning epidurals, only a more judicious approach. Epidurals are like any other obstetric intervention: they have their place, but they are a mixed blessing.

Notes: The British use extradural for epidural.

I have limited the abstracts to studies primarily of bupivacaine because that seems overwhelmingly to be the anesthetic of choice.

To show that adverse effects are not dose-dependent, I have listed concentrations after the citation.

Most articles refer to epidural *analgesia*, a softer word meaning "relief of pain." I use *anesthesia*, meaning "loss of sensation," because of its more serious connotation.

For a list of the generic and equivalent trade names of the medications used in epidurals, see Table 13.1.

SUMMARY OF SIGNIFICANT POINTS

- Epidurals substantially increase the incidence of oxytocin augmentation, instrumental delivery (which increases the incidence of deep perineal tears), and bladder catheterization, although the effect seems to depend on obstetric management. (Abstracts 2-9, 11-15, 17, 23, 26-28, 32-34)

- In primiparas, epidurals substantially increase the cesarean rate for dystocia. Here, too, the effect may depend on management. (Abstracts 2, 5-7, 10-15, 26, 33)

- Epidurals decrease the probability of an occiput posterior (OP) or occiput transverse (OT) baby's rotating. Oxytocin does not help. (Abstracts 2-3, 8-9, 13-14, 28)

- Having the epidural at 5 cm dilation or more greatly reduces excess incidence of OP and OT babies and cesarean for dystocia. (Abstracts 13-14)

- Epidurals may not relieve any pain or may not relieve all pain. (Abstracts 14, 20, 27)

- Innovations in procedure—lower dosages, continuous infusion, adding a narcotic—have not decreased epidural-related problems. (Abstracts 6-7, 10, 13-15, 19, 27, 32-35, 42)

- Delaying pushing until the head has descended to the perineum increases the chances of spontaneous birth.* Evidence is divided as to whether letting the epidural wear off increases spontaneous delivery. (Abstracts 3-5, 7)

- Maternal complications of epidurals include (Abstract 20, 1/3000 potentially life threatening; Abstract 22, 1/14,000 potentially life threatening; Abstract 36; 3-10/10,000 high spinal or intravascular):

    Maternal hypotension (Abstract 1, 1.4-12%; Abstract 7, 10%; Abstract 15, 16%; Abstract 17, 32% in high-risk population; Abstract 27, 5%). This reduces uteroplacental blood supply and can cause fetal distress. High-risk babies are at particular risk because they lack reserves to cope. (Abstracts 1, 7, 15, 17-19, 20, 32)

    Convulsions (Abstract 22, 4/100,000). (Abstracts 19-20, 22, 42)

    Respiratory paralysis (Abstract 22, 16/million). (Abstracts 19-20, 22)

    Cardiac arrest (Abstract 22, 6/million). (Abstracts 1, 16, 19-20, 22, 36)

    Allergic shock (Abstract 22, 2/million). (Abstracts 19, 22)

    Maternal nerve injury through injury by the needle or catheter, poor

---

*Two recent studies have claimed that delayed pushing did not increase the spontaneous birth rate, but in neither case was pushing truly delayed. The mean wait time was 52 minutes in one (Gleeson and Griffith 1991), and 72% began pushing less than one hour after full dilation in the other (Manyonda, Shaw, and Drife 1990).

positioning, forceps injury, infection, hematoma (bleeding at the site), or subarachnoid injection of chloroprocaine. The last three usually cause permanent damage (Abstract 21, 36.2/10,000 with epidurals versus 2.4/10,000 with no analgesia, all temporary; Abstract 22, 8/100,000, 4/million permanent; Abstract 40, 24% or more "nerve root irritation"). (Abstracts 1, 16, 18-22, 40-41)

Spinal headache, an incapacitating headache that can last days (Abstract 19, up to 50% with dural puncture; Abstract 22, 3/100,000; Abstract 24, 0.1% of all epidurals). (Abstracts 19, 22, 24)

Increased maternal core temperature, an additional stressor on both mother and fetus that may lead to a septic workup to rule out infection in the baby. (Abstracts 30-31)

Temporary urinary incontinence. (Abstract 22)

Long-term (weeks to years) backache (Abstract 24, 18.2% versus 10.2% nonepidural), headache (Abstract 24, 4.6% versus 2.9% nonepidural), migraines (Abstract 24, 1.9% versus 1.1% nonepidural), numbness or tingling. (Abstracts 20, 24)

- Serious complications occur despite proper procedure and precautions. The epinephrine test dose can cause complications. (Abstracts 16, 18-20, 26, 36-42)

- Epidural anesthetics "get" to the baby. (Abstracts 15-16, 19, 27-28)

- Epidurals do not protect the fetus from fetal distress. In fact, they cause abnormal fetal heart rate (FHR), sometimes severe, which may occur in association with or independent of maternal blood pressure (Abstract 7, 11%; Abstract 15, 43% bupivacaine, 16% chloroprocaine, 10% lidocaine; Abstract 17, 9.7% associated with maternal hypotension in a high-risk population; Abstract 26, 11%; Abstract 34, 20%). (Abstracts 7, 12-15, 17, 19-20, 26-27, 32-34, 37, 42)

- Epidurals may cause neonatal jaundice. (Abstracts 25, 28)

- Epidurals may cause adverse neonatal physical and behavioral effects. (These are both direct effects and indirect effects from the increased rate of labor complications and interventions.) The importance of the behavioral effects is debated. (Abstracts 1, 15, 28-29)

- Epidural anesthesia may relieve hypertension, but hypertensive women are at particular risk of epidural-induced hypotension, which reduces placental blood supply. (Abstracts 17-18)

ORGANIZATION OF ABSTRACTS

Risks and Benefits (Review)

Increase in Operative Delivery

    Forceps/Vacuum Extraction
    Cesarean

Complications

    Papers Including Complications in Both Mother and Baby
    Mother Only
    Baby Only
        Physical Adverse Effects
        Behavioral Adverse Effects
    Fever

Newer Techniques Offer No Improvement

    Continuous Infusion
    Anesthetic Plus Narcotic

Precautions Are Not Foolproof

    Test Dose
    Technique of Administration

Table 13.1: The 'Caine Family	
Generic Name	Trade Name
bupivacaine	Marcaine, Sensoricaine
2-chloroprocaine	Nesacaine
lidocaine	Xylocaine
mepivacaine	Carbocaine

RISKS AND BENEFITS (Review)

1. Avard DM and Nimrod CM. Risks and benefits of obstetric epidural analgesia: a review. *Birth* **1985;12(4):215-225.**
Based on a literature review, the authors conclude:

- Epidurals confer a higher degree of pain relief but not necessarily greater satisfaction with the birth.

- Epidurals may protect mother and fetus from the adverse effects of stress during birth.

- Epidurals allow women to be awake and alert.

- Epidurals may have a minimal, short-term adverse effect on newborn behavior. The association is stronger with greater dosages and with certain drugs, notably mepivacaine.

- Available evidence on the effect on labor is conflicting but is suggestive of a negative impact, especially in second stage.

- Complications reported are maternal hypotension (1.4-12% incidence rates), as well as case reports of permanent neurologic damage and cardiac arrest.

- "Most studies were fraught with methodological shortcomings."

INCREASE IN OPERATIVE DELIVERY

Forceps/Vacuum Extraction

2. Studd JWW et al. The effect of lumbar epidural analgesia on the rate of cervical dilatation and the outcome of labour of spontaneous onset. *Br J Obstet Gynaecol* **1980;87:1015-1021.** (no dosage given)
Outcomes were compared for 583 primiparas, of whom 80 had an epidural, and 1122 multiparas, of whom 46 had an epidural. All women had spontaneous onset of labor. Labor was augmented in 30% of primiparas and 16% of multiparas.
An epidural made no difference in cesarean rate (2.2% versus 2.5% in primiparas and 0.6% versus 0 in multiparas). Epidurals reduced spontaneous delivery rates among both primiparas (34.0% versus 79.0%, $p < 0.001$) and multiparas (67.0% versus 94.0%, $p < 0.001$). Rotational forceps were needed 20 times more often with an epidural (20.0% versus 0.8% in primiparas, $p < 0.001$; 4.3% versus 0.2% in multiparas, $p < 0.001$). When a subset of women in dysfunctional, augmented labor were compared, the trend was toward higher cesarean rates with an epidural (4.8% versus 5.8% in primiparas; 4.8% versus 7.5% in multiparas).

3. Phillips KC and Thomas TA. Second stage of labour with or without extradural analgesia. *Anesthesia* **1983;38:972-976.** (initial bolus 0.5%, first top-up 0.375%, other top-ups 0.25%)
Primigravidas with uncomplicated labors and epidurals were randomly allocated to two groups of 28. In group A, anesthesia was allowed to wear off when the mother was fully dilated and the fetal head descended below 0 station. The mother pushed when she felt the urge. In group B, anesthesia was continued, and the mother was directed to

push when the fetal head got below 0 station. Fifty percent of group A and 68% of group B had oxytocin augmention.

There was no difference in the incidence of malpositions at full dilation (43% in each group), but malposition was more likely to continue in group A (6 versus 2, $p < 0.05$). The forceps rate in group A was 43% versus 25% in group B, but the difference was not significant [possibly because of the small number of subjects]. Thus, allowing epidural anesthesia to wear off appears to increase both malpositions and forceps delivery rates while increasing the mother's experience of pain.

4. Maresh M, Choong KH, and Beard RW. Delayed pushing with lumbar epidural analgesia in labour. *Br J Obstet Gynaecol* **1983;90:623-627.** (no dosage given)

Primiparas with epidurals and uncomplicated labors ($N = 40$) were told to push as soon as they had the desire (early pushing), and outcomes were compared with 36 similar women who rested on their side and were told not to push until the head was visible (delayed pushing). Augmentation rates were 27.5% in the early pushing group versus 19.4% in the delayed pushing group.

Mean waiting time was 30 minutes for early pushing and two hours for delayed pushing. Delayed pushing was associated with more spontaneous deliveries (50% versus 35%, NS). The difference was wholly due to less need for rotational forceps (4% versus 11%). [This study may have been too small to demonstrate a significant difference.] Delayed pushing did not harm the baby.

5. Bailey PW and Howard MB. Epidural analgesia and forceps delivery: laying a bogey. *Anaesthesia* **1983;38:282-285.** (top-ups 0.25% in labor, 0.5% for perineal pain)

Comparing the year 1977, prior to introduction of an epidural service, with 1980, when 72.4% of primiparas had epidurals, little change in instrumental delivery (24.3% in 1977 versus 26.8% in 1980) or cesarean rates (7.9% in 1977 versus 10.4% in 1980) was found. Active pushing was encouraged only when the mother felt the urge to push or the fetal head had descended onto the perineum.

6. Diro M and Beydoun S. Segmental epidural analgesia in labor: a matched control study. *J Nat Med Assoc* **1985;78(1):569-573.** (0.25%)

Women in spontaneous labor who elected epidurals for pain relief ($N = 43$) were matched with respect to age range, parity, stage of gestation, and infant birth weight to the next patient who did not have an epidural. The clinicians were not aware of the study, and the investigators were not involved in patient care.

Augmentation was more frequent in the epidural group (74.4% versus 30.2%, $p < 0.001$). Among primigravidas, 7 of 35 (20%) had cesareans for failure to progress, all in the epidural group. All women having forceps deliveries were primigravidas—25.6% in the epidural group versus 9.3% in the nonepidural group ($p < 0.05$). "Segmental epidural anesthesia is reasonably safe for both mother and fetus. This is predicated on the premise that the patient is fully aware she would most likely undergo prolonged labor, necessitating oxytocin augmentation and eventual forceps delivery." [The 20% versus 0% cesarean rate among primigravidas is not mentioned.]

7. Chestnut DH et al. The influence of continuous epidural bupivacaine analgesia on the second stage of labor and method of delivery in nulliparous women. *Anesthesiology* **1987;66:774-780.** (initial bolus 0.25%, infusion 0.125%)

This trial randomly assigned 92 healthy nulliparous women with epidural anesthesia to one of two groups ($N = 46$ per group), one receiving bupivacaine as a top-up dose at 8 cm dilation, the other saline. (Five women were excluded who underwent cesarean section for dystocia before 8 cm). Ten percent of the women experienced "transient hypotension," and 11% of the fetuses had heart rate patterns alarming enough to prompt fetal scalp blood sampling.

Six women in each group underwent c-section for cephalopelvic disproportion (CPD) after the start of the study solution. Fifty-three percent of the bupivacaine group had an instrumental delivery versus 28% of the saline group ($p < 0.05$). While pain relief was superior with analgesia, letting the epidural wear off shortened second-stage labor and reduced the instrumental delivery rate. [The overall cesarean rate was 17.1%, all for dystocia. There is no discussion of this.]

8. Kaminski HM, Stafl A, and Aiman J. The effect of epidural analgesia on the frequency of instrumental obstetric delivery. *Obstet Gynecol* **1987;69(5):770-773.** (0.25%)

Women who elected epidural anesthesia for pain relief ($N = 155$) were matched with women who had either local or pudendal anesthesia [pudendal blocks can also interfere with pushing]. Both groups were instructed to push at full dilation.

Although birth weights did not differ, women who had epidurals had instrumental deliveries 2.5 times more often and midforceps procedures 3.4 times as often. White multigravidas who had epidurals were nine times more likely to have an instrumental delivery than white multigravidas who did not. OP presentations were found in 27% of those with epidurals versus 8% of controls. Of 103 women whose babies were born in the anterior (favorable) position, instruments were used three times as often and midforceps 3.7 times more often. All differences were significant ($p < 0.05$). Since birth weights were not different, this study refutes the theory that a bigger baby leads to a more painful labor, which leads to epidural anesthesia. It also refutes the theory that posterior babies lead to more painful labor and thus to epidurals because differences persisted when only anterior presentations were compared.

9. Saunders NJ et al. Oxytocin infusion during second stage of labour in primiparous women using epidural analgesia: a randomised double blind placebo controlled trial. *BMJ* **1989;299:1423-1426.** (0.375%)

This trial examined the effect of oxytocin on primiparous women with epidural anesthesia who reached full dilation without oxytocin. Women were given either oxytocin ($N = 108$) or saline ($N = 118$) at the onset of second stage. At this point 35% of babies were OP or OT. Oxytocin reduced the number of nonrotational instrumental deliveries (31% versus 47%, $p = 0.03$) and, because of this, the incidence of perineal trauma (episiotomy or second-degree tear [no information on deep tears]) (66% versus 79%, $p = 0.04$) but had no significant effect on rotational instrumental deliveries (18% oxytocin versus 9% controls).

Cesarean

Note: Neuhoff, Burke, and Porreco (1989) found that while indentical numbers of nulliparous women had epidural anesthesia (42%), the cesarean rate for failure to progress among clinic patients was 1.2% versus 20.2% for private patients (abstracted in Chapter 5). This suggests obstetric management plays an important role.

10. Thorp JA et al. The effect of continuous epidural analgesia on cesarean section for dystocia in nulliparous women. *Am J Obstet Gynecol* **1989;161(3):670-675.** (initial bolus 0.25%, infusion 0.125%)

The authors compared 447 nulliparous women in spontaneous labor who had epidurals with 267 nulliparous women who did not. The epidural was discontinued only for lack of progress in second stage.

Oxytocin use with epidural was more likely (73% versus 27%, $p < 0.05$). C-section for dystocia was more common with epidural (10.3% versus 3.8%, $p < 0.005$). Birth weights were greater ($p < 0.005$) in the epidural group; however, removing subjects whose babies weighed more than 4000 g did not decrease the cesarean rate discrepancy ($p < 0.002$), nor did removing six cesarean mothers with abnormal labor patterns prior to the epidural ($p < 0.005$). Oxytocin augmentation was "aggressively used to correct dysfunctional labor" (55.8% overall). The discrepancy in cesarean rates may be larger in hospitals taking a more conservative approach.

11. Philipsen T and Jensen NH. Epidural block or parenteral pethidine as analgesic in labour; a randomized study concerning progress in labour and instrumental deliveries. *Eur J Obstet Gynecol Reprod Biol* **1989;30:27:33.** (0.375%)

Women, almost all nulliparas (93%), with no evidence of CPD were randomly assigned in early labor to either pethidine (a narcotic) ($N = 54$) or epidural anesthesia ($N = 57$). So that the epidural could wear off, no top-ups were given after 8 cm dilation. All women were offered a pudendal block if they wished, and most accepted (86% in each group) [a confounding factor because pudendal blocks also interfere with pushing]. Equal numbers had oxytocin (33%).

The instrumental delivery rate was 25% versus 26%. The cesarean rate was 17% versus 11% for the epidural group versus control women (NS). [Surely no significance was achieved because the study too small.] Three times the number of women had cesareans for CPD in the epidural group (15.8% versus 5.5%). [Remember, there was no clinical evidence of CPD.] The authors concluded that epidural anesthesia did not increase the instrumental delivery rate and gave better pain relief. [The authors ignore the tripled cesarean rate for CPD.]

12. Gribble RK and Meier PR. Effect of epidural analgesia on the primary cesarean rate. *Obstet Gynecol* **1991;78(2):231-234.** (infusion 0.125%)

No differences were found when primary cesarean rates during the 15 months prior to availability of epidural anesthesia ($N = 1298$) were compared with the 15 months after its introduction ($N = 1084$, 48% opted for an epidural). Nor were there changes in cesarean indication. [Half the women did not have an epidural, which may have diluted the effect.] Overall cesarean rates were 9.0% prior to epidural availability versus 8.2% following epidural availability. Nulliparas had a 14.4% cesarean rate for dystocia and a 2.3% cesarean rate for fetal distress prior (16.7% total) and a 14.4% rate for dystocia and a 1.6% rate for fetal distress after (16.0% total). Multiparas had a 2.6% rate for dystocia and a 1.2% rate for fetal distress prior (3.8% total) versus a 1.5% rate for dystocia and a 1.7% rate for fetal distress after (3.2% total).

13. Thorp JA et al. Epidural analgesia and cesarean section for dystocia: risk factors in nulliparas. *Am J Perinatol* **1991;8(6):402-410.** (initial bolus 0.25%, infusion 0.125%) (This is a different population from Abstract 10.)

Nulliparas in spontaneous labor at dilation 5 cm or less were grouped as follows: (1)

dilation 1 cm per hour or more, no epidural (N = 117); (2) dilation 1 cm per hour or more, early epidural (N = 45); (3) dilation 1 cm per hour or more, late epidural (N = 44); (4) dilation 1 cm per hour or less, no epidural (N = 89); (5) dilation 1 cm per hour or less, early epidural (N = 170); (6) dilation 1 cm per hour or less, late epidural (N = 35). Active management of labor was used (see Chapter 5). To assess the effect of epidurals on cesareans for dystocia, it is important to exclude multiparas because dystocia is rarely a problem in this group.

Comparing group 4 versus 5 shows the effect of early epidural on dilating slowly. Group 5 women were more likely to have oxytocin (53% versus 86%, $p < 0.0009$) and cesareans for dystocia (3.4% versus 20.6%, $p < 00006$). Excluding macrosomic babies did not reduce the effect on cesarean (2.4% versus 20.9%, $p < 0.00005$), so selection bias is unlikely to explain the difference.

Comparing groups 4 and 6 shows the effect of late epidural on dilating slowly. Group 6 women were more likely to have oxytocin (53% versus 60%, NS) and cesareans for dystocia (3.4% versus 11.4%, NS), but comparisons probably did not reach significance because of small group size.

Comparing groups 1 and 2 shows the effect of early epidural on dilating rapidly. Group 2 women were more likely to have oxytocin (20% versus 49%, $p < 0.0004$), but not cesareans (1.7% versus 4.4%, NS). Again, the power of this comparison was low.

Comparing groups 1 and 3 shows the effect of late epidural on dilating rapidly. Group 3 was more likely to have oxytocin (43% versus 20%, $p < 0.005$) and cesareans for dystocia (1.7% versus 11.4%, $p < 0.02$).

Comparing all nonepidural (groups 1, 4) with all epidural groups (groups 2, 3, 5, 6), the authors found that women with epidurals were more likely to have oxytocin 34% versus 71%, $p < 0.00001$) and cesareans for dystocia (2.4% versus 15.6%, $p < 0.000001$). The cesarean rate for fetal distress in the nonepidural versus the epidural group was 1.9% versus 2.7%. [Epidurals do not protect against fetal distress.] The cesarean rate for dystocia correlated with time of placement of epidural (28% ≤ 3 cm, 16% 4 cm, 11% ≥ 5 cm, $p < 0.01$). Rate of dilation prior to epidural also correlated with cesarean for dystocia (23.3% ≤ 0.33 cm/hr, 11.5% 0.33-0.66 cm/hr, 6.8% ≥ 0.66 cm/hr, $p < 0.01$). Women with early epidurals were more likely to have OP or OT babies during second stage compared with women with no epidural (21.8% versus 9.0%, $p = 0.0002$) and early epidural (21.8% versus 5.2%, $p = 0005$), but incidence was similar for late epidural (5.2%) and no epidural (9.0%).

14. Thorp JA et al. The effect of intrapartum epidural analgesia on nulliparous labor: a randomized, controlled, prospective trial. *Am J Obstet Gynecol* **1993;169(4):851-858.** (initial bolus 0.25%, infusion 0.125%)

Nulliparas in spontaneous labor were randomly assigned to epidural (N = 48) or narcotic (N = 45) analgesia. Cesarean for dystocia was never performed during latent phase and was performed only after oxytocin augmentation and documentation by intrauterine catheter of adequate labor.

Epidurals associated with oxytocin use (26.7% versus 58.3%, $p < 0.05$), OP or OT baby persisting into second stage (4.4% versus 18.8%, $p < 0.05$) (RR 4.3 CI 1.8-6.8), cesarean rate (2.2% versus 25.0%, $p < 0.05$) (RR 11.4 CI 5.8-16.9), and cesarean for dystocia (2.2% versus 16.7%, $p < 0.05$) (RR 7.6 CI 2.8-12.4). The only woman who had a cesarean (for dystocia) in the nonepidural group was the sole woman who actually had an epidural. The risk of cesarean was 50% if the epidural was placed at 2 cm dilation, 33% if placed at 3 cm, 26% if placed at 4 cm, and nil if placed at 5 cm or more ($p < 0.05$). The cesarean rate for fetal distress for epidural versus nonepidural groups was 0 versus 8.3% (NS). The study was originally to have 100 women per group; however, it was discontinued when a significant increase in cesareans was demonstrated "because it would be unethical to continue randomization." [I wonder if they would have gotten a significant difference in cesareans for fetal distress if they had continued.] Before analgesia, women in both groups rated pain at about 7.8 on a scale of 1 to 10. After analgesia, scores in the narcotic group dropped to about 7 but increased to 9 as labor progressed. Scores in the epidural group dropped to about 2.8 and increased to 5 as labor progressed. [So women with epidurals were not pain free.] "Nulliparous patients who are offered epidural analgesia in labor should be informed that it may increase their risk of cesarean delivery."

COMPLICATIONS

Papers Including Complications in Both Mother and Baby

15. Abboud TK et al. Continuous infusion epidural analgesia in parturients receiving bupivacaine, chloroprocaine, or lidocaine—maternal, fetal, and neonatal effects. *Anesth Analg* 1984;63:421-428. (bupivacaine: initial bolus 0.5%; infusion 0.125%)

Healthy women in normal labor with continuous epidurals either with bupivacaine ($N = 23$), chloroprocaine ($N = 19$), or lidocaine ($N = 19$) were compared. Thirty percent of bupivacaine mothers had cesareans versus 11% of chloroprocaine women versus 5% with lidocaine. All were for failure to progress except one, done for fetal bradycardia. Adding forceps and vacuum extraction deliveries, operative delivery rates were 57% bupivicaine, 15% chloroprocaine, and 16% lidocaine ($p < 0.02$). Sixteen percent of the women developed hypotension in response to the anesthetic; incidence was similar among groups.

Umbilical vein lidocaine levels were approximately half that found in the mother's blood, and bupivacaine levels were one-third the mother's. Bupivacaine was significantly more likely to cause abnormal FHR patterns (43% versus 16% versus 10%, $p < 0.05$). Behavioral test scores were lowest in the lidocaine babies, and all scores were lower compared with unmedicated babies; however, differences did not reach significance [possibly due to the low numbers of subjects]. The authors attribute the excessive bupivacaine cesarean rate to CPD since six of the seven cesareans were for failure of descent in second stage and the anesthetic was allowed to wear off. [It seems unlikely that 26% (6/23) of the bupivacaine mothers coincidentally had CPD. That the epidural was discontinued is not a convincing rationale. Abstract 3 concluded that discontinuing the epidural may not help.]

16. Corke BC and Spielman FJ. Problems associated with epidural anesthesia in obstetrics. *Obstet Gynecol* 1985;65(6):837-839.

When a study that showed lidocaine and mepivacaine caused decreased muscle tone in newborns ("floppy, but alert") these drugs were replaced by bupivacaine and 2-chloroprocaine, although subsequent testing failed to confirm the effect with lidocaine.

"This happy situation was rudely interrupted in 1980 by a series of reports of permanent neurologic deficits after the use of 2-chloroprocaine," a problem subsequently discovered to occur with accidental injection of large amounts of any local anesthetic into the subarachnoid space.

Bupivacaine caused several deaths from cardiac arrest after accidental intravascular injection, something easy to do in pregnant women because they have "enormously dilated" epidural veins. Bupivacaine is more toxic than other local anesthetics; the margin of safety between the occurrence of relatively harmless seizures and the onset of cardiovascular collapse is much smaller. Also, cardiopulmonary resuscitation is particularly difficult in pregnant women.

Lidocaine, 2-chloroprocaine, and bupivacaine are still used, although the most concentrated solution of bupivacaine was banned. Safety measures are not foolproof. "Only personnel with appropriate skills should be responsible for the management of such blocks so the potential for catastrophes is minimal. Should they occur, the appropriate measures therefore can be undertaken promptly."

17. Nel JT. Clinical effects of epidural block during labour. A prospective study. *S Afr Med J* 1985;68(6):371-374. (0.5%)

On a high-risk delivery unit, 62 women, 21 of whom had hypertension, had an epidural after 4 cm dilation. Hypotension (defined as a fall in systolic pressure to below 100 mm Hg) occurred in 32% of the women after administration of the epidural; all were successfully treated. Women with hypertension experienced a greater mean fall in blood pressure, and 17 (81%) of them needed no other antihypertensive treatment during labor.

Of the fetuses, five (9%) showed improved FHR pattern and 16 (27%) worsened. Six (37%) of these 16 cases were associated with maternal hypotension, and four of the six improved when maternal hypotension was corrected. The cesarean rate was (19.4%), none for epidural-related fetal distress. Of women delivering vaginally, 44% had an instrumental delivery. Half of these (54%) were due to inadequate bearing-down efforts. Bladder atony resulted in a 19% catheterization rate. By lowering blood pressure, epidurals benefited hypertensive women but at increased risk of hypotension, which in this group may further reduce already inadequate placental perfusion. [FHR abnormalities were also common (6/21, or 29%), but with no hypertensive nonepidural control group, conclusions cannot be drawn.]

18. Cheek TG and Gutsche BB. Epidural analgesia for labor and vaginal delivery. *Clin Obstet Gynecol* 1987;30(3):515-529.

This clinical practice paper champions epidurals yet surrounds them with cautions and precautions:

- The person administering the epidural should be skilled in emergency management of the airway and toxic reactions and should have resuscitation equipment and medications on hand. Nursing staff should be sufficient for continuous one-on-one care. An anesthesiologist and obstetrician should be immediately available.

- "Epidural catheters occasionally migrate into both intravascular and subarachnoid spaces."

- With continuous infusions, the pump must be labeled and all injection ports taped so that nothing but the anesthetic gets into the epidural space.

- Maternal hypotension is the most common side effect; if ignored, it "can create significant maternal or fetal morbidity and mortality." Hypotension, by reducing uterine blood flow, is particularly dangerous for high-risk fetuses who may not tolerate even a 15% to 20% fall in maternal blood pressure. [Later the authors recommend epidural anesthesia in these very cases to provide the fetus a "stress-free labor."] Hypotension must be treated before the mother loses consciousness, lest vomiting and pulmonary aspiration occur.

- Since epidural veins are "often" entered during administration of epidural block, ways of diagnosing this are given. None is perfectly reliable, and an epinephrine-containing test dose can cause complications of its own.

- If the anesthetic is injected into the subarachnoid space, a high or total spinal results. "If managed properly, a high or total spinal block should not endanger the life of either the mother or fetus." If the anesthetic was chloroprocaine, "the risk of neural tissue toxicity can be decreased by draining the CSF [cerebrospinal fluid] and replacing it with an irrigant of preservative-free saline."

19. Uitvlugt A. Managing complications of epidural analgesia. *Internat Anesthes Clin* **1990;28(1):11-16.**

This detailed commentary on preventing and treating epidural complications stresses the importance of trained personnel, close monitoring of mother and baby, precautionary measures, and because precautions fail, the availability of resuscitation equipment and drugs.

Complications of procedure: Accidental subarachnoid injection causes high spinals; the woman loses the ability to speak, to breathe, and finally consciousness. Accidental intravascular injection causes central nervous system (confusion, muscle twitches, convulsions) and cardiovascular (hypotension, bradycardia, respiratory depression or arrest) toxicity. Hypotension, "a common effect," causes decreased uterine blood flow and fetal bradycardia. If the dura is punctured by a large-bore needle or catheter, the incidence of spinal headache approaches 50%. Since the catheter can migrate, precautions should be repeated at each top-up. [What about continuous infusions?]

Complications of drugs: In rare cases, anaphylactic shock occurs in reaction to the anesthetic. Lidocaine may accumulate in preterm or distressed fetuses, possibly impairing their ability to adapt to asphyxia. Bupivacaine is more cardiotoxic than lidocaine or chloroprocaine and is more likely to cause cardiac arrest if injected vascularly. With bupivacaine, the patient may not be able to be resuscitated. Chloroprocaine should be given "only after a test dose with another agent shows unequivocally that the catheter is not in the intrathecal space [because it does permanent nerve damage]." Epinephrine can cause hypotension, which decreases placental blood flow. Epinephrine should be avoided in preeclamptic or eclamptic patients because they are especially sensitive to catecholamines. The addition of narcotics causes itching or nausea and vomiting in 10% to 30% of patients and can cause respiratory depression or even arrest.

Nerve injury: The needle or catheter may injure a nerve. Recovery may take as long as 12 weeks. Most neurologic problems after the birth (numbness, pain, or muscle weakness in leg or buttock) are due to faulty positioning or forceps trauma. [These occur without epidural anesthesia, but if the mother is not numbed, she would be more likely to shift from an uncomfortable position and less likely to need forceps]. If the mother has a blood-borne infection or is taking anticoagulants, an abscess or hematoma may form. These often do irreversible nerve damage even when promptly recognized and treated.

Mother Only

20. Crawford JS. Some maternal complications of epidural analgesia for labour. *Anaesthesia* **1985;40(12):1219-1225.**

"[T]here appears to be no reliable data relating to the incidence of complications of [epidural anesthesia] and to the grades of severity of such complications." This review of 26,490 consecutive cases was undertaken to fill that gap. [Yet epidurals have achieved immense popularity, and millions of women have been assured of their safety without this information.] The review excluded elective c-section, complications of anesthesia failure, and brief episodes of hypotension, backache, and bladder problems. Case histories were presented of life-threatening, serious, and moderately serious complications.

The authors found nine (1:3000) potentially life-threatening complications, of which three (1:9000) caused a "relatively protracted period of real concern." These were intravenous or intrathecal injection causing loss of consciousness, convulsions, cardiopulmonary arrest, hypotension, or respiratory difficulty and fetal distress. There were as well two serious but not life-threatening complications: (1) foreign matter provoked cyst formation, which impinged on a nerve, causing foot drop (surgery effected a cure), and (2) an abscess formed due to an undetected strep infection (surgery effected a cure). There were 13 moderately serious complications, including prolonged hypotension; severe hypertension; persistent postpartum backache, leg ache, numbness, or weakness; and 17 mildly disturbing complications. A number of moderate and mild complications were blamed on the epidural but turned out to have other causes. The test dose did not prevent intrathecal or intravenous injection, and all the major problems occurred with experienced anesthesiologists.

21. Ong BY et al. Paresthesias and motor dysfunction after labor and delivery. *Anesth Analg* **1987;66:18-22.**

Reviewing the charts of 23,827 births over a 9-year period gave occurrence rates for paresthesias [abnormalities of sensation] and motor dysfunction [abnormalities of muscle control] of 36.2 per 10,000 for patients with epidurals versus 18.9 per 10,000 for deliveries overall, 2.4 per 10,000 for women with no analgesia, and 6.3 per 10,000 for women with inhalational analgesia. [Charts are likely to underreport problems.] The epidural rate was 40%. These injuries were more likely among primiparas than multiparas ($p < 0.02$) and with instrumental compared with spontaneous deliveries ($p < 0.03$). All were minor and resolved with supportive therapy. [They may not have been minor to the mother.] The authors believe that the increased instrumental delivery rate associated with epidurals was the likely cause of the difference rather than the epidural itself.

22. Scott DB and Hibbard BM. Serious non-fatal complications associated with extradural block in obstetric practice. *Br J Anaesth* **1990;64:537-541.**

All United Kingdom obstetric units were sent a questionnaire requesting information on the incidence and nature of serious complications following an epidural. Of the 271 obstetric units, 203 responded, representing 78% of British births. This study reports on 505,000 extradural blocks given between 1982 and 1986—84% for pain relief in labor and 16% for cesarean section.

Adverse events included (1) three cases of cardiac arrest, one leading to brain damage; (2) 39 cases of nerve damage, two with permanent effect; (3) one case of spinal abscess and one of hematoma, both listed as "still improving"; (4) six cases of urinary problems "of sufficient severity to be remembered"; (5) five cases of severe backache; (6) one case of memory loss; (7) 22 cases of dural tap, 16 causing severe headache, five leading to cranial nerve palsy, and one to subdural hematoma; (8) 20 cases of convulsions; (9) eight high or total spinals leading to paralysis of the respiratory muscles; and (10) one case of allergic shock. [It is a safe bet that with self-reporting on a voluntary basis, complications were underreported.]

23. Yancey MK et al. Maternal and neonatal effects of outlet forceps delivery compared with spontaneous vaginal delivery in term pregnancies. *Obstet Gynecol* **1991;78(4):646-650.** (infusion 2% chlorprocaine or 0.25% bupivacaine)

When the fetal head had descended to +2 station in the anterior position, women were randomly assigned to spontaneous birth ($N = 168$) or outlet forceps delivery ($N = 165$). Women who had epidurals made up half the group (7 of 14) that had to be excluded from the spontaneous arm because they required forceps. No woman who had an epidural was in the group (none of 13) that was excluded from the forceps arm because spontaneous birth was imminent. Infant outcomes were similar, but more women in the forceps group had episiotomy (93% versus 78%, $p < 0.05$) and tears into or through the rectal sphincter (24% versus 10%, $p < 0.05$). [See Chapter 14 for the consequences of deep tears.]

24. MacArthur C, Lewis M, and Knox EG. Investigation of long term problems after obstetric epidural anaesthesia. *BMJ* **1992;304:1279-1282.**

Data on long-term postpartum effects (meaning began at 3 months or less after birth, lasted 6 or more weeks, never experienced prior to birth) of epidurals were gathered from hospital case notes and postal questionnaires mailed to mothers. Data ranged from 13 months to 9 years postpartum. No information on severity was obtained. The 11,701 women represented 78% or more of those mailed questionnaires. Of them, 4766 had epidurals, and 6935 did not. Discriminant analysis was used because it eliminates associations with epidurals that might arise because epidurals associate with more interventive deliveries. [But since epidurals cause operative delivery, they could be an indirect cause of problems in such cases.]

Symptoms that were more likely to be reported after epidural were backache (18.2% versus 10.2%, $p < 0.001$), frequent headaches (4.6% versus 2.9%, $p < 0.001$), migraines (1.9% versus 1.1%, $p < 0.001$), neckache (2.4% versus 1.6%, $p < 0.01$), tingling in the hands (3.0% versus 2.2%, $p < 0.01$), dizziness or fainting (2.1% versus 1.6%, $p < 0.05$), and visual disturbances (1.7% versus 1.3% [no p value given]). Spinal headache occurred in 34 women as a result of accidental dural puncture (0.1% of all epidurals) or spinal anesthesia (2.5% of all spinal blocks). Although this headache is believed to subside within a week even without treatment, nine women reported the headache lasted more than 6 weeks and five that it lasted more than 1 year. Headache, neckache, and tingling related to epidural only when reported in association with backache. Visual disturbances related only to migraine. In response to an open-ended question, 26 women reported numbness or tingling in lower back, buttocks, or leg, of whom 23 had an epidural—a "highly significant" difference. Most symptoms had lasted much longer than the six weeks of the study definition. "About two thirds were still present at the time of our inquiry. It was clear that many problems had become chronic."

Baby Only

Physical Adverse Effects

25. Clark DA and Landaw SA. Bupivacaine alters red blood cell properties: a possible explanation for neonatal jaundice associated with maternal anesthesia. *Pediatr Res* 1985;19(4):341-343.
"Neonatal jaundice has been correlated with epidural anesthesia. Bupivacaine has been especially suspect." This study confirms through in vitro and in vivo experiments that bupivacaine, compared with lidocaine, mepivacaine, or buffer, shortens neonatal red blood cell lifetime. [Neonatal jaundice results when the infant cannot cope with the breakdown products of dead red blood cells, so shortened survival time increases the likelihood of jaundice. See also Chapter 11. IV fluids, especially nonisotonic solutions given in bolus amounts, as is done prior to an epidural, cause swelling and rupture of red blood cells from osmotic pressure.]

26. Stavrou C, Hofmeyr GJ, and Boezaart AP. Prolonged fetal bradycardia during epidural analgesia. *S Afr Med J* 1990;77:66-68. (initial bolus 0.375%, top-ups of 0.25% or infusion 0.08%)
The fetal monitor tracings of 207 women in normal labor with epidural anesthesia were analyzed. Prolonged bradycardia (defined as a fall in FHR of at least 50 beats per minute below the previous rate and lasting 3 minutes or more) occurred in 11% of the fetuses. In two cases, this led to an emergency cesarean and in three cases to an instrumental delivery. The cesarean rate was 31.4%, and 26.1% of those delivering vaginally had assisted deliveries. (Primiparas made up 79% of the population.) Since maternal hypotension "did not seem to play an important role" in this study, the authors theorized that the adrenaline-containing test dose was the culprit. The authors concluded that although epidurals associated with fetal bradycardia, this was not of clinical significance because all babies were fine. [Apparently the authors consider the two epidural-caused cesareans to be trivial.]

27. Eddleston JM et al. Comparison of the maternal and fetal effects associated with intermittent or continuous infusion of extradural analgesia. *Br J Anaesth* 1992;69:154-158. (intermittent bolus 0.25% versus infusion 0.125%)
To examine the effect of epidurals on FHR in first-stage labor, 80 healthy primigravidas in established labor with normal FHR who wanted epidural anesthesia were randomly and evenly assigned to either intermittent bolus (group A) or continuous infusion with top-ups as required (group B). Two women in the bolus group and three in the infusion group (6.2%) got no pain relief from the epidural. Five EFM tracings were missing. [This may be an important omission.]
The cesarean rate was 15% (six women per group) and 40% of group A had instrumental delivery versus 53% of group B (NS). Five percent of the women in each group

experienced hypotension (systolic arterial pressure < 100 mm Hg or drop > 30 mm Hg) after top-ups. Most babies experienced FHR decelerations (72.7%) after the epidural was given, and almost half (47.9%) of these decelerations were associated with top-ups or an increase in the infusion rate. None was associated with maternal hypotension. Group A had 20 deceleratory episodes lasting more than 10 minutes on 38 tracings (53%), of which 11 (55%) were related to top-ups. Group B had 27 similar events on 37 tracings (73%), of which 13 (35%) were related to top-ups or increase in infusion rate. "Fetal myocardial uptake is the proposed mechanism to explain a proportion of fetal decelerations observed within a relatively short time interval (30 min) after . . . injection of bupivacaine."

Behavioral Adverse Effects

28. Murray AD et al. Effects of epidural anesthesia on newborns and their mothers. *Child Develop* 1981;52:71-82.

The effects of an epidural on newborn behavior were assessed among women having vaginal births. Twenty mothers had a bupivacaine epidural, 20 mothers a bupivacaine epidural plus oxytocin, and 15 control mothers "little or no medication." Bupivacaine was found in umbilical vein plasma. Five women were excluded from the control group because fetal blood levels of lidocaine from the local perineal injection for episiotomy were so high. These babies exhibited the same "worrisome" symptoms as the epidural babies. Those conducting neonatal behavioral tests and evaluating mother-baby inter-actions were blinded to groups.

Epidural mothers were more likely to have malpositions (0 unmedicated, 25% epidural, 40% oxytocin and epidural, $p < 0.02$) and forceps deliveries (0 unmedicated, 60% epidural, 80% oxytocin and epidural, $p < 0.01$). They were also more likely to be separated from their babies (0 unmedicated, 20% epidural, 30% oxytocin and epidural, $p < 0.07$ [probably did not reach significance because the groups were so small]). During the first 24 hours, medicated babies performed poorly compared with control babies. Oxytocin and forceps delivery further depressed scores. By the fifth day, scores had improved, but medicated babies still showed poor state organization [crying, feeding, alertness, sleeping]. The mother's observations of behavior and feedings agreed with scores. A higher incidence of neonatal jaundice in the oxytocin-epidural group may have contributed to lowering scores. Twenty percent needed phototherapy versus none in the unmedicated group and 5% in the epidural-only group. By one month, few differences between groups persisted, but mothers of medicated babies perceived them to be more difficult to care for. The authors theorize that the first days of life may have an imprinting effect on the mother's perceptions.

29. Kuhnert BR, Linn PL, and Kuhnert PM. Obstetric medication and neonatal behavior. *Clin Perinatol* 1985;12(2):423-439.

Confined to recent studies, this review paper focuses on the difficulties of conducting studies on behavioral effects of labor medications in the newborn and evaluating the results. Epidural anesthetic medications do affect the newborn, but the significance of the effect is debated.

Fever

30. Fusi L et al. Maternal pyrexia associated with the use of epidural analgesia in labour. *Lancet* **Jun 3, 1989;1250-1252.** (0.375%)

Fifteen healthy women in spontaneous labor who had no evidence of infection and used pethidine [a narcotic] for pain relief were compared with a similar group of 18 women who had epidurals. Temperatures were taken both orally and vaginally. The body temperature of the pethidine group remained constant; the vaginal temperature of the epidural group rose roughly 1° centigrade every seven hours ($p < 0.001$). Vaginal and oral temperatures correlated. In the mother, pyrexia [fever], even in the absence of uterine infection, can lead to hypertonic [overly contracted] uterus, hypotension, tachycardia [rapid heartbeat], and metabolic acidosis. Maternal fever can cause fever in the fetus, leading to tachycardia, and reduced ability to adapt to the stress of labor [also separation from the mother after birth and a septic workup to rule out infection]. Persistent fetal fever can lead to hypotension and acidosis.

31. Macaulay JH, Bond K, and Steer PJ. Epidural analgesia in labor and fetal hyperthermia. *Obstet Gynecol* **1992;80(4):665-669.** (0.5%)

An intrauterine probe was used to measure uterine wall and fetal skin temperature in laboring women, of whom 33 had epidurals and 24 used other methods of pain control. Maternal oral temperatures were also taken. Only two women had oral temperatures over 37.5° C, but uterine temperatures rose above this point in 45% of the epidural versus 8% of the nonepidural group. Among the fetuses, 30%, all from the epidural group, had skin temperatures over 38° C. Maximum fetal skin temperature correlated with time since epidural induction ($p = 0.012$), but there was no correlation with time in the nonepidural group. Anesthetic dosage also did not correlate with temperature. An estimated 5% of fetuses reached a core temperature more than 40° C, all in association with an epidural. "[T]he fetus whose mother has a long labor using epidural analgesia in a hot environment may reach a temperature at which heat-induced neurologic injury can occur."

NEWER TECHNIQUES OFFER NO IMPROVEMENT

Continuous Infusion

32. Bogod DG, Rosen M, and Rees GAD. Extradural infusion of 0.125% bupivacaine at 10 Ml H^{-1} to women during labour. *Br J Anaesth* **1987;59(3):325-330.** (initial bolus 0.5%, top-ups 0.5% or 0.25%, infusion 0.125%)

Outcomes were compared between primigravidae assigned to continuous infusion ($N = 50$) or to intermittent top-ups ($N = 50$). Twenty percent of the infusion group versus 18% of the top-up group had cesareans. Fifty-two percent of the infusion group versus 46% who had top-ups had instrumental deliveries. Eighty-two percent of the infusion group had bladder catheterizations versus 84% of the top-up group. The mean maximum decrease in systolic blood pressure was 16 mm Hg in the infusion group versus 17 mm Hg in the top-up group and the mean slowest fetal heart rate was 122 beats per minute in the infusion group versus 118 beats per minute among top-ups. [The lower limit of normal is 120 beats per minute. The mean does not tell how many babies experienced bradycardia or how severely.]

33. Smedstad KG and Morison DH. A comparative study of continuous and intermittent epidural analgesia for labour and delivery. *Can J Anaesth* **1988;35(3):234-241.** (initial bolus 0.25%, top-ups 0.25%, infusion 0.25%)

Twenty-eight women had continuous infusions, of whom 29% had a cesarean, 11% had mid-forceps, and 43% had low forceps. Twenty-nine women had an initial bolus and top-ups, of whom 24% had cesarean sections and 7% had mid-forceps, and 17% had low forceps. Continuous epidural anaesthesia offers no improvement over top-ups with regard to cesarean section and mid-forceps. Top-ups reduced the need for low forceps ($p < 0.05$).

Anesthetic Plus Narcotic

34. Chestnut DH et al. Continuous infusion epidural analgesia during labor: A randomized, double-blind comparison of 0.0625% bupivacaine/0.0002% fentanyl versus 0.125% bupivacaine. *Anesthesiol* **1988;68:754-759.** (see article title)

When 41 healthy nulliparous women with a fentanyl-bupivacaine epidural were compared with a similar group of 39 women with a bupivacaine epidural, outcomes were similar. Cesarean rates were 15% and 18% and forceps rates were 27% and 21%, respectively. [These forceps rates were despite discontinuing the infusion at full dilation and delaying pushing one hour if the mother felt no urge to push.] Of the fentanyl-bupivacaine group, 27% were augmented with oxytocin after the epidural started (37% were already on IV oxytocin) versus an 18% augmentation rate among the bupivacaine epidural group (33% were already on IV oxytocin). Eight fetuses in each group had FHR patterns alarming enough to prompt fetal scalp blood pH determinations (20% total fetal distress rate), and 39% fentanyl-bupivacaine babies versus 31% bupivacaine babies had meconium-stained amniotic fluid. Fentanyl-bupivacaine women were more likely to experience pruritis [mild itching] (22% versus 5%).

35. Naulty JS. Continuous infusions of local anesthetics and narcotics for epidural analgesia in the management of labor. *Int Anesthes Clin* **1990;28(1):17-24.**

Naulty reviews the literature on narcotic-bupivacaine epidurals and pure narcotic epidurals. He favors narcotic-bupivacaine epidurals because there is less total dosage and less motor blockade (leg paralysis). Even so, he reports on two studies where this did not increase the percentage of spontaneous deliveries.

PRECAUTIONS ARE NOT FOOLPROOF

Test Dose

36. Prince G and McGregor D. Obstetric test doses. *Anaesthesia* **1986;41:1240-1249.**

This review article answers several questions:

Is the test dose necessary? The test dose helps avoid "two potentially lethal complications": total spinal block and intravascular injection. The incidence of each is 3 to 10 per 10,000 epidurals. Three fatal cases of spinal block have been reported in the U.K. since 1984. Twenty-two cases of maternal cardiac arrest following intravascular injection of bupivacaine were reported, of which 15 were fatal and led to the banning of 0.75% bupivacaine. A two-stage safety check—aspiration to check for blood or cerebrospinal fluid and injection of a small test dose—minimizes these risks.

Is the test dose safe? When placental blood flow is inadequate, "even small intravenous injections of adrenaline can be dangerous to the fetus."

Is the test dose effective? The aspiration test can fail if (1) the catheter is blocked; (2) if aspiration is done through the needle, but then the catheter punctures a blood vessel (occurs ≤ 9% of the time) or the dura (occurs "less frequently"); (3) there is an air lock; or (4) cerebrospinal fluid is misidentified as saline injected during localization of the epidural space. Intravascular injection can occur if (1) the aspiration test is not done; (2) an inadequate amount of anesthetic is injected in the test dose or adrenaline is not used; (3) the test dose is misinterpreted; or (4) the catheter migrates later in labor. Failure of the test dose to predict subarachnoid injection can occur if (1) the aspiration test is not done; (2) the test dose is inadequate; (3) the test dose is misinterpreted; or (4) the catheter migrates.

Despite all precautions, intravascular and subarachnoid injection occur. "It is emphasized that these complications should not cause fatalities if trained personnel and adequate resuscitation facilities are available."

37. Leighton BL et al. Limitations of epinephrine as a marker of intravascular injection in laboring women. *Anesthesiology* **1987;66:688-691.**

Epinephrine marks accidental intravascular epidural catheter placement by increasing maternal heart rate. In this randomized double-blind study of unanesthetized healthy laboring women, 10 had saline injected intravenously and 10 had 15 Ugm epinephrine. Investigators were able to determine which mothers had received epinephrine but only after careful study of maternal heart tracings, something not feasible under clinical conditions. Identification was difficult because maternal heart rate normally varies in response to contractions. Other precautions also fail. In one study, aspiration failed to detect 65 of 194 intravascularly placed catheters, and fractionating the anesthetic dosage produced no symptoms in 12 of 51 of these patients. Epinephrine also caused two episodes of fetal distress. One woman became hypertensive, then profoundly bradycardic, which raises the question of risk in a hypertensive mother or an already compromised baby.

38. Dain SL, Rolbin SH, and Hew EM. The epidural test dose in obstetrics: is it necessary? *Can J Anaesth* **1987;34(6):601-605.**

This article reviews the controversies surrounding test doses and makes practical recommendations. The drawbacks of a test dose for intravenous placement are: (1) false positives and false negatives and (2) test dose amounts of epinephrine entering maternal circulation could decrease uterine blood flow and pose a risk to a compromised fetus. The authors recommend fractionating the dose so that each fraction acts as its own test dose. [Abstract 37 mentions that fractionation too has false negatives.]

Injecting fluid prior to catheter insertion is not recommended because it clouds the aspiration test for cerebrospinal fluid. Dry insertion results in "an acceptable incidence of paraesthesia and return of blood in the catheter." The authors also recommend inserting the catheter no more than 3 cm to minimize the risk of perforating a blood vessel or of kinking and knotting. "Until a controlled study is performed, test doses should be done . . . with the understanding that they are neither 100 per cent sensitive nor specific in preventing complications," and that epinephrine in test doses may be "detrimental to fetal wellbeing."

Technique of Administration

39. Phillips DC and Macdonald R. Epidural migration during labour. *Anaesthesia* **1987;42:661-663**
The catheter used in 100 women with epidural anesthesia was marked in centimeters. As usual, the catheter was looped, covered with gauze, and taped to the skin. At the time of removal, the catheter had migrated outward in 18 women and inward [toward the subarachnoid space] in 36, more than one third. One woman in whom it migrated inward developed a spinal headache indicative of concealed dural tap and another the "signs and symptoms of an intravenous injection" at the final top-up for episiotomy repair.

40. Rolbin SH and Hew E. A comparison of two types of epidural catheters. *Can J Anaesth* **1987;35(5):459-461.**
In a study of catheter type in 150 women with epidurals, one type of catheter had about half the rate of blood vessel injuries and nerve root irritation compared with the other, but the better catheter still had a 24% rate of nerve root irritation and a 6.7% incidence of vascular injury.

41. Rolbin SH et al. Fluid through the epidural needle does not reduce complications of epidural catheter insertion. *Can J Anaesth* **1990;37(3):337-340.**
Some anesthesiologists inject fluid through the epidural needle prior to catheter insertion either to separate the epidural tissues and permit easier passage of the catheter or as a test dose. The authors compared inserting the catheter without fluid injection ($N = 77$) versus injecting a test dose of lidocaine ($N = 68$) versus injecting saline ($N = 55$). The incidence of blood vessel trauma ranged from 9% to 10% and paresthesia [abnormal sensation] ranged from 50% to 56%. However, persisting neurologic deficits are very rare. No differences were significant. But when fluid is injected, the significance of clear fluid upon aspiration [normally a sign of dural puncture] becomes difficult to interpret.

42. McLean BY, Rottman RL, and Kotelko DM. Failure of multiple test doses and techniques to detect intravascular migration of an epidural catheter. *Anesth Analg* **1992;74(3):454-456.** (bolus 0.25%; infusion 0.0625% with 2 Ug/ml fentanyl)
A healthy primigravida had a 3-minute episode of fetal bradycardia after a top-up [see Abstracts 26 and 27 for data on the causal relationship between epidurals and bradycardia], at which time the doctor decided to perform a cesarean for fetal distress and macrosomia. Although aspiration and a test dose revealed no problems with the catheter, when lidocaine was administered for the cesarean, the mother had a grand mal seizure and a fetal bradycardia that continued until the infant was delivered by cesarean under general anesthesia eight minutes later. Mother and baby recovered.

REFERENCES

ASA. Anesthesia & You . . . Planning Your Childbirth. 1992.

Bates RG et al. Uterine activity in the second stage of labour and the effect of epidural analgesia. *Br J Obstet Gynaecol* 1985;92(12):1246-1250.

Brownridge P. Treatment options for the relief of pain during childbirth. *Drugs* 1991;41(11):69-80.

Clark RB. Fetal and neonatal effects of epidural anesthesia. *Obstet Gynecol Ann* 1985;14:240-252.

Cohn V. *News and numbers.* Ames: Iowa State University Press, 1989.

Fuchs AR. Personal communication, 1990.

Gleeson NC and Griffith AP. The management of the second stage of labour in primiparae with epidural analgesia. *Br J Clin Prac* 1991;45(2):90-91.

Goodfellow CF et al. Oxytocin deficiency at delivery with epidural analgesia. *Br J Obstet Gynaecol* 1983;90(3):214-219.

Humenick SS. Mastery: The key to childbirth satisfaction? A review. *Birth* 1981;8(2):79-83.

Humenick SS and Bugen LA. Mastery: The key to childbirth satisfaction? A study. *Birth* 1981;8(2):84-89.

Jimenez S. Supportive pain management strategies. In *Childbirth education: practice, research, and theory.* FH Nichols and SS Humenick, eds. Philadelphia: Saunders, 1988.

Johnson M and Everitt B. *Essential reproduction.* 3d ed. Cambridge, MA: Blackwell Scientific Publications, 1988.

Lagercrantz H and Slotkin T. The "stress" of being born. *Sci Am* 1986;254(4):100-107.

Manyonda IT, Shaw DE, and Drife JO. The effect of delayed pushing in the second stage of labor with continuous lumbar epidural analgesia. *Acta Obstet Gynecol Scand* 1990;69:291-295.

Oriol NE. "Report of a study on 'walking epidurals.'" Presented at Innovations in Perinatal Care: Assessing Benefits and Risks, tenth conference presented by *Birth*, Boston, Oct 31-Nov 1 1992.

Reynolds F. Epidural analgesia in obstetrics. *BMJ* 1989;299:751-752.

Richardson T. Epidural anaesthesia for obstetrics: where are we? *N Z Med J* 1988;101(856 Pt 1):657-658.

San Jose Mercury News. The natural pain of giving birth. Aug 25, 1993.

Simkin P. Stress, Pain, and catecholamines in labor: Part 1. A review. *Birth* 1986;13(4):227-233.

Simkin P. Just another day in a woman's life? Women's long-term perceptions of their first birth experiences. Part 1. *Birth* 1991;18(4):203-210.

Simkin P and Dickersin K. Control of pain in labour. In *A guide to effective care in pregnancy and childbirth.* Enkin M, Keirse MJNC, and Chalmers I, eds. Oxford: Oxford University Press, 1989.

Wuitchik M, Bakal D, and Lipshitz J. Relationships between pain, cognitive activity and epidural analgesia during labor. *Pain* 1990;41:125-132.

14

Episiotomy

Myth: *A nice clean cut is better than a jagged tear.*

Reality: *"Like any surgical procedure, episiotomy carries a number of risks: excessive blood loss, haematoma formation, and infection. . . . There is no evidence . . . that routine episiotomy reduces the risk of severe perineal trauma, improves perineal healing, prevents fetal trauma or reduces the risk of urinary stress incontinence."*

Sleep, Roberts, and Chalmers 1989

Routine or prophylactic episiotomy (as opposed to episiotomy for specific indication such as fetal distress) is the quintessential example of an obstetrical procedure that persists despite a total lack of evidence for it and a considerable body of evidence against it. All the authoritative pronouncements in favor of episiotomy descend from a 75-year-old article (DeLee 1920) that produced not a shred of evidence in its support. Most recently, *William's Obstetrics* (Cunningham, MacDonald, and Gant 1989) states, "The reasons for [episiotomy's] popularity among obstetricians are clear. It substitutes a straight, neat surgical incision for the ragged laceration that otherwise frequently results. It is easier to repair and heals better than a tear." *Human Labor and Birth* (Oxorn-Foote 1986) adds that it averts "brain damage" by "lessen[ing] the pounding of the head on the perineum." An earlier edition of *William's Obstetrics* (Pritchard, MacDonald, and Gant 1985) claims that it reduces the incidence of cystocele (a herniation of the posterior bladder through the anterior rectal wall), rectocele (a herniation of the anterior rectal wall through the posterior vaginal wall), and stress incontinence (involuntary loss of urine in response to laughing, sneezing, etc., although the 1989 edition admits this benefit is unproved). It then lists "important questions for the obstetrician concerning episiotomy," none of which is whether to do one at all.

In a branch of medicine rife with paradoxes, contradictions, inconsistencies, and illogic, episiotomy crowns them all. The major argument for episiotomy is that it protects the perineum from injury, a protection accomplished by slicing through perineal skin, connective tissue, and muscle. Obstetricians presume spontaneous tears do worse damage, but now that researchers have finally done some studies, every one has found that deep tears are almost exclusively extensions of episiotomies. This makes sense, because as anyone who has tried to tear cloth knows, intact material is extremely resistant until you snip it. Then it rips easily.

By preventing overstretching of the pelvic floor muscles, episiotomies are also supposed to prevent pelvic floor relaxation. Pelvic floor relaxation causes sexual dissatisfaction after childbirth (the concern was the male partner, of course, hence, the once-popular "husband's knot," an extra tightening during suturing that made many women's sex lives a permanent misery), urinary incontinence, and uterine prolapse. But older women currently having repair surgery for incontinence and prolapse all had generous episiotomies. In any case, episiotomy is not done until the head is almost ready to be born. By then, the pelvic floor muscles are already fully distended. Nor has anyone ever explained how cutting a muscle and stitching it back together preserves its strength.

Perhaps the most absurd rationale of all is brain damage from the fetal head's "pounding on the perineum." A woman's perineum is soft, elastic tissue, not concrete. No one has ever shown that an episiotomy protects fetal neurologic well-being, not even in the tiniest, most vulnerable preterm infants, let alone a healthy, term newborn (Lobb, Duthie, and Cooke 1986; The 1990, both abstracted below).

Meanwhile, as the authors of this chapter's "Reality" quotation point out, episiotomy, like any other surgical procedure, carries the risk of blood loss, poor wound healing, and infection. Infections are painful. Sutures must be removed to drain the wound, and later the perineum must be restitched. In their literature survey Thacker and Banta (1983, abstracted below) found wound infections and abscess rates ranging from 0.5% to 3%.

Moreover, there are two extremely rare gangrenous infections called necrotizing fasciitis and clostridial myonecrosis reported in the literature. These infections *kill* many of the women who contract them and maim the survivors. *William's Obstetrics* (Cunningham, MacDonald, and Gant 1989) says of them in boldface type, "Mortality is virtually universal without surgical treatment, and it approaches 50% even if aggressive excision is performed." While these infections are rare, they make a substantial contribution to maternal mortality. Between 1969 and 1976 they caused 27% (3/11) of the maternal deaths in Kern County, California (Ewing, Smale, and Eliot 1979). A fourth woman survived, spending 23 days in the hospital. Shy and Eschenbach (1979) report on four cases in King County, Washington, between 1969 and 1977. Three women died, representing 20% of the maternal mortality rate during those years. The fourth woman survived, losing most of her vulva to surgical excision and debridement. Nine additional cases are also reported, of which seven women died and two had extensive surgeries and prolonged hospitalizations (Soper 1986; Sutton et al. 1985; Ewing, Smale and Elliott 1979; Golde and Ledger 1977). Since all fatalities were in healthy women who had uncomplicated labors, their episiotomies literally killed them!

Obviously an infection could start in a repaired tear, but substantial numbers of women who do not have episiotomies have intact perineums. There also appears to be an association between the extent of the wound and these deadly infections. Nine of the 17 cases, or more than half, involved third- or fourth-degree injuries (tears or deliberate cuts into or through the anal sphincter). It bears repeating that women with no episiotomy hardly ever suffer deep tears.

Despite two decades of evidence to the contrary, most doctors and some midwives still cling to the liberal use of episiotomy. The Canadian multicenter randomized controlled trial (Klein et al. 1992, abstracted below) could not get doctors to abandon it. Episiotomy rates were reduced by only one-third in the so-called restricted arm of the study. More than half of primiparas in the restricted group (57%) still had episiotomies, as did nearly one-third of multiparas (31%). "The intensity with which physicians adhere to the belief that episiotomy benefits women is well illustrated by the behavior of many of the participating physicians in this trial. Many were unwilling or unable to reduce their episiotomy rate according to protocol."

If episiotomy lacks scientific rationale, what drives its use? As Robbie Davis-Floyd (1992), medical anthropologist, writes, episiotomy fits underlying cultural beliefs about women and childbirth. It reinforces beliefs about the inherent defectiveness and untrustworthiness of the female body and the dangers this poses to women and babies. So DeLee (1920), imbued with these beliefs, writes:

> Labor has been called, and still is believed by many, to be a normal function. . . . [Y]et it is a decidedly pathologic process. . . . If a woman falls on a pitchfork, and drives the handle through her perineum, we call that pathologic—abnormal, but if a large baby is driven through the pelvic floor, we say that is natural, and therefore normal. If a baby were to have its head caught in a door very lightly, but enough to cause cerebral hemorrhage, we would say that it is decidedly pathologic, but when a baby's head is crushed against a tight pelvic floor, and a hemorrhage in the brain kills it, we call this normal.

Having invented the problem, he proffers a solution: as soon as the head passes through the dilated cervix, anesthetize the woman with ether, cut a large mediolateral episiotomy, pull the baby out with forceps, and manually remove the placenta, then give the woman scopolamine and morphine for the lengthy repair work and to "prolong narcosis for many hours postpartum and to abolish the memory of labor." Repair involves pulling down the cervix with forceps to examine it and stitch any tears and laboriously reconstructing the vagina to restore "virginal conditions." While few modern obstetricians are willing to go as far as DeLee, these beliefs about women still pervade obstetrics, and they fuel episiotomy.

Episiotomy serves another purpose. Davis-Floyd observes that surgery holds the highest value in the hierarchy of Western medicine, and obstetrics is a *surgical* specialty. Episiotomy transforms normal childbirth—even natural childbirth in a birthing suite—into a surgical procedure.

Davis-Floyd also points out that episiotomy, the destruction and reconstruction of women's genitals, allows men to control the "powerfully sexual, creative, and male-threatening aspects of women." This is what lurks behind DeLee's emphasis on surgically restoring "virginal conditions." It also partially explains why most trials of episiotomy have been done in European countries where normal birth is conducted by female midwives, not in the U.S. or Canada, where birth is conducted (until recently) by male doctors: women are not subconsciously threatened by birth. Klein et al. attribute the greater success of a British "restricted" versus "liberal" use of episiotomy trial in achieving fewer episiotomies and more intact perineums to "the increased comfort of British midwives in attending births with the intention of preserving an intact perineum."

In short, routine episiotomy has a ritual function but serves no medical purpose. If any reader believes otherwise, I challenge him or her to find a credible study done in the past 15 years that supports that belief.

Note: There are two types of episiotomies: *midline* or *median* (straight down toward the rectum) and *mediolateral* (down and off to one side) U.S. and Canadian doctors usually do midline episiotomies while European doctors and midwives prefer mediolateral ones. According to *William's Obstetrics* (Cunningham, MacDonald, and Gant 1989), midline episiotomies are less painful, heal better, are less likely to cause dyspareunia (coital pain), and cause less blood loss, but they are more likely to extend into the rectum. Mediolateral episiotomies are the opposite. Because of these differences, I will note which type was performed after the abstract citation.

Also, because of these differences, I have excluded studies of mediolateral episiotomy where data were available on median episiotomies. For many areas of interest, however, they were unavailable. (For those living in countries where mediolateral episiotomy is the norm, conclusions about the benefits and risks of episiotomy were similar regardless of type.) This is because until very recently, U.S. and Canadian doctors were so convinced of episiotomy's value that they did not feel it necessary to test their theory. This was less true of European midwives, and by extension, the doctors with whom they work.

SUMMARY OF SIGNIFICANT POINTS

- Episiotomies do not prevent tears into or through the anal sphincter or vaginal tears. In fact, deep tears almost never occur in the absence of an episiotomy. (Abstracts 1-12, 16, 19-20, 23-28)

- Even when properly repaired, tears of the anal sphincter may cause chronic problems with coital pain and gas or fecal incontinence later in life. In addition, anal injury predisposes to rectovaginal fistulas. (Abstracts 11, 15, 21-22)

- If a woman does not have an episiotomy, she is likely to have a small tear, but with rare exceptions the tear will be, at worst, no worse than an episiotomy. (Abstracts 1, 2, 5, 8-10, 14, 16, 24-25)

- Episiotomies do not prevent relaxation of the pelvic floor musculature. Therefore, they do not prevent urinary incontinence or improve sexual satisfaction. (Abstracts 1-4, 7, 12-16)

- Episiotomies are not easier to repair than tears. (Abstracts 1, 3, 9)

- Episiotomies do not heal better than tears. (Abstracts 1, 5-6, 12-15, 21)

- Episiotomies are not less painful than tears. They may cause prolonged problems with pain, especially pain during intercourse. (Abstracts 1, 2, 7, 12, 14-15, 19-20)

- Episiotomies do not prevent birth injuries or fetal brain damage. (Abstracts 1, 3, 5-7, 12, 14, 17-18, 27)

- Episiotomies increase blood loss. (Abstracts 1, 12, 19)

- As with any other surgical procedure, episiotomies may lead to infection, including *fatal* infections. (Abstracts 1, 12, 19, 22)

- Epidurals increase the need for episiotomy. They also increase the probability of instrumental delivery. Instrumental delivery increases both the odds of episiotomy and deep tears. (Abstracts 5, 11-12, 21, 25-26)

- The lithotomy position increases the need for episiotomy, probably because the perineum is tightly stretched. (Abstracts 10, 25, 27)

- The birth attendant's philosophy, technique, skill, and experience are the major determinants of perineal outcome. (Abstracts 2, 5-7, 9-10, 25-27)

- Some techniques for reducing perineal trauma that have been evaluated and found effective are: prenatal perineal massage, slow delivery of the head, supporting the perineum, keeping the head flexed, delivering the shoulders one at a time, and doing instrumental deliveries without episiotomy. (Others, such as perineal massage during labor or hot compresses have yet to be studied.) (Abstracts 23-24, 28)

- Independent of specifically contracting the pelvic floor muscles (Kegels), a regular exercise program strengthens the pelvic floor. (Abstract 13)

ORGANIZATION OF ABSTRACTS

Episiotomies Do Not Perform as Advertised (Reviews)

Episiotomies Do Not Perform as Advertised (Studies)

Episiotomies Do Not Prevent Deep Tears
Episiotomies Do Not Heal Better Than Tears
Episiotomies Do Not Prevent Pelvic Floor Muscle Relaxation
Episiotomies Do Not Prevent Fetal Brain Damage

The Downside of Episiotomies

Pain and Dyspareunia
Anal Incontinence

Factors That Reduce the Probability of Tears

EPISIOTOMIES DO NOT PERFORM AS ADVERTISED (Reviews)

1. Thacker SB and Banta HD. Benefits and risks of episiotomy: an interpretive review of the English language literature, 1860-1980. *Obstet Gynecol Surv* **1983;38(6):322-338.**
The authors reviewed more than 350 articles, reports, and book chapters published between 1860 and 1980 and found no convincing evidence that episiotomy prevented tears into the rectum, damage to the pelvic wall, or trauma to the fetal head or that episiotomies were easier to repair than tears. Like any other surgery, episiotomy has risks, including extension of the incision, blood loss, dyspareunia, pain, poor healing, and infection, including *fatal* infection, all of which are documented in the literature. "[T]he risks of episiotomy are more severe than many might appreciate. Although rarely associated with a life-threatening problem, the complications of this procedure can be a source of serious morbidity to young mothers who already have major personal

and social adjustments to undergo." In some cases, episiotomy is justified but not as a routine procedure. Based on rates reported at birth centers and home births, 20% seems a reasonable episiotomy rate. "If [women] were fully informed as to the evidence for benefit and risk in the face of demonstrable risks, it is unlikely that women would readily consent to having routine episiotomies."

2. Bromberg MH. Presumptive maternal benefits of routine episiotomy. *J Nurse Midwifery* **1986;31(3):121-127.**

"A survey of the available literature is remarkable for the astonishing dearth of valid data to support long-held beliefs about episiotomy." This review focuses on two of them: preservation of pelvic floor integrity and prevention of lacerations.

Episiotomy is supposed to prevent overstretching of the muscles, which is believed to be the cause of poor perineal tone. (Poor perineal tone increases the risk of cystocele, rectocele, uterine prolapse, and stress incontinence.) What little evidence exists in favor of episiotomy is over 60 years old and of poor methodology. Some causes of pelvic floor relaxation may be iatrogenic: poor episiotomy repair or pulling the cervix down for inspection [see DeLee's protocol above]. As for prevention of lacerations, at best women do no worse without an episiotomy with respect to pain and lacerations, and some studies show an association between episiotomy and deep tears. Iatrogenic factors contributing to lacerations may include: use of techniques to shorten second stage (e.g. fundal pressure or strenuous pushing), failure to wait for shoulder rotation before delivering them, faulty repair of a previous episiotomy, and possibly injecting local anesthetic but not doing an episiotomy. "Review of the literature on episiotomy indicates the likelihood that it is over used, with shaky justification at best. It seems reasonable to infer that a median episiotomy has no great advantage over a first- [into the skin] or second-degree [into the underlying muscle] laceration when there are no overriding fetal indications." [An episiotomy is equivalent to a second-degree laceration.]

3. Hofmeyr GJ and Sonnedecker EW. Elective episiotomy in perspective. *S Afr Med J* **1987;71(6):357-359.**

This article summarized recent clinical studies and concluded that episiotomy did not prevent genital prolapse or fetal damage, was not easier to repair than a second-degree tear, did not heal better, and did not prevent third-degree laceration or impairment of coital function. The authors observed that if episiotomy is to prevent overstretching of the perineum and protect the fetal head, it must be done early, but episiotomies are not done until maximal stretching has already occurred. "If elective episiotomy does indeed confer any of the benefits conventionally ascribed to the procedure, properly controlled evidence for such benefit is yet to emerge. . . . It is the responsibility of the proponents of elective episiotomy to provide such evidence."

4. Thorp JM and Bowes WA. Episiotomy: Can its routine use be defended? *Am J Obstet Gynecol* **1989;160(5 Pt 1):1027-1030.**

The literature is reviewed for support of the two main rationales for routine episiotomy: reduction of perineal trauma and prevention of pelvic musculature relaxation. No study found that midline or mediolateral episiotomy reduced the incidence of third- or fourth-degree tears. Many found midline episiotomy associated strongly with deep tears. Some studies in the 1920s and 1930s concluded that episiotomy reduced pelvic relaxation, but they were flawed. Moreover, their conclusions do not apply to modern practice. For example, in order to prevent stretching of the pelvic floor, episiotomy would have to be performed prior to distension of the levator muscles; modern episiotomies are done much later. "[T]here is little evidence to support routine use of episiotomy. This procedure may well increase the incidence of third- and fourth-degree lacerations. There are few data to support the premise that this procedure prevents pelvic relaxation." Studies should be done to ascertain whether routine episiotomy is truly beneficial. [How much more evidence do we need that it is not?]

EPISIOTOMIES DO NOT PERFORM AS ADVERTISED (Studies)

5. Reynolds JL and Yudkin PL. Changes in the management of labour: 2. Perineal management. *Can Med Assoc J* **1987;136(10):1045-1049.** (mediolateral)

Vaginal births of singleton, vertex babies born between 1980 and 1984 were analyzed ($N = 24,439$). Changes in second stage management included more midwife-attended births, longer second stages, fewer epidurals, more spontaneous births, and, especially, fewer episiotomies. The episiotomy rate fell from 72.6% to 44.9% among primiparas and from 36.8% to 15.4% among multiparas. The percentage of intact perineums rose from 7.4% to 13.7% among primiparas and from 26.1% to 33.8% among multiparas ($p < 0.001$ for both). The incidence of first- and second-degree tears increased, but third-degree tears did not. [In other words, women were more likely to have a small tear, at most no worse than an episiotomy, but were not more likely to have a deep tear.] Third-degree tears were more common with forceps delivery compared with spontaneous birth (5.8% versus 2.6%, $p < 0.01$). Nearly all forceps deliveries included an episiotomy. Whether this is necessary has never been addressed. Rates of infection, wound breakdown, labial tears, and vulval bruising were unchanged (incidence in all cases < 0.5%). Neonatal outcomes were unchanged. Epidurals associated with episiotomy, and not having an epidural associated with intact perineum "likely due to the well-known effect of epidural analgesia on the woman's ability to push."

6. Wilcox LS et al. Episiotomy and its role in the incidence of perineal lacerations in a maternity center and a tertiary hospital obstetric service. *Am J Obstet Gynecol* **1989;160(5 Pt 1):1047-1052.** (both, but presume mostly midline because this is a U.S. study)

The study compared two groups of women of similar characteristics, 686 attended by midwives at a maternity center and 576 delivered by obstetric residents at a nearby hospital. No differences in incidence or type of laceration were found by episiotomy type, so results were combined.

At the maternity center, the episiotomy rate was less than that at the hospital for both primigravidas (82.7% versus 95.6%, $p < 0.001$) and multigravidas (44.9% versus 76.8%, $p < 0.001$). [These numbers are high for midwives.] After adjusting for institutional differences in other variables related to use of episiotomy, women were "less than half as likely" to have an episiotomy at the maternity center. Women with episiotomies suffered a marked increase in the probability of third-degree tear (OR 4.29 CI 1.58-11.69). Neither the number of days of maternal fever [a measure of infection] nor the incidence of birth injuries differed by use of episiotomy. Since place of birth was a strong predictor of episiotomy, "[i]t is not unreasonable to assume that this difference . . . is related to . . . institutional differences in philosophies." Given these results, serious questions are raised about the frequent use of episiotomy.

7. Klein M et al. Does episiotomy prevent perineal trauma and pelvic floor relaxation? *Online J Curr Clin Trials* **1992;1(Document 10).** (midline)

Between 1988 and 1990, women were randomly assigned to "restricted" (try to avoid an episiotomy) or "liberal" (try to avoid a tear) episiotomy groups. Enrollment was limited to low-risk women past 34 weeks gestation (N = 1044). Randomization took place late in second stage labor. Ultimately, 359 primiparas and 344 multiparas were randomized. Among those randomized, only 32% of primiparas and 48% of multiparas gave birth without oxytocin augmentation, epidural anesthesia, or forceps [!]. The study had 90% power to detect a 7% difference in intact perineums among primiparas and a 15% difference among multiparas, assuming a 30% dropout rate.

No infant in either group required special care or had a 5-minute Apgar less than 6. Among primiparas, the episiotomy rate was reduced by one-third in the restricted group for both primiparas (57.2% versus 81.4%) and multiparas (30.7% versus 47.0%). The reasons given for episiotomy in the restricted group were severe tear anticipated (40%), fetal distress (29%), and perineum not distending (23%). "Accustomed to the liberal or routine use of episiotomy, and despite being presented with a population of healthy, low-risk women, many physicians had difficulty in withholding episiotomy in the [restricted] arm of the trial." Among primiparas, 52 (14.5%) had episiotomy extensions, of which 46 were third or fourth degree, and six were tears into the upper vagina. Only one woman had a spontaneous deep tear. Among multiparas, 1.8% had third- or fourth-degree episiotomy extensions, and no one had a spontaneous deep tear. As measured by electromyographic perineometry, no differences were found between groups for pelvic floor functioning three months postpartum. Values related to parity, size of baby, and antepartum status. Episiotomy had no effect. No differences were found between groups for anterior vaginal trauma, pain, pain at resumption of intercourse, or female sexual satisfaction. Urinary incontinence was more prevalent in primiparous women in the restricted group (21.1% versus 14.5%, NS) and among multiparous women in the liberal group (12.9% versus 21.5%, NS). [Because outcomes are reported by group, instead of according to whether the woman had an episiotomy, we do not know how these findings relate to episiotomy.] Based on the results, the authors recommend that liberal or routine use of episiotomy be abandoned. This recommendation can be implemented only where the birth attendant has learned how to protect the perineum. Such training should be part of normal education and practice. At least some instrumental deliveries could be done without episiotomy, and doctors should be trained in that too.

Episiotomies Do Not Prevent Deep Tears

8. Gass MS, Dunn CD, and Stys SJ. Effect of episiotomy on the frequency of vaginal outlet lacerations. *J Reprod Med* **1986;31(4);240-244.** (midline)

To examine the effect of episiotomy on laceration, women having spontaneous births who either had or did not have an episiotomy were matched for age (range 18-24), parity (range 0-2), and birth weight (within 200 g) (N = 205 pairs). Commonly lacerations are considered only when they occurred in addition to an episiotomy. "[This] implie[s] that an intact perineum with no episiotomy or lacerations is equivalent to a perineum with an episiotomy and no lacerations. The validity of that statement may be questioned. To the patient they are not equivalent since she must undergo the incision, incision repair and recovery." If an episiotomy is counted as a second-degree laceration, then women with no episiotomy had fewer lacerations ($p < 0.0001$). Analyzing lacerations this way, the woman with an episiotomy will have fewer lacerations $6 \pm 3\%$ of the time, whereas the woman with no episiotomy will have fewer lacerations $78 \pm 5\%$ of the time. The 2% of women who had third- or fourth-degree lacerations all had episiotomies (17% para 0, 3% para 1, 0 para 2). However, since the study was not randomized, it is possible that episiotomy was done to forestall a tear or for fetal distress, which might raise the third- and fourth-degree tear rate. "The results of this study do not support routine use of episiotomy."

9. Thorp JM et al. Selected use of midline episiotomy: effect on perineal trauma. *Obstet Gynecol* **1987;70(2):260-262.** (midline)

One author, attending 113 women, limited his use of episiotomy to instrumental deliveries or when there was fetal distress. His episiotomy rate was 14%. He compared his outcomes with the rest of the residents, who, attending 265 women, had an unrestricted policy. Their episiotomy rate was 63%. Among all women, the incidence of third- or fourth degree tears in the unrestricted group was 13.2% versus 1.8% ($p \le 0.05$) in the restricted group. Both nulliparas (22.1% versus 1.6%, $p \le 0.001$) and multiparas (5.6% versus 1.8%, NS) were less likely to have deep tears in the restricted group. All third- and fourth- degree lacerations were preceded by an episiotomy. Deep tear rates agree with other published reports. In no case was there injury to the urethra or bladder, and there were no differences in periclitoral or periurethral tears. The only difference in perineal trauma in the restricted group was that nulliparas were more likely to have a first-degree tear. All lacerations that occurred in the absence of episiotomy were easy to repair.

10. Green JR and Soohoo SL. Factors associated with rectal injury in spontaneous deliveries. *Obstet Gynecol* **1989;73(5 Pt 1):732-738.** (midline)

Logistic regression was done on 2706 spontaneous cephalic births to determine factors associated with rectal injury (third and fourth degree). The rectal injury rate was 13.0%. Ninety percent occurred with episiotomy. The episiotomy rate was 45.5% among doctors versus 27.4% among midwives ($p < 0.0001$). The intact perineum rate among women who did not have an episiotomy ($N = 760$) was 47.7%. The adjusted odds ratio for rectal injury was 8.9 for episiotomy versus no episiotomy, 3.3 for nulliparity versus multiparity, 2.4 for physician versus midwife, and 2.0 for delivery room birth versus a labor bed. (Birth in the delivery room was in the lithotomy position; in the labor bed, a variety of positions were used, with semirecumbent the most common.) "It seems likely that midwives have the patience to allow for slow stretching of the perineum . . . and this may be an important factor that distinguishes them from many physicians." Although cause and effect cannot be proved in an observational study, the magnitude of the difference makes noncausal explanations unlikely.

11. Shiono P, Klebanoff MA, and Carey JC. Midline episiotomies: more harm than good? *Obstet Gynecol* **1990;75(5):765-770.** (both)

The association between episiotomy and severe (third and fourth degree) lacerations was studied in 24,114 women having a singleton, vertex birth of a baby weighing over 500 g. The severe tear rate was 8.3% among primiparas and 1.5% among multiparas.

Women with midline episiotomies were 50 times more likely to have a severe tear (OR 12.5 among primiparas; OR 32.3 among multiparas), and women with mediolateral episiotomies were eight times more likely to have a severe tear (OR 1.2 among primiparas; OR 5.3 among multiparas) compared with women with no episiotomy. Forceps increased the odds eightfold. All differences were significant. After statistical adjustment for confounding factors, midline episiotomy increased the risk of deep tears 4.2-fold among primiparas and 12.8-fold among multiparas. Mediolateral episiotomy reduced the risk of deep tears 2.5-fold among primiparas and increased it 2.4-fold among multiparas (NS) compared with no episiotomy. Forceps use tripled the probability of severe lacerations. Although mediolateral episiotomy offered some protection against severe tears for primiparas, studies have found they have other problems, including increased pain, poorer cosmetic results, and more dyspareunia. Since most rectovaginal fistulas occur after severe tears, reducing the rate of these tears would result in fewer fistulas and less morbidity.

Episiotomies Do Not Heal Better Than Tears

12. McGuiness M, Norr K, and Nacion K. Comparison between different perineal outcomes on tissue healing. *J Nurse Midwifery* 1991;36(3):192-198. (both but presumably mostly midline because this is a U.S. study)

The article begins with a brief literature review concluding that episiotomy does not improve healing, prevent pelvic floor relaxation, prevent lacerations, or protect the fetus. Episiotomy increases the risk of infection, including fatal infection, causes short-term and long-term pain and dyspareunia, and causes "considerable" blood loss.

Perineal healing was compared one to two weeks postpartum between 181 women with episiotomies and 186 women without them (episiotomy rate 49%). All women were indigent low-risk women who had spontaneous births. Only 2% of the no-episiotomy group had third-degree lacerations versus 15% of the episiotomy group (third- and fourth-degree tears were collapsed into one category). In the episiotomy group 7.7% of women experienced delayed healing versus 2.2% in the no-episiotomy group ($p < 0.05$). The difference persisted when women with intact perineums (53% of the no-episiotomy group) were excluded. None of the four third-degree lacerations that occurred without episiotomy exhibited delayed healing versus 18.5% of the 27 deep tears that occurred with epsiotomy. Both infections occurred in women with episiotomies (midline with first-degree periurethral tear; mediolateral with third-degree extension). Women who had instrumental deliveries were excluded. However, this group had a 35% third-degree extension rate, and delayed healing occurred in 17.6%, confirming that instrumental delivery increases perineal trauma. "This suggests that women without episiotomies exhibit better perineal healing than women with episiotomies."

Episiotomies Do Not Prevent Pelvic Floor Muscle Relaxation

13. Gordon H and Logue M. Perineal muscle function after childbirth. *Lancet* 1985;2:123-125. (unstated, but presumably mediolateral because this is a British study)

The strength of the perineal muscles was measured in primiparas one year after delivery. Women with an intact perineum, a second-degree laceration, an episiotomy, and a forceps delivery with episiotomy were compared with women who had a cesarean and nulliparas. No differences were found among groups. Women were also grouped by whether they exercised regularly, had done only postpartum exercises, or never exercised. Regardless of perineal history, women who exercised regularly fared best, those who did postpartum exercises fell in the middle, and those who did not exercise did worst ($p < 0.0001$ for no exercise compared with postpartum exercise and regular exercise). Exercise regimens included fitness classes, walking, jogging, running, swimming, dancing, and yoga. Few women specifically did pelvic floor contractions [Kegels]. "This study does not support the theory that episiotomy results in improved healing and better perineal muscle function."

14. Sleep J et al. West Berkshire perineal management trial. *Br Med J*;289:587-**590.** (mediolateral)

Women were allocated to either "avoid episiotomy" [restricted group] ($N = 498$) or "prevent a tear" [liberal group] ($N = 502$). The study had 90% power to detect a significant difference if restricted policy doubled the incidence of an outcome expected in 5% of cases.

The episiotomy rate was 10% in the restricted group versus 51% in the liberal group. The restricted group experienced more perineal tears and labial tears and had more intact perineums. "Severe maternal trauma" (defined as extension through the anal sphincter, the rectal mucosa, or to the upper third of the vagina) occurred in four cases in the restricted group versus one case in the liberal group (NS). More women in the liberal group required suturing (78% versus 69%, $p < 0.01$). Neonatal outcomes were similar. There were no differences in reporting of pain [which may reflect only that pain relief measures were effective] or in the use of analgesics at 10 days postpartum (3% versus 2%). Twelve percent of each group sought medical advice for perineal problems. However, 37% of the restricted group versus 27% of the liberal group resumed sexual intercourse within one month after birth ($p < 0.01$). By three months postpartum, the prevalence of dyspareunia was similar (22% versus 18%). Equal numbers of women were breastfeeding at 10 days (70%) and 3 months (48%). [This is a confounding factor for dyspareunia. Breastfeeding women may experience vaginal dryness due to low estrogen levels.] No differences were found for stress incontinence. "A large proportion of women (19%) had involuntary loss of urine three months after delivery, but there is no evidence from this study that the liberal use of episiotomy prevents this problem."

15. Sleep J and Grant A. West Berkshire perineal management trial: Three year follow up. *Br Med J* 1987;32(3):181-183. (mediolateral)

Of the original 1000 women [see Abstract 14], 674 filled out a questionnaire three years later. The response rate was 91% among those still at the same address. Dyspareunia was reported by 16% of the restrictive episiotomy group versus 13% of the liberal group. Stress incontinence was reported among 34% of the restrictive versus 36% of the liberal group. For 9% and 8%, respectively, problems were severe enough to wear a pad. Three of the four women in the restrictive group with severe trauma had minor degrees of urinary incontinence and/or dyspareunia. The one woman with severe trauma in the liberal group reported no problems. "There was no clear difference between the groups with respect to dyspareunia. There was also no difference in the prevalence of urinary incontinence, even when the severity and nature of the incontinence, and subsequent deliveries, were taken into account."

16. Rockner G, Jonasson A, and Olund A. The effect of mediolateral episiotomy at delivery on pelvic floor muscle strength evaluated with vaginal cones. *Acta Obstet Gynecol Scand* **1991;70(1):51-54.** (mediolateral)

Pelvic floor muscle strength pre- and postpartum was evaluated by measuring the mother's ability to retain vaginal cones of various weights for one minute while upright. The population was 87 primigravidas, of whom 16 had elective c-section. Among vaginal births, 30% had episiotomy, 36% had spontaneous tears, and 34% had intact perineums. Two women had third-degree tears in the episiotomy group versus one in the spontaneous tear group. Compared with spontaneous tear ($p < 0.001$) and intact perineum ($p < 0.01$), pelvic floor strength was weakest in the episiotomy subgroup (mean decrease in muscle strength 30.0 ± 11.8). Those with spontaneous tears (mean decrease 18.9 ± 9.1) were similar to intact perineum (mean decrease 19.2 ± 10.2). Those who had elective cesareans (mean decrease 0) faired the best compared with all subgroups of vaginal birth ($p < 0.01$). [Median episiotomy may give different results compared with mediolateral episiotomy because fewer muscle groups are cut. In any case, spontaneous laceration and intact perineum were similar, which means not doing an episiotomy does no harm and that the major effect on pelvic floor function may be intrinsic to vaginal birth.] "[T]he present results do not support the concept that [episiotomy] reduces the risk of damage to pelvic floor muscles."

Episiotomies Do Not Prevent Fetal Brain Damage

Note: If episiotomy has no protective effect in low- and very-low-birth-weight babies, a population highly vulnerable to brain damage from stress or trauma, benefits for a full-term, healthy baby seem unlikely.

17. Lobb MO, Duthie SJ, and Cooke RW. The influence of episiotomy on the neonatal survival and incidence of periventricular haemorrhage in very-low-birth-weight infants. *Eur J Obstet Gynecol Reprod Biol* **1986;22(1-2):17-21.**

The protective effect of episiotomy on infants weighing 1500 g or less and free of lethal abnormalities was examined. Some doctors routinely did episiotomy in such cases ($N = 43$ infants), others did not ($N = 51$ infants). When all very-low-birth-weight (VLBW) babies were compared, episiotomy appeared to improve survival rates and decrease incidence of periventricular hemorrhage. "However, . . . when VLBW babies of similar weight and age are considered, the use of episiotomy appears to hold no advantages."

18. The TG. Is routine episiotomy beneficial in the low birth weight delivery? *Int J Gynaecol Obstet* **1990;31(2):135-140.**

The protective effect of episiotomy was analyzed for 439 singleton, vertex, spontaneous births of babies weighing less than 2500 g. Preexisting pregnancy complications were excluded. Since episiotomy rate depends on parity, primiparas and multiparas were analyzed separately. Neonatal mortality rates were similar for episiotomy versus no episiotomy among both nulliparas (6.7% versus 8.6%) and multiparas (10.0% versus 9.3%) as were 5-minute Apgar scores. One of the two postulated protective effects of episiotomy is reduced pressure on the fetal head. However, to achieve this, episiotomy would have to be done before the head distended the perineum. The other protective effect is shortening second stage. However, length of second stage does not correlate consistently with outcome. "The results of this . . . study suggest that routine episiotomy has little, if any beneficial effect on . . . neonatal outcome."

THE DOWNSIDE OF EPISIOTOMIES

Note: As you read this, consider that the most common way doctors describe episiotomy to women is as a "little cut," which implies episiotomy is a trivial matter.

19. Varner MW. Episiotomy: techniques and indications. *Clin Obstet Gynecol* **1986;29(2):309-317.** (both, but I confine the abstract to midline)
   This clinical practice paper discusses how to perform and repair both types of episiotomies. [Indications that Varner lists that are not supported by the literature include "prolonged second stage of labor" and "premature infant," as indications distinct from "fetal distress," the potential problem with prematurity or long pushing phase. He also lists "prevention of maternal lacerations." The illogic of lacerating the perineum in order to protect it from laceration needs no further comment from me.]

- "Caution must be observed in both techniques that the rectum is not entered inadvertently."

- "If it is performed too early, excess blood loss will probably occur."

- "The sutures should be placed tightly enough to ensure hemostasis, but not so tightly as to occlude capillary perfusion." [The episiotomy should be stitched tightly enough to prevent bleeding but loosely enough for blood flow in the tissue.]

- "If the knot is placed at or inside the hymenal ring, postpartum dyspareunia can be minimized."

- "[P]ostpartum discomfort or dyspareunia can be minimized by avoiding suture knots at the fourchette [the fold connecting the two inner labia (labia minora) at the base of the vulva]."

- "A gentle rectal examination should be performed to ascertain that no sutures were inadvertently placed through the rectal mucosa. Such sutures could serve as a nidus of infection or fistula formation."

- "A sponge and needle count should also be routinely performed at the conclusion of the repair. Besides being embarrassing, a sponge retained in the vagina may be the nidus for an infection. Likewise, a needle retained or broken off in the episiotomy repair mandates exploration of the wound."

- "Perineal extensions of midline episiotomies frequently involve the rectal sphincter or mucosa."

- "[In repairing a third-degree extension] the importance of attention to anatomic reapproximation and hemostasis as well as the use of interrupted sutures cannot be overemphasized for successful repair."

- "Successful repair of . . . vaginal extensions can challenge the most experienced surgeon."

- "Severe hemorrhage is possible with episiotomy."

- "Excessive perineal pain should raise the possibility of a perineal, vulvar, vaginal, or ischiorectal hematoma [a blood-filled swelling]."

- "As with any surgical procedure, infection is a potential complication of episiotomy. . . . A rare but extremely serious and sometimes fatal infectious complication of episiotomy is necrotizing fasciitis."

- "Many patients receiving episiotomies require oral analgesics for several days afterward."

- "Most patients with postepisiotomy pain gradually recover over the ensuing several months."

- "Postepisiotomy pain that is catamenial [synchronized to the menstrual cycle] in nature may represent endometriosis [within the episiotomy scar]."

- "Another aspect of episiotomy pain that should not be underestimated is its psychosexual impact."

"Relative contraindications" include the "patient's absolute refusal to consent to the procedure."

Pain and Dyspareunia

20. Abraham S et al. Recovery after childbirth: a preliminary prospective study. *Med J Aust* 1990;152(1):9-12. (both)

Primiparas who gave birth vaginally ($N = 93$) were studied to evaluate factors influencing perineal pain. In 62% an episiotomy was performed. Women having spontaneous births (67%) "predominantly" had midline episiotomies. Those with forceps deliveries mostly had mediolateral episiotomies. Sixteen percent had an episiotomy and an extension or vaginal tear, of which one involved the anus. Of those who had no episiotomy, 31% did not require stitches. One tear involved the anus.

At one month postpartum, 41% reported perineal pain, 12% at two months, 7% at three months, 2% at four months, and 0% by six months. Pain during intercourse was reported by 91% at one month, 59% at two months, 33% at three months, 18% at four months, and 15% at five months. A gradual decrease followed until at one year 1% reported dyspareunia. The median time for perineal comfort was one month and three months for comfortable sexual intercourse. [The authors did not adjust for breastfeeding, a confounding factor for dyspareunia because low estrogen levels can cause vaginal dryness.] Of 20 women who reported no discomfort the first few days, 13 were using pain-relief methods. [Their evaluation may reflect only the effectiveness of those methods.] Factors associated with longer than average perineal pain or dyspareunia were a vaginal but not perineal tear; forceps delivery [forceps may cause vaginal tears or bruising]; and mediolateral rather than midline episiotomy [but women with mediolateral episiotomies were also the women with forceps]. Women who had spontaneous births with episiotomy had similar outcomes compared with women without episiotomy. Performing an episiotomy did not prevent vaginal tears.

Anal Incontinence

Note: Episiotomy predisposes to rectal tears.

21. Snooks SJ et al. Risk factors in childbirth causing damage to the pelvic floor innervation. *Br J Surg* **1985;72(Suppl):S 15-S 17.** (unstated but presumably mediolateral because this is a British study)

The effect of childbirth on the pudendal nerve and the external anal sphincter was studied in 62 primiparas and 60 multiparas. Twenty women (16%) had elective cesareans. Results were compared with 34 nulliparous controls. Most women (90%) who had an elective epidural had forceps deliveries. Vaginal birth in and of itself, adversely affected these measurements as did forceps use in primiparas, bigger babies, and longer second stage [but women with bigger babies and/or longer second stages would be more likely to have forceps deliveries]. Episiotomies and tears were equivalent, providing the tear did not involve the anal sphincter. In these cases, injury was not more than that due to vaginal birth. Third-degree tears, on the other hand, showed evidence of greater long-term injury. The authors believe that women who still had evidence of nerve damage to the pelvic floor musculature two months after delivery were at greater risk for anal incontinence later in life, especially, since damage is cumulative, if they went on to have more children. Two multiparas, neither with a third-degree tear, experienced fecal soiling postpartum.

22. Haadem K et al. Anal sphincter function after delivery rupture. *Obstet Gynecol* **1987;70(1):53-56.**

Of 63 women who had partial or total tears of the anal sphincter, 59 (95%) responded to a questionnaire sent two to seven years later. Two women had postoperative infections: one developed a rectovaginal fistula, the other a necrosis and rerupture of the sphincter. Both required further surgery. Despite prompt surgical repair, 28 (45%) reported symptoms: 19 of incontinence "especially for gas," five of dyspareunia, and four of perineal pain. Women with problems were offered an evaluation of anal sphincter function, and 14 accepted. The reference group was 10 women of similar age and parity who had no sphincter rupture or anal disease.

The women with anal sphincter injury showed reduced muscle strength compared with controls. Since reduced strength had persisted for years, it should be considered permanent. Slight impairment does not necessarily result in incontinence, but the margin between continence and incontinence is reduced. Since anal sphincter strength decreases with age, women with sphincter injuries are at increased risk for incontinence later in life. [Testing was not offered to women who were symptom free, but it would be interesting to know how strength would compare in these women. If they had weaker anal sphincters, they could be headed for trouble down the line.]

FACTORS THAT REDUCE THE PROBABILITY OF TEARS

23. Avery MD and Van Arsdale L. Perineal massage: effect on the incidence of episiotomy and laceration in a nulliparous population. *J Nurse Midwifery* **1987;32(3):181-184.**

Perineal outcomes were compared between 29 nulliparous women who practiced perineal massage and 26 similar control women. Women in the massage group were instructed to massage the vaginal opening 5 to 10 minutes daily with a natural vegetable oil beginning at 34 weeks. They were to massage the oil into the perineum and lower vaginal wall. Then they, or their partner, were to massage using a "U" or "sling" movement, stretching enough to produce a slight burning sensation. Pelvic floor contractions [Kegels] were also recommended.

In the massage group, 52% had an intact perineum or first-degree laceration, and 48% had an episiotomy and/or second-degree or deeper tears. Among controls, 24% had an intact perineum or first-degree laceration and 76% had an episiotomy and/or second-degree or deeper tears ($p < 0.05$). The episiotomy rate was 38% in the massage group versus 65% among controls. All third-degree tears were preceded by episiotomy. [Keep in mind that the study was not blinded and births were mostly attended by midwives with a commitment to avoiding episiotomy.]

24. Thompson DJ. No episiotomy?! *Aust N Z J Obstet Gynaecol* **1987;27(1):18-20.**
This clinical practice paper recommends that as the birth commences, support the perineum, keep the fetal head flexed, have the mother push gently or pant, gently push the anterior vagina over the back of the baby's head, wait until the mother pushes the anterior shoulder into view, and deliver the shoulders one at a time. By proceeding in this fashion, distension of the perineum and risk of injury are minimized. Comparing 100 consecutive deliveries in 1985 using this technique to 100 deliveries in 1983, the episiotomy rate was 7% versus 78% and the incidence of intact perineum was 68% versus 16%. All episiotomies accompanied forceps deliveries, but 55% of forceps deliveries were over an intact perineum. The majority of tears were first degree; there were three second-degree tears and no third-degree tears.

25. Nodine PM and Roberts J. Factors associated with perineal outcome during childbirth. *J Nurse Midwifery* **1987 May-June;32(3):123-130.**
Perineal outcomes of 275 spontaneous vaginal births of term occiput anterior infants were examined. The episiotomy rate was 34.2%, of which 4.4% had extensions. Overall 17.8% had intact perineums; 19% had spontaneous first-degree tears; 15.8% had second-degree tears; and 12.8% had periurethral or labial tears. No one had a spontaneous third- or fourth-degree tear. Factors associated with episiotomy were use of analgesia ($p < 0.001$) and maternal position for birth ($p < 0.001$). In particular, women with no analgesia had the highest rate of intact perineums (34.1%), and women with epidurals had the highest episiotomy rate (65.2%). Episiotomy rates by birth position were: 14% semisitting; 20% dorsal [supine with legs flexed but not in stirrups]; 33.3% Sims [side lying]; and 55.3% lithotomy [supine, legs in stirrups]. Intact perineum rates by position were: 31.6% semisitting, 17.5% Sims, 15% dorsal, and 12.8% lithotomy. (Too few women squatted to provide data.) Women who gave birth in the dorsal position were most likely to have a spontaneous second-degree tear. However, relationships are complex. For example, the lithotomy position is more likely to be used when an episiotomy is anticipated. First-time mothers were more likely to have an episiotomy, but the association disappeared when birth position was factored in because they were more likely to give birth in the lithotomy position. Attendant's experience may also be a factor. Maternal position is related to perineal outcome only when student midwives attend the birth.

26. Legino LJ et al. Third- and fourth-degree perineal tears. 50 years' experience at a university hospital. *J Reprod Med* **1988;33(5):423-426.** (midline)
Currently 82% of all women at this U.S. hospital have episiotomies. Since 1980 the percentage of third-degree tears and fourth-degree tears has been stable at 10.7% and 6.4%, respectively. Between 1982 and 1985 all women with third- and fourth-degree tears ($N = 743$) were compared with women without such tears ($N = 3,893$). The following associated with deep tears: nulliparity (82% versus 38%, $p < 0.0001$), use of

oxytocin (47% versus 29%, $p < 0.0001$), epidural anesthesia (22% versus 7%, $p < 0.01$), and forceps delivery (34% versus 7%, $p < 0.0001$). Residents had higher deep tear rates than staff doctors ($p < 0.001$) (experience counts). Two or more predisposing factors were present in 91% of cases and three or more in 51%. [This is not surprising; for example, a woman with an epidural is likely to have oxytocin and forceps.] A big baby (≥ 4000 g) was not associated with a greater risk of tear, probably because such babies are likely to be cesarean deliveries [!].

27. Borgatta L, Piening SL, and Cohen WR. Association of episiotomy and delivery position with deep perineal laceration during spontaneous delivery in nulliparous women. Am J Obstet Gynecol 1989;160(2):294-297. (midline)
    The study group was 241 nulliparous women having spontaneous, vertex, singleton births. The episiotomy rate was 46.1%. Midwives attended 65.1% of births and obstetricians the rest. Doctors were more likely to use stirrups ($p < 0.01$). Of the 174 women known to give birth in an alternative position, the most common was semisitting ($N = 153$). Apgar scores did not relate to episiotomy.
    "Deep lacerations" (third or fourth degree) were fewest (0.9%) in women without episiotomy who were not in the lithotomy position and highest (27.9%) in women with both. Women with one factor but not the other had intermediate rates. Episiotomy correlated strongly with deep tears (OR 22.46 CI 7.81-64.61, $p < 0.003$) as did the lithotomy position (OR 14.01 CI 4.18-47.28, $p < 0.029$). The role played by birth attendant is unclear. Doctors had a higher tear rate, but they were more likely to do episiotomies and to use stirrups. This may reflect that they would be called in when there were problems. When data are adjusted for stirrups and episiotomy, the association between doctor and deep tears disappeared. [Still, doctors are more likely to do episiotomies and use the lithotomy position regardless of labor complications.] One possible explanation for the relationship between stirrups and deep tears is that the position overstretches the perineum.

28. Helwig JT, Thorp JM, and Bowes WA. Does midline episiotomy increase the risk of third- and fourth- degree lacerations in operative vaginal deliveries? Obstet Gynecol 1993;82(2):276-279. (midline)
    The records of all instrumental deliveries were examined ($N = 392$) to determine the relationship between episiotomy and third- and fourth-degree lacerations. Sixty percent of instrumental deliveries were performed without an episiotomy. After adjusting for birth weight and primiparity, episiotomy more than doubled the risk of a deep tear during instrumental delivery (RR 2.4 CI 1.7-3.5). For primiparas, the deep tear rate for episiotomy versus no episiotomy was 48.5% versus 20.3% and the rates for intact perineum or lesser tears were 51.5% versus 79.7%. Similarly, for multiparas, the deep tear rates were 21.4% versus 8.7%, and the rates for intact perineum or lesser tears were 78.6% versus 91.3%.

REFERENCES

Cunningham FG, MacDonald PC, and Gant NF, eds. *Williams Obstetrics*. 18th ed. Norwalk, CT: Appleton and Lange, 1989.

Davis-Floyd RE. *Birth as an American rite of passage*. Berkeley: University of California Press, 1992.

DeLee JB. The prophylactic forceps operation. *Am J Obstet Gynecol* 1920;1:34-44.

Ewing TL, Smale LE, and Elliott FA. Maternal deaths associated with postpartum vulvar edema. *Am J Obstet Gynecol* 1979;134:173-179.

Golde S and Ledger WJ. Necrotizing fasciitis in postpartum patients: a report of four cases. *Obstet Gynecol* 1977;50(6):670-673.

Oxorn-Foote H. *Human labor and birth*. 5th ed. Norwalk, CT: Appleton-Century-Crofts, 1986.

Pritchard JA, MacDonald PC, and Gant NF, eds. *Williams Obstetrics*. 17th Edition. Norwalk: Appleton, Century, Crofts, 1985.

Shy KK and Eschenbach DA. Fatal perineal cellulitis from an episiotomy site. *Obstet Gynecol* 1979;54(3):292-298.

Sleep J, Roberts J, and Chalmers I. The second stage of labour. In *A guide to effective care in pregnancy and childbirth*. Enkin M, Keirse MJNC, and Chalmers I, eds. Oxford: Oxford University Press, 1989.

Soper DE. Clostridial myonecrosis arising from an episiotomy. *Obstet Gynecol* 1986;68(3 Suppl):26S-28S.

Sutton GP et al. Group B streptococcal necrotizing fasciitis arising from an episiotomy. *Obstet Gynecol* 1985;66(5):733-736.

Part III

THE CASE FOR AN ALTERNATIVE SYSTEM

Doctors point out that one-quarter of the admissions to neonatal intensive care units come from babies born to low-risk women, and more than half of the complications in childbirth occur in low-risk women. "This seems to be a damning defense of the present system of obstetric care," said Doris Haire, president of the American Foundation of Maternal and Child Health. "It compels one to ask what proportion of these complications, which had their onset during labor and birth, are the direct result of aggressive obstetric procedures."

Diana Korte and Roberta Scaer, *A Good Birth, a Safe Birth,* 1992

15

Midwives

> Myth: *You don't want a midwife when you can have the best—an obstetrician.*
>
> Reality: *"Analysis of national perinatal statistics from Holland, 1986, demonstrates that for all births after 32 weeks' gestation mortality is much lower under the non-interventionist care of midwives than under the interventionist management of obstetricians at all levels of predicted risk. This finding confirms . . . the conclusions of all earlier impartial analyses from . . . other countries."*
>
> Tew and Damstra-Wijmenga 1991

Defining an obstetrician as "the best" has strictly to do with the definer's beliefs about pregnancy and childbirth. Since the definers are obstetricians, who believe these processes to be inherently difficult and dangerous, it follows that obstetricians, by virtue of their surgical and medical training, will consider themselves the best qualified to relieve the difficulties and reduce the dangers.

In the medical model, the doctor's expertise is all that stands between mother and baby and disaster. Childbearing women are viewed as unreliable and often defective machinery (Davis-Floyd 1992). The obstetrician's job becomes to keep the "machine" running efficiently, a task made heroic by its frequent tendency to fail. Thus, doctors frequently intervene in the normal process, considering their numerous tests and manipulations to be right and necessary to produce a quality "product" (baby).

The mother, who in most cultures plays the central role as birth giver, is relegated to the sidelines. As a "patient," her responsibilities, as with the sick or injured, begin and end with doing what she is told and being grateful for the doctor's keeping (or making) her or her baby well. Treatment is something done to her, and her actions are irrelevant to successful outcome, unless she questions her doctor's decisions or fails to follow orders. Then she will be accused of not caring about her baby's welfare, and she may even be subjected to court proceedings in an attempt to force her compliance (San Jose Mercury News 1993).*

This model could hardly be worse for preparing women to be mothers, for it portrays women as incompetent or even obstacles to their child's well-being. Even the lone element intended to address the woman's psychological needs, epidural anesthesia, teaches that women cannot cope with the pain unaided and their participation is not required for the birth (Davis-Floyd 1992). Barbara Katz Rothman (1986) quotes a mother who described birth with an epidural as like seeing a rabbit pulled from a hat. Comments Katz Rothman, "Being the hat is a far cry from being the magician."

By contrast, the midwifery model aims to empower women by helping them master the challenges of pregnancy and birth (Sakala 1988; Lehrman 1981, both abstracted below). Midwives traditionally view pregnancy and birth as healthy, normal events, albeit ones demanding supervision and care. In the midwifery model, the childbearing woman has the central role. The midwife watches over her, serves her, supports her, provides information, and facilitates the natural process. Decision making is collaborative, and treatment, in most cases, begins with what the woman can do for herself (Sakala 1988, abstracted below; Lichtman 1988; Flanagan 1986). So, for example, if cervical dilation were slow, the midwife might suggest walking or ask if anything was troubling the mother, whereas the obstetrician would order IV oxytocin.

To the criticism that obstetric management disempowers women, obstetricians reply, "Which do you want: a healthy baby or a nice experience?" Doctors justify their management by claiming it averts perinatal deaths and injuries. The medical model's claim to validity—that it is based on scientific measurement of objective outcomes—is itself a belief and not a fact. The evidence presented in this book proves that obstetric management has not produced better outcomes even when evaluated on its own grounds, the medical literature. Indeed, it could not. As Michel Odent stresses, "[O]ne cannot help an involuntary process. The point is not to disturb it" (Odent 1987). As we shall now see, midwifery promotes both healthy babies and nice experiences. It succeeds on both counts where obstetrics fails.

This is not to say that midwives have a lock on a particular approach. Family practitioners tend to act and think more like midwives than obstetricians (Smith, Ruffin, and Green, abstracted below; Tilyard et al. 1989; Adams 1983; Brody and Thompson, abstracted below). Even a few obstetricians do the same. Midwives, too, have widely varying intervention rates. However, as a

---

*Doctors told a Chicago woman her baby would die or be born brain damaged if she did not have a cesarean. She refused. They took her to court. She won her case and gave birth via natural childbirth to a healthy 4 lb 12 oz boy several weeks later. The court-appointed lawyer for the fetus, obviously unwilling to admit the doctors were wrong, "warned" that it may take months to tell if the baby is really normal.

general rule, midwives and obstetricians split according to oppositional viewpoints of birth.

Every culture develops rituals around major transformational life events that reinforce the core beliefs of the culture. Our culture's core beliefs relevant to birth are that technology is superior to nature and that women are inferior and untrustworthy. Thus, our dominant maternity care system reflects those beliefs and does its best to make them appear to be a reality (Davis-Floyd 1992). Anyone wanting a different type of care must choose a practitioner who works from a different model; as one wit put it, "If you don't want to get cut, don't go to a surgeon."

Transforming the obstetric model to a healthier paradigm is no easy matter. Appeals to logic and evidence will not work; belief systems are not amenable to alteration by such means. Underlying beliefs must be changed first, or attempts at innovation will fall prey to sabotage.

The rise and fall of hospital alternative birth centers in the 1970s and early 1980s illustrates that taking the doctor out of the delivery room did not take the delivery room out of the doctor. Said one obstetrician, "I treat the birth center as a normal delivery room. . . . I use monitors, I use IVs, I use whatever is necessary" (DeVries 1983). In-hospital birth centers were grudgingly introduced in response to concern about losing business, not better births. Most women never found out they existed; many who did were discouraged from using them; those who persisted were often disqualified; and intervention rates for the few who managed to give birth there were mostly unchanged (Klein et al. 1984; DeVries 1983; Saldana et al. 1983). These days, no one even pretends that reducing intervention in normal labor is a goal.

Another consequence of dealing with faith, rather than fact, is the ridicule, suppression, and persecution of those espousing different beliefs. The virulence and hysteria with which midwifery has been attacked by doctors is a giveaway that the driving force is not a rational assessment of the facts but the threat to beliefs, power, and income (Wertz and Wertz 1979).

Recently, however, midwives have begun making a comeback in the U.S. Again, this has been for economic reasons, not belief in the superiority of midwifery care. Midwives are increasingly caring for the poor, whom few others want, delivering more cost-efficient care in clinics and health maintenance organizations (HMOs), and helping to attract customers to private obstetric practices (LeVeen 1988).

Once again, unlike "improved maternity care," good economics is congruent with the obstetric belief system and has nothing to do with the welfare of women. While cost containment may back midwives and midwifery practices, it can equally well be used to justify management completely contrary to women's interests. Chambliss et al. (1992, abstracted below) cite "space constraints" and "lack of assisting personnel" as reasons for denying women freedom of activity, choice of birth position, and the right to the companionship and help of a loved one, despite acknowledging their value. In other chapters we have seen doctors justify labor induction for ruptured membranes because of the expense of in-hospital observation, even though induction did not improve outcomes (Guise, Duff, and Christian 1992; Duncan and Beckley 1992). We have even seen doctors argue for elective induction because it is not "cost-effective" to waste an obstetrician's time and training "observing one normal woman in labor" (Macer, Macer, and Chan 1992).

Because the obstetric model holds sway, the acceptance of midwifery into the mainstream has a price: co-optation. Enormous social, political, and economic pressures constrain midwives from practicing midwifery (as opposed to obstetrics).

First, although there is no reason a midwife must first become a nurse or that accredited midwifery schools should train midwives in tertiary care centers, this is the only legally sanctioned route to midwifery almost everywhere in the U.S. This route ensures socialization into the medical model and the loss of some, sometimes all, of the philosophy and knowledge that distinguish midwifery from obstetrics.

When midwifery and obstetrics conflict, midwifery loses because doctors have authority positions in institutional power structures. Some of the hallmarks of midwifery are continuity of care, education, and support, but hospital-based midwives are rarely allowed to provide these. Most hospital programs mandate fragmented care. In one hospital where midwives tried to get compensation and obstetrician backing for outreach education programs, longer prenatal appointments, and labor sitting, they failed. "The most sympathetic [obstetricians] believed that the midwives were inefficient; the least sympathetic referred to them as . . . 'mollycoddling' [women], 'providing Cadillac care when a Chevy would do'" (LeVeen 1988). One study compared women cared for by midwives in freestanding birth centers with similar women cared for by hospital-based midwives. When all women with complications were excluded, women in the hospital group consistently had higher rates of intervention (electronic fetal monitoring [(EFM], IVs, oxytocin use, episiotomy, etc.) and lower rates of supportive care (shower/bath in labor, food in labor, etc.) (Fullerton and Severino 1992). A comparison of statistics will show that intervention rates for hospital-based midwives generally considerably exceed those of out-of-hospital-based midwives (see also Chapters 16 and 17).

Midwives increasingly are relegated to being employees of obstetricians instead of independent practitioners. The American College of Obstetricians and Gynecologists (ACOG) opposes full autonomy for midwives. ACOG's (1982) official position, unchanged as of January 1994, is that while the doctor need not be present during the labor or birth, "[T]he maternity care team should be directed by a qualified obstetrician/gynecologist."

Unfortunately, doctors have the power to enforce this statement. HMOs and preferred provider organizations (PPOs) often do not accept midwives as providers. Malpractice insurance companies, whose policies are determined mostly by doctors, may stipulate that only patients regularly seen by the doctor are covered. This effectively blocks doctors from backing midwives. Imagine the reaction if malpractice insurance companies refused to cover patients referred to surgeons or other specialists except under these same conditions. Indeed, in all other areas, primary care providers are becoming gateways to the specialist, not vice versa.

Even the midwife in independent practice is not immune from obstetric control. She is kept in line by the scarcity of obstetric backup. The pool of doctors who will accept referrals of midwifery patients with complications is vanishingly small, so her practices had better be agreeable to those who will. She is denied hospital privileges. The committees that grant privileges are made up of doctors. She is kept from attending home births too. The company insuring members of the American College of Nurse-Midwives recently dropped home birth coverage ("News" 1992).

We have every reason to believe that these measures are working. Midwives imbued with the true philosophy of midwifery find their commitment eroding in the struggle to make a living; they end up going along to get along. And many of the labor and delivery nurses now becoming nurse-midwives are all too comfortable with the medical model and all too disinclined to challenge it where it conflicts with midwifery philosophy and practices. A growing fund of anecdotal evidence tells me that one danger of the acceptance of midwifery is that we may well end with the form but little of the content.

The authors of *Effective Care in Pregnancy and Childbirth* (1989) concluded, "It is inherently unwise, and perhaps unsafe, for women with normal pregnancies to be cared for by obstetric specialists." To have obstetricians care for all pregnant women wastes the specialist's skills and mismatches the woman's needs with what the obstetrician best provides. "Optimal care can only occur when both primary and secondary caregivers recognize their complementary roles." Until that particular lion lies down with the lamb, the woman who wants the fullest benefits of midwifery care would do best to birth outside the hospital to minimize, as one study put it, "a natural tendency for high-risk care to spill over into the . . . management of [low-risk women]" (Klein et al. 1983) and to find out her prospective midwife's policies, philosophy, and statistics to make sure she is not hiring an obstetrician in midwife's clothing. Finally, as a society, we would all do well to remember that for most births, the best "obstetrician" is a midwife.

SUMMARY OF SIGNIFICANT POINTS

- Midwifery care differs from obstetric care in philosophy, style, and practices. It promotes the normal, speaks to psychological care as well as physical care, is woman rather than doctor centered, empowers women, and looks to simple, noninterventive remedies before resorting to technology. (Abstracts 4-9, 11-16, 19-20)

- Midwifery care is safe. (Abstracts 7-10, 12, 14-20)

- Routine obstetric management does not produce benefits and may increase risks. (Abstracts 1-3, 6-7, 11-13, 16, 18-20)

- Intervention rates depend on philosophy of practice, not medical risk. (Abstracts 1-2, 6-9, 11-17, 19-24)

- Midwifery reduces intervention rates, but how much and which ones varies widely. (Abstracts 8-24)

- One reason midwives have lower intervention and cesarean rates is their clients have fewer epidurals. (Abstracts 19-20)

- When obstetricians control policies and protocols, midwives' intervention rates tend to go up. Conversely, intervention rates are lower where midwives operate independently. [See also Chapters 16 and 17, which report exclusively on out-of-hospital births.] (Abstracts 10, 16-18, 21-24)

- Midwifery care benefits medically and demographically high-risk women as well as low-risk women. (Abstracts 7, 10, 12-18)

- Midwifery care costs less. (In addition, although cost comparisons are not given, the fact that midwives intervene less often and their clients have more spontaneous births means other birth-related costs are lower.) (Abstracts 7, 9)

ORGANIZATION OF ABSTRACTS

Obstetricians Do Too Much Too Often

How Midwifery Care Differs

Prenatal Care
Intrapartum Care

Studies of Midwifery Care

Review Paper
Reports of Midwifery Outcomes

Studies Comparing Obstetricians with Midwives
Studies Showing Midwifery Care Benefits Medically and
Demographically High-Risk Women
Studies Showing Obstetrician Control Deforms Midwifery Care

OBSTETRICIANS DO TOO MUCH TOO OFTEN

1. Brody H and Thompson JR. The maximin strategy in modern obstetrics. *J Fam Pract* 1981;12(6):977-986.
The "maximin" approach, from games theory and military strategy, is defined as "choosing the alternative that makes the best of the worst possible outcome, regardless of the probability that that outcome will occur." This approach is "subtly or overtly" encouraged in obstetrics because of these assumptions:

- "[T]he hallmark of obstetric quality is the prevention or adequate management of the rare disaster rather than the optimal conduct of the many normal cases."

- "The best hope for prevention or adequate management lies with modern medical technology."

- "[P]hysiological variables are much more important than psychological or emotional variables."

- "[A]dopting [the strategy] does not in itself change the probabilities of the outcomes," making it more likely that the worst possible case will occur.

The literature is reviewed on certain issues in order to test the validity of these assumptions.

Prenatal risk scoring and prediction systems are intended to isolate a high-risk group. Instead, because they discriminate poorly (episodes of abnormal fetal heart rate [FHR] patterns in healthy babies, for example), they lead obstetricians to treat every pregnancy and labor as high risk. They also fail to distinguish problems where intervention can help from problems such as fetal growth retardation or congenital anomalies where it cannot.

As for specific interventions, some studies documented risks with oxytocin, and no evidence could be found that its liberal use improved outcomes. Amniotomy may speed labor but at increased risk of cord prolapse, infection, and possibly elimination of protective cushioning. Laboring supine "typifies the 'sins' of maximin obstetrics" by placing staff convenience and the ease of intervention ahead of both the mother's comfort and the adverse effects of the position itself. Pain relievers may cause problems, some of which are relieved by yet other risk-bearing interventions (e.g., oxytocin with an epidural). EFM has not been shown to improve outcomes compared with frequent auscultation, may require other interventions such as supine positioning or amniotomy, and may increase the odds of a cesarean. Nor does EFM's ability to predict abnormal outcome mean it can be averted by intervening. The benefits of episiotomy have never been documented, which "is striking given the wide disparity between the 80 percent episiotomy rate in standard obstetrical units and the nearly zero precent rate among some midwives." While prophylactic low forceps delivery does not pose a serious hazard to the baby, neither is it beneficial.

Few firm conclusions can be reached, but several are *not* warranted:

- A physician who does not use the latest technology routinely is practicing second-rate obstetrics.

- The maximin approach increases morbidity. [This fails to consider the impact of the maximin approach on the cesarean rate, which had already tripled from 5% to 15% during the previous decade.]

- Conclusions will have to wait for more data. The kinds of studies that would settle the matter cannot be done, either because they require too many subjects or random assignment would be impractical or unethical.

"To the maximin way of thinking, progress in the management of labor and delivery can come only through more technology. Furthermore, the power of maximin thinking can impede nontechnological progress by raising ungrounded fears that neonatal and maternal safety are being sacrificed in exchange for 'mere' emotional satisfaction." These assumptions must not be accepted without testing.

2. Davis L and Riedmann G. Recommendations for the management of low risk obstetric patients. *Int J Gynaecol Obstet* 1991;35(2):107-115.
The study reviewed current recommendations for five common interventions used in managing low-risk women:

Amniotomy: In three of the better-done studies amniotomy shortened labor by one hour. Other studies found no difference. No study showed that short labors were better. Amniotomy introduced the risk of infection, cord prolapse, and possibly increased stress on the fetus. "Amniotomy should not be done to merely 'hurry things up a bit,' or to satisfy a need to 'do something.'"

IV fluids: IV fluids do not supply adequate nutrition, maternal overhydration is common, and they slow labor by interfering with mobility and increasing the mother's pain. Neonatal problems include hypoglycemia, which increases the incidence of jaundice. Failure to use balanced electrolyte solutions can cause fetal hyponatremia.

Third-stage oxytocics: Purported benefits are decreased blood loss, less need for intensive postpartum monitoring, and prevention of hemorrhage. The first benefit has not been documented, and the second benefits only staff. Women with risk factors should be given oxytocics prophylactically, but considering the rarity of uterine atony among low-risk women and the pain and cost of routine administration, the policy of routine oxytocics should be reconsidered.

Episiotomy: The most common surgical procedure today, "episiotomy has never been shown to be of benefit in controlled clinical trials." Prophylactic episiotomy does not prevent damage to the pelvic floor, improve neonatal outcome, or prevent lacerations. Episiotomy increases the likelihood of deep tears.

EFM: The American College of Obstetricians and Gynecologists stated in 1989 that EFM had "no benefit over intermittent auscultation in both high and low risk pregnancies." [The papers on which that conclusion was based were summarized.]

"A unique feature of modern medicine is that techniques and therapies designed to provide benefits for specific groups of patients often are applied to patients who have no indication for the specific intervention. This phenomenon is especially common in the United States where technological resources are widely available, viewed as evidence of superior medical care, and applied to low risk obstetric patients as well as high risk patients." This practice should be reevaluated.

3. Smith MA, Ruffin MT, and Green LA. The rational management of labor. *Am Fam Physician* **1993;47(6):1471-1481.**

This review paper examines labor protocols:

IVs versus oral intake: Forbidding oral intake produces dehydration, ketosis, hunger, and thirst. The rationale behind it is gastric inhalation during anesthesia. However, this is neither "a major [n]or a significant cause of maternal death. A factor repeatedly associated with deaths from aspiration of gastric contents, however, is an inexperienced anesthetist using improper techniques." IVs have adverse effects: restricted movement, pain, infection, fluid overload, induction of fetal acidosis, maternal and fetal hyperglycemia, followed by neonatal hypoglycemia. "[T]he routine withholding of food and oral liquids and the consequent use of [IV] fluids lack supporting evidence and pose potential risks to both mother and infant. . . . Oral fluids should be given to women in labor unless there is a demonstrated need for intravenous fluids."

Analgesia: Narcotics cross the placenta, causing lower Apgar scores and, possibly, respiratory depression and "impaired neuroadaptive capabilities." These effects may be stronger in an acidotic baby because acidosis increases the concentration of narcotics in the fetus. Adverse effects associated with epidurals are prolonged labor, increased rates of instrumental and cesarean delivery, increased use of oxytocin, and maternal fever. "Narcotics . . . should be used with caution." If epidural anesthesia is offered, a skilled person must be available and "the physician should be prepared to intervene as necessary with oxytocin . . . or instrumental or surgical delivery."

Continuous EFM: Studies have failed to find benefits from routine EFM. Doctors cite malpractice as a reason to persist, but "[t]he plaintiff's expert witness can readily portray trival findings . . . as ominous; therefore the monitor recording strip may be more harmful than helpful. . . . [EFM's] routine use appears to increase the risk for operative delivery without the justification of improved outcome."

Amniotomy: Adverse effects include cord prolapse, infection, and fetal laceration. Randomized trials find amniotomy shortens labor by one to two hours. The benefits must be weighed against the risks.

Positioning: "Women should be informed about positions during labor and encouraged to find the positions that work best for them, both to maximize comfort and improve labor progress and efficiency."

Episiotomy: "Risks of episiotomy include excessive bleeding, hematoma formation, infection, and trauma involving the anal sphincter and rectal mucosa, which may result in rectovaginal fistulae, loss of rectal tone, and perineal abscess." No data support episiotomy's supposed benefits (protection of the perineum, prevention of pelvic relaxation, protection of fetal well-being). "A restrictive policy towards episiotomy should be adopted."

HOW MIDWIFERY CARE DIFFERS

Prenatal Care

4. Lehrman E. A descriptive study of prenatal care. *J Nurse Midwifery* **1981;26(3):27-41.**

Audiotapes of 40 prenatal visits conducted by 23 nurse-midwives scattered throughout seven western states were analyzed with respect to the following aspects of midwifery care: continuity of care, family-centered care, education and counseling as part of care, noninterventionist care, flexibility in care, participative care, consumer advocacy, and time spent. Within the limitations of self-selection by the participating midwives and with caution about generalizing on the basis of a few visits with a few midwives, midwifery prenatal care lived up to its promise.

5. Aaronson LS. Nurse-midwives and obstetricians: alternative models of care and client "fit." *Res Nurs Health* **1987;10(4):217-226.**
This study explored personality differences among 244 women getting prenatal care at a facility offering both obstetricians and certified nurse-midwives (CNM). CNM and obstetrician clients were similar in most demographic and psychological factors, but while both were highly motivated to comply with their care provider, CNM clients scored higher on "internal locus of control" scales and obstetrician patients scored higher on "powerful others" and "chance locus of control" scales. Midwifery clients were more adventurous, not unexpected since obstetric care is the norm.

Marked differences, most exceeding a full scale point on a nine-point scale, also emerged in how women viewed their care provider. Midwifery clients believed their midwife held significantly stronger opinions on their engaging in health-promoting behaviors (prenatal care, diet, exercise, abstinence from caffeine, alcohol, and cigarettes) and were more supportive.

Intrapartum Care

6. Sakala C. Content of care by independent midwives: assistance with pain in labor and birth. *Soc Sci Med* **1988;26(11):1141-1158.**
"In an environment of limited understanding of the process of midwifery care and of the great cultural authority associated with medical approaches, midwifery care has been trivialized and even suppressed. Such an environment discourages formal, reasoned evaluation of midwifery approaches." This report compared labor pain control strategies used by U.S. obstetricians versus midwives.

Information on the obstetric approach to pain relief was gathered from medical textbooks and articles. Anesthetic and analgesic drugs were the only viable labor pain-relief options, and women were to be encouraged to use them. Childbirth preparation was welcomed but only as a complement to pain medication and because "preparation leads to better, more co-operative patients." Obstetric medicine showed "minimal interest in, awareness of, and expectations for the efficacy of alternatives." Yet, despite this, the medical literature extensively documented numerous risks associated with the use of pain medications.

Information on the midwifery approach was gathered from interviewing 15 actively practicing, experienced direct-entry Utah midwives who were asked how they would assist a specific hypothetical low-risk woman. Recommendations were diverse, flexible, and innovative and stressed individualizing care to the woman's needs. They encompassed:

- *Prenatal preparation*: formation of a trust relationship, empowerment through knowledge, mobilization of the mother's and family's psychosocial resources.

- *Physical manipulation*:   massage, reflexology, acupressure, and counter-pressure.

- *Hydrotherapy*: tub baths; hot, wet towels on the abdomen or perineum.

- *Oral intake*: food and drink, herbal medicines.

- *Breathing and relaxation techniques*: eye contact; slow, deep breathing; progressive relaxation.

- *Psychological techniques*: focused support and attention of all present; positive, supportive language; visualization, creation of a peaceful environment; vocalization of pain.

In summary, obstetricians believed pain medication to be necessary and alternatives ineffective; midwives found medications unnecessary and risky. Midwives stressed responsiveness to the individual; medical institutions were bureaucratic and stressed routine and protocol. Midwives emphasized continuity of care and time to build a relationship; obstetric care was brief and fragmented. Midwives respected the knowledge, resources, and capability of the mother; the medical approach stressed her limitations and the importance of professional expertise. Midwives were committed to innovation and experimentation; medical practice adhered to protocol and routine. Finally, midwifery techniques did not require special equipment or training, were inexpensive, and introduced negligible risk, whereas obstetric techniques were the reverse.

STUDIES OF MIDWIFERY CARE

Review Paper

7. Thompson JE. Nurse-midwifery care: 1925 to 1984. *Ann Rev Nurs Res* 1986;4:153-173.
A brief historical overview is given followed by an examination of nurse-midwifery practice based on 50 selected studies of nurse-midwifery care. Although there were methodological problems, the studies showed improved outcomes among underserved or disadvantaged women for both home and hospital births and at least similar outcomes when compared with obstetric care, as well as reduced use of interventions (IVs, EFM, episiotomy, analgesia, and anesthesia) and reduced cost. Evidence also supported the efficacy of some aspects of noninterventive care, such as freedom of activity and position during labor, pushing with the urge, and skin-to-skin contact with the newborn. Women were satisfied with midwifery care, as evidenced by increased numbers of prenatal visits and a higher return rate for postpartum care.

Reports of Midwifery Outcomes

Note: Unlike the obstetrician-attended in-hospital birth centers cited in the chapter introduction, midwifery care in birth centers differed from obstetric management, achieving good outcomes with lower intervention rates.

8. Hewitt MA and Hangsleben KL. Nurse-midwives in a hospital birth center. *J Nurse Midwifery* **1981;26(5):21-29.**

Data were reported on 496 singleton births during 1978-1979 to women cared for by a Minneapolis midwifery group. Enrollment exclusions were major medical or obstetrical complications or planned cesarean delivery. The majority of births (79%) took place in an in-hospital birth center where labor was managed in a flexible, noninterventive manner. Midwives attended 86% of the births; the rest were forceps, cesareans, vaginal breech, or premature births.

Most women (72%) had no analgesics, while 7% had regional or general anesthesia, primarily for cesareans. Births were 89% spontaneous, 4.8% instrumental, and 6.4% cesarean section. For midwife-managed births, the episiotomy rate was 27%; 58% had no episiotomy or laceration requiring repair, and 15% had lacerations requiring repair despite the fact that 27% of birth weights were above the ninetieth percentile. The breastfeeding rate was 87%.

As for postpartum complications, four women had endometritis, and six had a postpartum hemorrhage. Twenty-eight babies were admitted to the special care nursery, but in a teaching institution, inexperienced clinicians tend to overdiagnose. Five babies died: three were less than 28 weeks gestation, one had anomalies incompatible with life, and one was a term fetal death from unknown causes.

"This Nurse-Midwife Service based in an in-hospital birth center, has demonstrated that highly individualized care for normal childbearing women can be provided with good results."

9. Stewart RB and Clark L. Nurse-midwifery practice in an in-hospital birthing center: 2050 births. *J Nurse Midwifery* **1982;27(3):21-26.**

This study described an Atlanta midwifery practice of one obstetrician and four midwives and reported outcomes for 2050 women. The midwives attended 80% of the births, which occurred in an in-hospital birth center. Estimated costs for an uncomplicated vaginal birth at eight area hospitals ranged from $806 to $1300 for a 24-hour stay and from $1000 to $1600 for a 3-day stay. Birth center costs were $640 and $850, respectively.

Management was midwifery style. Prenatal care included emotional support and education. Freedom of position and activity and eating and drinking were encouraged in labor, and midwives were actively involved in labor support. Enemas and perineal shaves [still common at this time] were not done nor were membranes routinely ruptured. EFM was done only for suspected or actual fetal distress. Analgesia and anesthesia rates for vaginal births were 3% and 5%, respectively. Women could choose their birth position and touch the baby during the birth. Labor and birth occurred in the same room [a rarity then]. The episiotomy rate was 27%, 36% had a laceration requiring repair, and 37% had an intact perineum. The baby was placed skin-to-skin with the mother after birth, and oxytocics were not given routinely. Anyone could attend, including the baby's siblings. The father could spend the night.

Birth statistics were primary cesarean rate 7.9%, forceps rate 5.0%, and 85.6% spontaneous births. Half of women with a previous cesarean were allowed to labor of whom 76% gave birth vaginally. Breech presentation occurred in 3.4% of clients of whom two-thirds gave birth vaginally.

Neonatal mortality rates for 1977-1980 were about half the Georgia rates, which were similar to the U.S. rates. The perinatal mortality rate was slightly more than half the U.S. rate. (Georgia rates were not available.) The sole maternal death was a woman with medical problems who was comanaged by and gave birth in a tertiary care hospital.

10. van Alten D, Eskes M, and Treffers PE. Midwifery in the Netherlands. the Wormerveer study; selection, mode of delivery, perinatal mortality and infant morbidity. *Br J Obstet Gynaecol* 1989;96(6):656-662.

In Holland, midwives are independent practitioners. They provide primary maternity care, referring to the specialist obstetrician as needed. Outcomes were analyzed for pregnant women booked at a Dutch midwifery practice between 1969 and 1983. An estimated 92% of all nulliparas and 79% of all multiparas in the catchment area booked with this practice. Excluding miscarriages, women who moved, and referrals to an obstetrician before 20 weeks gestation, 7980 women (8055 children—75 sets of twins) remained. During most of the time period, women could give birth in a small maternity center or at home. During the last year, the center closed, and the women could choose home or hospital.

The perinatal mortality rate (PMR) was 11.1 per 1000 versus 14.5 per 1000 nationally. The cesarean rate was 1.4%. (It increased over time from 1.0% in nulliparas and 0.4% in multiparas in 1969 to 3.5% and 0.5%, respectively, in 1980.) Among a low-risk subgroup (defined as all women starting labor under the care of a midwife), the PMR was 2.3 per 1000 and the cesarean rate was 0.4%. Most infant admissions during the first week of life were infants weighing less than 2500 g admitted for observation. The rates were 8.2% overall, 4.3% in the low-risk subgroup, and 3.8% for infants born under the midwife's sole care. In this last category, emergency admission for birth asphyxia occurred in 0.4% of cases. Of these 23 infants, 21 were born before 1977. The incidence of neonatal convulsions before 48 hours was 0.9 per 1000 overall, 0.8 per 1000 in the low-risk group, and 0.7 per 1000 in the group born under the midwife's sole care. In 1982 a study proposed that the incidence of convulsions before 48 hours in low-risk infants be used as an index of the quality of perinatal care. The rate in that study was 1.7 per 1000.

Studies Comparing Obstetricians with Midwives

11. Mayes F et al. A retrospective comparison of certified nurse-midwife and physician management of low risk births. A pilot study. *J Nurse Midwifery* 1987;32(4):216-221.

All 29 midwifery clients who gave birth vaginally between April and June 1985 at a Michigan tertiary care center were matched to 29 low-risk obstetric patients for time of delivery, parity, age, and birth weight.

Intrapartum care for CNM versus physician differed for IV (38% versus 72%, $p <$ 0.02), Pitocin (22% versus 56%, $p < 0.01$), amniotomy (35% versus 66%, $p < 0.05$), EFM (34% versus 100%, $p < 0.01$), analgesia (10% versus 45%, $p < 0.02$), anesthesia (45% (local only) versus 93% (59% local, 7% pudendal block, 24% epidural, 3% general), p for no anesthesia < 0.01), episiotomy (24% versus 76%, $p < 0.01$), lacerations (all third- and fourth-degree tears occurred with episiotomy) (7% third degree versus 10% third degree, 10% fourth degree, and 14% periurethral tear). "The findings . . . indicate that women who seek care from nurse-midwives do tend to experience labor and delivery in ways that differ from women cared for by physicians, even in a tertiary care in-hospital setting. . . . If various procedures . . . are not necessary for low-risk births, then payors can question whether they should be reimbursable expenses; and those paying their own bills may question whether they should be used at all."

12. Baruffi G et al. Patterns of obstetric procedures use in maternity care. *Obstet Gynecol* **1984;64(4):493-498.** (See also Abstract 13 below and Abstract 9 in Chapter 16, which use data from the same populations.)

This study compares two populations with similar demographics and medical history who had live-born singleton births. One group (N = 804) received care from Thomas Jefferson University Hospital (TJUH), a tertiary care center staffed by obstetricians, and the other (N = 796) from Booth Maternity Center (BMC), a midwife-staffed maternity hospital. Women were grouped by risk into four groups: low prenatal-low intrapartum (L-L), high prenatal-low intrapartum (H-L), low prenatal-high intrapartum (L-H), and high prenatal-high intrapartum (H-H).

In general, women managed at TJUH were more likely ($p < 0.0001$) to have prenatal diagnostic X rays (4.5% versus 16.0%), labor augmentation (22.2% versus 32.1%), EFM (42.7% versus 63.3%), analgesia/anesthesia (analgesia only, 24.7% versus 7.1%; anesthesia only, 8.9% versus 53.6%; both, 15.6% versus 25.0%), episiotomy (43.1% versus 64.8%), and nonspontaneous delivery (spontaneous birth, 83.0% versus 53.9%; outlet forceps, 6.4% versus 22.0%; primary cesarean, 4.3% versus 12.9%). Induction rates were similar (9.7% versus 12.1%).

Interventions were more tightly associated with risk at BMC, and in most cases interventions were more likely to be used at TJUH regardless of risk category. For example, for L-L women, X-ray rates were 5.6% versus 15.6%; augmentation, 12.1% versus 33.9%; EFM, 24.3% versus 60%; episiotomy, 56.4% versus 90.5%; anesthesia, 8.6% versus 73.6%; outlet forceps, 2.7% versus 26.8%; cesarean section, 0.3% versus 2.7%. The cesarean section rate for H-L women was 0% versus 13%, for L-H women it was 6.8% versus 29.4%, and for H-H women it was 19.3% versus 33.7%. Odds ratios for intervention use at TJUH compared with BMC were calculated for low and high intrapartum risk for X rays (low 4.2, high 3.7), augmentation (low 3.7, high no difference), EFM (low 4.0, high no difference), analgesia (no difference), anesthesia (low 22.3, high 7.1), and more interventive delivery (low 12.6, high 3.5). Neonatal and maternal morbidity rates favored BMC, suggesting that the greater use of intervention at TJUH conferred risks. In conclusion, differences in practice did not reflect differences in risk status, and differences in practices at BMC appear to reduce morbidity for mothers and babies. Other aspects of midwifery care untested here—the relationship between care providers and women, the environment, the women's participation in decision making—may also prove beneficial to outcomes.

13. Baruffi G, Strobino DM, and Paine LL. Investigation of institutional differences in primary cesarean birth rates. *J Nurse Midwifery* **1990;35(5):274-281.**

The same populations as in Abstract 12 were used to explore reasons for differences in primary cesarean rates (4.3% BMC versus 13.7% TJUH). After adjustment for differences in demographics and risk factors, the odds of having a cesarean at BMC were half that of TJUH (OR 0.49 CI 0.36-0.67).

Age less than 20 or greater than or equal to 30 increased the odds of cesarean at TJUH compared with ages 20 to 29, but age had no effect at BMC. Primiparas were

80% more likely to have a cesarean at TJUH compared with multiparas, but the relationship of parity to cesarean "only approached statistical significance" at BMC. At TJUH 15.4% of women were diagnosed prenatally as having an abnormally small pelvis versus 6.6% at BMC. Women with this diagnosis were twice as likely to have a cesarean at BMC, but the diagnosis had no effect at TJUH. Cesarean birth was not associated with birth weight or neonatal morbidity at either institution, nor did it improve infant outcomes.

It seems clear from our results and from other studies that divergence in management of labor and delivery is a likely explanation for the differences in cesarean birth rates. The continued rise in cesarean births must be questioned in the face of these differing labor and delivery management styles as well as the higher risk of morbidity among women with primary cesarean deliveries and the uncertain benefits to the newborn.

Studies Showing Midwifery Care Benefits Medically and Demographically High-Risk Women

14. Schreier AC. The Tucson nurse-midwifery service: the first four years. *J Nurse Midwifery* **1983;28(6):24-30.**

This study reports on 823 midwifery clients between 1978 and 1982, of whom almost one-third were teenagers and almost half nulliparas. Prenatal transfers were not included. Birth place was a community hospital.

"More than one-half" had no analgesia and no internal EFM (monitoring was mostly intermittent external EFM) and gave birth in the labor room. "More than one-third" had no IV. Oxytocin was given to 28% (17% induction, 11% augmentation). Of women attended by midwives (86%), 31% had an episiotomy, 37% had an intact perineum, 28% had a first- or second-degree laceration, 3.5% had a third- or fourth-degree extension, and less than 1% had a cervical laceration. Obstetricians delivered 5% by forceps and 5% by cesarean section.

The most common complication was postpartum hemorrhage (8%). Only 3% of babies were transferred to a tertiary care center. The neonatal death rate was 7.2 per 1000. One baby had multiple anomalies; one developed fetal distress in labor, was delivered by emergency cesarean, and was transferred; and one was born at home with no attendant (autopsy revealed no cause of death). The other three babies weighed less than 1500 g.

15. Platt LD et al. Nurse-midwifery in a large teaching hospital. *Obstet Gynecol* **1985;66(6):816-820.**

The midwifery service operated in a Los Angeles tertiary care center serving mostly indigent women. All low-risk women were eligible. Almost 15% of women attended by midwives had no prenatal care. Except for the teen clinic, women receiving prenatal care from midwives were not necessarily attended by them in labor. During 1979 and 1980 midwives attended about 3600 births—13.5% of all births.

Most births were with no anesthesia (42%) or local anesthesia only (42%). The epidural rate was 2%. EFM was routine. The cesarean rate for the last half of 1980 was 2% (18 of 863). (The departmental hospital primary cesarean rate was 8.7%.)

Meconium staining occurred in 15% of births, but only two infants aspirated meconium. Only 0.3% of infants had a 5-minute Apgar below 7. One neonatal death and one stillbirth occurred in 1979 and none in 1980 for a perinatal mortality rate of 1.8 per 1000.

16. Haire D. Improving the outcome of pregnancy through increased utilization of midwives. *J Nurse Midwifery* **1981;26(1):5-8.** (This study and Abstract 17 are about the same midwifery program.)

"Evidence is accumulating rapidly that our basic system of providing obstetric care is not in the best interests of normal pregnant and parturient women and their offspring, nor, in many cases, in the best interests of high-risk mothers and their offspring." Amniotomy (cord compression, cord prolapse, and pressure on the fetal head), confinement to bed (lengthens labor, increases need for intervention, increases perinatal complications), and drugs ("[t]here is no obstetric drug that has been proven safe for unborn children") are cited as examples.

The North Central Bronx Hospital serves indigent women, of whom 30% are medically high risk. Midwives are the primary care providers, with physician backup, and there is no obstetric residency program. Intervention rates and outcomes for the 2608 births during 1979 were detailed. Women were encouraged to walk, to eat and drink, and to bring one or two companions. Vaginal exams were few. Amniotomy was not done. Women with a previous cesarean were allowed to labor, and 37% gave birth vaginally. No labors were electively induced; only 3% were augmented. Fewer than half (including the 30% high risk) had EFM. More than 70% of women had neither analgesia nor anesthesia. Episiotomy was performed in only 26% of births, and 45% of women had an intact perineum. Four percent had third- or fourth-degree tears, all episiotomy extensions during forceps deliveries. The midwives attended 83% of women, and 88% of births were spontaneous. Place of birth was delivery table 15%, labor bed in the delivery room 21%, and labor rooms 64%. The instrumental delivery rate was 2.3% and the cesarean rate was 9% (7% primary and 2% repeat). Of infants weighing more than 1000 g, only 1.7% had 5-minute Apgars below 7. The neonatal mortality rate for infants weighing over 1000 g was 4.2 per 1000. "There is no doubt in my mind that ultimately the midwife will be recognized as the health professional most capable of improving the outcome of pregnancy throughout the United States."

17. Haire DB and Elsberry CC. Maternity care and outcomes in a high-risk service: the North Central Bronx Hospital experience. *Birth* **1991;18(1):33-37.**

In 1988, the hospital served 3500 women in a service designed for 2200. The high-risk rate was 70%; 11% had no prior care; and 10% of the babies were low birth weight. Policies were the same as in 1979 (see Abstract 16). Despite allowing women to eat and drink, the hospital has had no cases of aspiration in 30,000 births. Other policies not mentioned previously were gentle bearing down, choice of birth position, skin-to-skin contact with baby, ethnic or religious observances permitted, and breastfeeding encouraged (60% left the hospital breastfeeding).

In 1988 midwives attended 86.1% of the births, all spontaneous, of which 64.4% occurred in the labor room and 32.1% in the bed in the delivery room. Another 2.1% of spontaneous births were attended by obstetricians, for a total rate of 88.2%. The instrumental delivery rate was 0.3%, and the cesarean rate was 11.8% (70% were primary and 30% repeat). The induction rate was 4.2% and the augmentation rate 6.4%.

Of those giving birth vaginally, 13% had analgesia and 7% an epidural. The episiotomy rate was 7.1% and 52.5% had an intact perineum. Tear rates were 29.0% first degree, 8.7% second degree, and 2.3% third- and fourth-degree extensions of episiotomies. The neonatal mortality rate for infants weighing 1000 g or more was 3.7 per 1000, and 89.8% of infants had 1-minute Apgars above 7.

18. Tew M and Damstra-Wijmenga SMI. Safest birth attendants: recent Dutch evidence. *Midwifery* 1991;7:55-63.

In all economically developed countries except Holland, maternity care has come to be organised so as to give full effect to the theory that child-birth is always safer if it takes place under the management of obstetri-cians in a hospital provided with the technological equipment for carrying out interventions in the natural process. It is a remarkable fact that obste-tricians have never at any time had valid evidence to support the theory they have so successfully propagated.

In Holland, midwives are autonomous practitioners. They train directly as midwives and are not required to have a prior nursing degree. They are the primary care providers of maternity care, and they do not practice under obstetrical supervision. About one-third of the population gives birth at home. This unique situation allows an evaluation of perinatal mortality rate (PMR) by midwife versus obstetrician in a system where obstetricians do not control maternity care. Since high-risk births are transferred to in-hospital obstetric care, the effect of this on the PMR for obstetrician-attended hospi-tal births must be taken into account. Data covered all Dutch births during 1986.

In descending order, the PMR was 18.9 per 1000 for obstetricians in hospital, 4.5 per 1000 for general practitioners at home, 2.1 per 1000 for midwives in hospital, and 1.0 per 1000 for midwives at home ($p < 0.0005$ for adjacent pairs). The same gradient is found for all subgroups of parity and age ranges except for mothers over age 34, where PMRs for midwives did not differ for home versus hospital. The PMR for all obstetri-cians (hospital) versus all midwives (home or hospital) was 18.9 per 1000 versus 1.5 per 1000 ($p < 0.000001$). Differences were significant for all gestational ages except below 33 weeks (185.5 per 1000 versus 169.8 per 1000, $p < 0.6$). At term (> 36 wks), the PMRs for obstetrician versus midwife were 8.1 per 1000 versus 0.8 per 1000 ($p < 0.000001$). For the 98.2% of babies born after 32 weeks gestation, PMRs are nearly 12 times lower (11.9 per 1000 versus 1.0 per 1000) for midwife-attended births, and [as shown above] for babies before 32 weeks, place of birth and attendant made no differ-ence. No possible confounding factor can explain the 10-fold difference in PMR for obstetricians versus midwives. "At a stretch" it might account for a three- or four-fold difference. "Indeed, [the data] support the contrary hypothesis, that obstetricians' care actually provokes and adds to the dangers."

19. Chambliss LR et al. The role of selection bias in comparing cesarean birth rates between physician and midwifery management. *Obstet Gynecol* 1992;80(2):161-165.

At this Los Angeles hospital, low-risk women were randomly assigned to either physician ($N = 253$) or midwifery ($N = 234$) care. Care providers were blinded to study group members because low-risk women were normally assigned to a service based on bed availability. Most women (75%) were multiparous. The physician service used epidurals [no percentage given]. Unlike the midwifery service, the physician service usually forbade women labor support and confined them to bed, and they gave birth in the lithotomy position on a delivery table because of "space constraints, lack of assisting personnel, and use of epidural anesthesia."

The cesarean rate for physician versus midwifery groups was 0.4% versus 2.1% (NS). [Remember, 75% were multiparous.] The department primary cesarean rate for the physician service is 9%. However, the physician group did have a higher oxytocin augmentation rate (37% versus 12%, $p < 0.0004$), internal EFM use (38% versus 16%, $p < 0.00005$), episiotomy rate (35% versus 24%, $p < 0.0005$), third- and fourth-degree tear rate (0.8% versus 0.09%, $p < 0.0003$), and instrumental delivery rate (7.5% versus 0, $p < 0.006$). Episiotomy associated with deep tears ($p < 0.0005$), and half occurred in women with instrumental deliveries. [Differences in intervention rates may reflect epidural use on the physician service.] Neonatal outcomes were similar. "A low cesarean rate (2-3%) can be achieved by either the physician- or midwife-managed service." [Obstetricians can achieve low cesarean rates, but they usually do not. Here, the midwifery cesarean rate was typical, but the physician rate was not. Even the physicians' departmental rate was half the national rate. Moreover, midwifery clients still came out ahead because midwives had lower intervention rates, although here, too, rates were lower than usual for physicians. Women also undoubtedly had more pleasant experiences because unlike physician-managed births, they were allowed freedom of activity, birth position, and labor support.]

20. Butler J et al. Supportive nurse-midwife care is associated with a reduced incidence of cesarean section. *Am J Obstet Gynecol* **1993;168(5):1407-1413.**
At this San Francisco hospital, women managed by doctors ($N = 3551$) were compared with similar women cared for by midwives ($N = 1056$). Although women self-selected the midwifery service, a long list of exclusionary medical conditions ensured comparable populations of low-risk women at time of labor. [It seems unlikely that self-selection could confound results if the populations were similar at onset of labor.] The decision for operative delivery was made by the same consulting faculty on both services. The hospital cesarean rate was 19.8%, and the rate for the low-risk cohort was 11.7%.

The cesarean rate for the midwifery group was 9.75% versus 12.3% for the doctor group ($p = 0.02$) (crude OR 0.77 CI 0.61-0.96). This was despite the midwifery group's having more nulliparas (63.4% versus 57.5%, $p < 0.001$) and more large-for-gestational-age babies (10.2% versus 8.0%, NS). After adjusting for age, race, parity, and year of birth, the OR became 0.71 with CI 0.55-0.91. Midwifery clients were half as likely to be diagnosed with fetal distress and 25% less likely to be diagnosed with labor abnormalities. Midwifery clients were less likely to have epidurals (22.8% versus 42.2%, $p < 0.001$), and epidurals were strong predictors of c-section (cohort OR 9.58 CI 7.5-12.2). However, comparing subgroups with no epidural, the midwifery cesarean rate was still lower (2.4% versus 4.1%, $p = 0.02$). Fewer midwifery group babies were admitted to intensive care (1.0% versus 1.8%, OR 0.47 CI 0.24-0.95). Elements of midwifery care improving outcomes could be one-to-one support throughout labor reduces stress, ambulation improves progress and increases comfort, and less use of EFM reduces diagnosis of distress. "Our study provides additional evidence that [midwifery] care, characterized by personal one-on-one support, improves the outcome of labor. . . . [T]hese findings . . . suggest a far less interventional approach to reduce cesarean section than current strategies of active management of labor."

Studies Showing Obstetrician Control Deforms Midwifery Care

21. Beal MW. Nurse-midwifery intrapartum management. *J Nurse Midwifery* **1984;29(1):13-19.** (Abstract 22 also reports statistics from the Yale midwives.)

The records of low-risk adolescent mothers at Yale University Hospital were reviewed, of whom 53 were managed by CNM and 32 by an obstetrician. Labor management statistics for CNM versus obstetrician were: IV (83.0% versus 87.5% [error in table; percentages do not match numbers]), amniotomy (69.2% versus 77.2%), EFM (90.6% versus 100%), analgesia "mean number of times medicated" (0.81 versus 0.88) epidural (15.1% versus 43.8%), episiotomy (58.5% versus 90.6%), and third- or fourth-degree laceration (9.4% versus 32.3%). Modes of birth were as follows: spontaneous (81.1% versus 56.3%), instrumental (17.0% versus 40.6%), and cesarean (1.9% versus 3.1%). [The major differences were epidural rates, episiotomy rates, severe laceration rates, spontaneous birth rates, and instrumental delivery rates, although much was made of the fact that midwives intervened later in labor than did obstetricians. And although episiotomy and deep tear rates were lower, they were still unusually high for midwives.] "The results of this study lend support to the expectation that nurse-midwives do in fact give patient care that involves more selective use of technology. This is especially significant given that this study was carried out in a tertiary care center with a population considered to be at risk for complications." [Ignoring that the study population was actually low risk and that the style of care was very much like the doctors, the authors congratulated themselves on the success of midwifery care at reducing interventions.]

22. Nichols CW. The Yale nurse-midwifery practice: addressing the outcomes. *J Nurse Midwifery* **1985;30(3):159-165.** (Abstract 21 also reports statistics from the Yale midwives.)

Outcomes are reported for 175 consecutive clients of the Yale CNM private practice. Clients were mostly middle-class, married women of prime childbearing age. Only 20% were primiparous; only 2% had a prior cesarean (all three gave birth vaginally); and 7% had either planned or unplanned home births. Statistics were: induction 11.2%, augmentation 17.8%, IV 43%, EFM 43.0%, analgesia 13.1%, epidural 11.4%, episiotomy or laceration repair 57.0% [no information on episiotomy rate], fourth-degree laceration 3.4%, instrumental delivery 9.1%, and primary cesarean rate 5.1%. Meconium staining occurred in 36% of primiparas and 28% of multiparas, and the neonatal mortality rate was two per 1000.

23. Keleher KC and Mann LI. Nurse-midwifery care in an academic health center. *J Obstet Gynecol Neonatal Nurs* **1986;15(5):369-72.**

Among 1852 low-risk women managed by midwives within a Vermont tertiary care center, almost half had continuous EFM, the spontaneous birth rate was 84.0%, the forceps rate 5.6%, and the primary cesarean rate was 10.4%. Obstetricians or pediatricians were called in almost half of the time, the indications, in order of frequency, being dysfunctional labor, meconium staining, and fetal distress. The authors concluded that the frequency of physician involvement, EFM, and cesarean proved that birth needed to take place in a hospital. [I interpret it as showing how proximity bred overuse.]

24. Kaufman K and McDonald H. A retrospective evaluation of a model of midwifery care. *Birth* **1988;15(2):95-99.**

Because midwifery was illegal in Canada, this tertiary care center set up midwifery services by "delegating" nurses (several of whom had midwifery degrees) to deliver babies. The article compared 79 low-risk women managed by the midwifery service with 373 low-risk women managed by obstetricians. Somewhat fewer amniotomies were done (33% versus 47%, $p < 0.026$) and somewhat fewer epidurals (34% versus 49%, $p < 0.016$). Rates were similar for episiotomy (40% versus 49%), third- and fourth-degree extensions (13% versus 8%), spontaneous birth (75% versus 77%), forceps (20% versus 16%), and cesarean (5% versus 7%). "This occurred despite hospital policies that support noninterventive, family-centered care. . . . [The difficulties of practicing low-risk obstetrics in a tertiary care center] are underscored when the midwife functions under physician supervision."

REFERENCES

ACOG. Joint Statement of Practice Relationships between Obstetrician/Gynecologists and Certified Nurse-Midwives. Nov 1, 1982.

Adams JL. The use of obstetrical procedures in the care of low-risk women. *Women Health* 1983;8(1):25-35.

Davis-Floyd RE. *Birth as an American rite of passage.* Berkeley: University of California Press, 1992.

DeVries RG. Image and reality: an evaluation of hospital alternative birth centers. *J Nurse Midwifery* 1983;28(3):3-9.

Duncan SLB and Beckley S. Prelabour rupture of the membranes—why hurry? *Br J Obstet Gynecol* 1992;99:543-545. (abstracted in Chapter 10)

Enkin M, Keirse JNC, and Chalmers I, eds. *A guide to effective care in pregnancy and childbirth.* Oxford: Oxford University Press, 1989.

Flanagan JA. Childbirth in the eighties: What next? When alternatives become mainstream. *J Nurse Midwifery* 1986;31(4):194-199.

Fullerton JT and Severino R. In-hospital care for low-risk childbirth: comparison with results from the National Birth Center Study. *J Nurse Midwifery* 1992;37(5):331-340. (abstracted in Chapter 16)

Guise JM, Duff P, and Christian JS. Management of term patients with premature rupture of membranes and an unfavorable cervix. *Am J Perinatol* 1992;9(1):56-60. (abstracted in Chapter 10)

Katz Rothman B. The social construction of birth. In *The American way of birth.* Eakins, PS, ed. Philadelphia: Temple University Press, 1986.

Klein M et al. A comparison of low-risk pregnant women booked for delivery in two systems of care: shared care (consultant) and integrated general practice unit. II. Labour and delivery management and neonatal outcome. *Br J Obstet Gynaecol* 1983;90:123-128.

Klein M et al. Care in a birth room versus a conventional setting: a controlled trial. *Can Med Assoc J* 1984;131:1461-1466.

LeVeen D. Unionizing midwifery in California. In *Childbirth in America.* Michaelson, KL, ed. Amherst, MA: Bergin and Garvey, 1988.

Lichtman R. Medical models and midwifery: The cultural experience of birth. In *Childbirth in America.* Michaelson, KL, ed. Amherst, MA: Bergin and Garvey, 1988.

Macer JA, Macer CL, and Chan LS. Elective induction versus spontaneous labor: a retrospective study of complications and outcome. *Am J Obstet Gynecol* 1992;166(6 Pt 1):1690-1697. (abstracted in Chapter 5)

"News." *Birth* 1992;19(2):107-108.

Odent M. The fetus ejection reflex. *Birth* 1987;14(2):45-46.

Saldana LR et al. Home birth: negative implications derived from a hospital-based birthing suite. *South Med J* 1983;76(2):170-173.

San Jose Mercury News. Dec 13, 15, 17, 30, 1993.

Tilyard MW et al. Is outcome for low risk obstetric patients influenced by parity and intervention? *N Z Med J* 1989;102:523-526.

Wertz RW and Wertz DC. *Lying-in: A history of childbirth in America.* New York: Schocken Books, 1979.

16

The Freestanding Birth Center

> Myth: *A freestanding birth center may seem attractive, but it isn't safe.*
>
> Reality: *"[Low risk] women in hospital were more likely to receive an interventive style of labor and birth management [than similar women in birth centers]. Neonatal outcomes were . . . similar, although the incidence of sustained fetal distress, prolapsed cord, and difficulty in establishing respirations were significantly greater in the hospital sample. Hospital care did not offer any advantage . . . , and it was associated with increased intervention. The results of this study provide support for the National Birth Center Study's conclusion that birth centers offer a safe and acceptable alternative for selected pregnant women."*
>
> Fullerton and Severino 1992

Freestanding birth centers arose in the mid-1970s in response to women's dissatisfaction with hospital births. They were—and are—primarily vehicles for midwifery care or at least midwifery-style care. At the typical birth center, prescreened, low-risk laboring women eat and drink and move around freely. They have whomever and however many people they wish with them, including children. They give birth in the position of their choice. Electronic fetal monitoring (EFM), episiotomies, and pain-relief medication are not routine. Common obstetric interventions such as oxytocin, epidurals, instrumental deliveries, and cesareans are not used, and those who need them are transferred to a hospital.

The primary argument against freestanding birth centers is that because obstetric emergencies occur even in prescreened low-risk populations, no labor should occur outside a hospital (Permezel, Pepperell, and Kloss 1987). It is true that obstetric risk assessment tools cannot adequately predict who will need hospital care during labor (Marshall 1989), but it does not follow that all women should give birth in hospitals. Few obstetric problems are situations in which time is of the essence. Those that are, such as postpartum hemorrhage or a baby who fails to breathe, are correctable or can be at least stabilized with low-tech equipment or medications available in birth centers. In fact, birth center studies uniformly report outcomes equivalent or superior to those of comparable women giving birth in the hospital. Turning the tables, the routine interventions practiced in hospitals introduce risks. Birth center studies also uniformly report much lower rates of these interventions. Furthermore, if a hospital lacks 24-hour blood banking and in-house, around-the-clock anesthesiologists and pediatricians—and many do—it offers no greater margin of safety in an emergency than an out-of-hospital birth. It may even offer less because nurse-to-patient ratios, and thus, patient supervision, are likely to be better at a birth center.

An in-hospital birth center would seem the ideal, but the entrenched medical model of childbirth swamps attempts to introduce reforms. The in-hospital alternative birth centers and family birth rooms of the 1970s and early 1980s died and were revived in the late 1980s as the highly successful "single-room maternity units" of the current day. Here, however, it is business as usual, albeit without the trip to the delivery room (except for the one in four women who has a cesarean). Polly Perez (1994), nurse consultant on maternity care, says all too many of these units practice "designer obstetrics—the same old pair of jeans with a fancy new label."

Mainstream medical practitioners fervently hope freestanding birth centers will go away. In 1983, the same year that *Guidelines for Perinatal Care*, jointly published by the American College of Obstetricians and Gynecologists (ACOG) and the American Academy of Pediatrics (AAP), stated there were not enough studies to evaluate the safety of freestanding birth centers, the American Public Health Association (APHA) published a set of guidelines for licensing and regulating freestanding birth centers. Citing four references, it said, "Births to healthy mothers can occur safely in birth centers outside the setting of an acute care hospital" (APHA 1983). Several more studies were done in the next five years. Nonetheless, ACOG and the AAP did not change its mind; the 1988 edition said the same thing. Despite the definitive Rooks et al. report published in 1989 (abstracted below), an ACOG (1982) policy statement—"[U]ntil scientific studies are available to evaluate safety and outcome in free-standing . . . birth centers, such centers cannot be encouraged"—still holds as of summer 1994.

Doctors also have done all they could to make freestanding birth centers disappear. Doctors own or control most of the malpractice insurance companies (Shearer and Eakins 1988). Despite the safety record and low incidence of malpractice suits, five out of eight malpractice insurance companies in California (all eight doctor owned) said they would not insure birth centers unless they were located on hospital grounds, had only obstetricians delivering, and had cesarean capability (Shearer and Eakins 1988; Eakins 1988). For several years no company would insure freestanding birth centers.

However, because birth center births cost substantially less than hospital births and cost containment is increasingly an issue, cracks are appearing in the dam. Liability insurance is once more available. The National Association of Childbearing Centers (NACC) reports that there are about 140 freestanding birth centers scattered around the U.S., and 60 more are under development. And, regardless of ACOG's official position, obstetricians are beginning to make inquiries to the NACC (Ernst 1994).

This development has both positive and negative potential. Because birth centers operate independently of hospital-based medicine, they have a real chance to introduce an alternative, healthier model into the maternity care system that has the potential of leavening the whole lump. Yet as with midwifery itself, acceptance into the mainstream carries a danger. Kitty Ernst (1991), executive director of the NACC, describes freestanding birth centers as "maxi-homes" rather than "mini-hospitals." But if mainstream obstetricians begin to own and operate birth centers, the reverse may come to be true, unless their thinking undergoes a radical change. Let us hope that such will be the case.

SUMMARY OF SIGNIFICANT POINTS

- The freestanding birth center is safe providing: (1) women are prescreened for risk, (2) care providers are trained professionals, (3) physician backup is available, (4) rapid transport to the hospital is available, and (5) emergency equipment is available on-site. (Abstracts 1-12)

- Birth center care costs substantially less than hospital care. (Abstracts 2-4, 7, 10)

- Compared to low-risk hospital obstetric patients, women choosing a free-standing birth center are much less likely to undergo any of the common obstetric interventions (which themselves introduce risk). In particular, birth center women were two to three times less likely to undergo cesarean sections. (Abstracts 2-12)

- Women opting for hospital birth are more likely to have interventions than similar women opting for birth centers even when both groups are cared for by midwives. (Abstract 12)

- The good outcomes and lower intervention rates among birth center women are not due to intrinsic differences from low-risk hospital counterparts. (Abstracts 5, 9-12)

- Women electing birth center care should know how practices differ, especially regarding pain medication. For example, none of the birth centers offered epidurals. (Abstracts 2-4, 8, 10-12)

- Care providers new to the birth center approach may have higher transfer rates and intervention rates than their more experienced colleagues. (Abstract 7)

- Qualifying for a birth center at an initial visit does not mean a woman will give birth and recover there. The proportion of women "risking out" during pregnancy or labor or being transferred postpartum ranges up to one-fourth or even one-third. (Abstracts 1-8, 10-12)

- Mainstream practitioners oppose freestanding birth centers on political, economic, and philosophical grounds but express their opposition as medical concerns. (Abstracts 1, 6-7)

ORGANIZATION OF ABSTRACTS

Reports of Statistics from Individual Birth Centers

Self-Selection to Birth Center Care Does Not Make a Difference

Multiple Birth Center Studies   ·

Comparisons between Birth Centers and Hospitals

REPORTS OF STATISTICS FROM INDIVIDUAL BIRTH CENTERS

Note: However useful and interesting, data from individual birth centers cannot settle the question of safety because incidences of poor outcome and emergencies occur at very low rates, especially in low-risk populations.

1. Faison JB et al. The childbearing center: an alternative birth setting. *Obstet Gynecol* **1979;54(4):527-532.** (This is the same birth center as in Abstract 11.)
    The New York City Maternity Center Association developed a freestanding birth center as a demonstration project. It was located outside the hospital "to attempt to reach a population that rejects and distrusts hospitals . . . to avoid staff bias within a hospital setting that often makes it difficult if not impossible to implement pilot programs of this kind . . . to avoid the pressures encountered within teaching institutions for student physician experience that can prevent the fulfillment of birth management promises made to families." Nurse-midwives provided care.
    Of 714 women registering at the birth center, 119 (15.1%) risked out during pregnancy for medical reasons. Others were ineligible at the first visit, had spontaneous

abortions, or moved. The intrapartum transfer rate was 19.1% for the 304 women who began labor at the birth center. Of the 244 women who gave birth there, 2% of the mothers and 3.7% of the babies were transferred postpartum. There was one neonatal death that was unrelated to birth center care. The safety factors of the birth center were (1) prescreening, (2) good backup by obstetricians, (3) a system for rapid transfer to the hospital in emergencies, (4) emergency equipment at the birth center, and (5) in-depth education of the families. Belief among medical professionals that women opting out of the hospital represent a "lunatic fringe" is not true. "In our experience, opting-out families are well aware of the risks of out-of-hospital birth; they are equally aware of what to them, are the risks of in-hospital birth."

2. Reinke C. Outcomes of the first 527 births at the Birthplace in Seattle. *Birth* 1982;9(4):231-238.
Run by nurse-midwives, the Birthplace offered prenatal classes and home postpartum follow-up in addition to prenatal care and birth services. Friends and family were welcome at the labor. Women were free to eat, drink, move around, and take showers or baths. Fetal heart tones were auscultated once every hour in early labor, every 30 minutes in active first-stage labor, and after almost every contraction during pushing. The cost was $750 to $825 from 1978 to 1981 and $1400 in 1982.

Of the initial 527 registrants, 12.6% risked out during pregnancy for medical reasons. Others were ineligible at the first visit, moved, or dropped out. Of 385 women who started labor at the birth center, 21% were intrapartum transfers. Of the 303 mothers who gave birth at the birth center, the postpartum maternal and neonatal transfer rates were 3.6% and 3.3%, respectively. The midwives delivered 35.4% of the hospital transfers. The cesarean rate for women who began labor at the center was 4.7%, and the forceps rate was 5.4%. Of the 385 who began labor at the center, 89.7% used only a local anesthetic (to repair a tear or an episiotomy) or no medication at all. (The 10.3% who used pain medication includes the 4.7% who had an epidural for their cesarean.) Of the 303 women who gave birth at the center, 20% had episiotomies. An ambulance was used an average of twice yearly for such problems as fetal distress or severe hemorrhage. There were five perinatal deaths, none attributable to birth center management. "The results confirm the safety and effectiveness of the management of pregnancy, birth, and the postpartum periods at the Birthplace, and suggest that additional benefits to parents . . . are its low cost, assistance in getting appropriate intermediate and intensive perinatal care when needed, and support and education in birth and new parenthood."

3. Zabrek E, Simon P, and Benrubi GI. Nurse-midwifery prototypes: clinical practice and education. The alternative birth center in Jacksonville, Florida: the first two years. *J Nurse Midwifery* 1983;28(4):31-36.
Nurse-midwives provided perinatal care, including education. An obstetrician and pediatrician consulted at the center. Fetal heart tones were auscultated at least every 30 minutes in first stage and every 5 to 15 minutes (as indicated) in second stage. Women had freedom of activity and oral intake during first stage. Narcotic analgesia was available.

Between 1980 and 1982, 111 women met the birth center criteria for care. Of them, 22 (20%) were antepartum transfers (only three for medical reasons). Of the 89 women admitted in labor, 18 (20%) were intrapartum transfers. However, seven were for rupture of membranes longer than 12 hours and no active labor, and one woman wanted an epidural. The cesarean rate was 3.4%. The episiotomy rate was 35%, and 80% of those who had no episiotomy had an intact perineum. No woman giving birth at the center had a third- or fourth-degree laceration. The only maternal complication among the 71 women giving birth at the center was a case of postpartum uterine atony, which was successfully treated with oxytocics at the center. [No neonatal transfers are mentioned.] The total cost was $950 versus $2000 or more for a physician-attended birth in the hospital. "With the appropriate physician and hospital affiliation, and with the strictest adherence to protocol for screening, acceptance, and transfer, alternative birthing centers provide the clients with a safe environment for a meaningful birth experience."

4. Eakins PS et al. Obstetric outcomes at the Birth Place in Menlo Park: the first seven years. *Birth* **1989;16(3):123-129.**

This San Francisco-area birth center differs from the typical in that 46% of births were attended by an obstetrician, 29% by nurse-midwives, and 25% by family practitioners. Policies and philosophy were typical for birth centers. There was no EFM, but medical staff auscultated fetal heart tones every 15 minutes in first stage and every 5 minutes during pushing. Analgesia and anesthesia, other than local anesthesia for episiotomies and repairs, were not available.

Seventeen percent of the 898 registrants risked out before labor. Of the 690 admitted in labor, 18% were intrapartum transfers, most of them primiparas (86%). Of the 563 women who gave birth at the center, 1% were postpartum maternal transports, and another 1% were infant transports. Few transfers were emergencies. Because of on-site emergency equipment, staff training, and the proximity to a tertiary care hospital, birth center emergency care and the ability to arrange for a cesarean were about the same as at nontertiary care hospitals. The cesarean rate for those admitted to the birth center was 3%. The forceps rate was also 3%. At the birth center, only 11% of the women had an episiotomy. Two-thirds of the women had no (36%) or only first-degree tears (28%). There were four third-degree tears and one fourth-degree tear. There was no neonatal morbidity or mortality related to birth site. "It appears from the growing number of studies that, for an appropriately risk-screened population, the [freestanding birth center] alternative, at two-thirds the price of hospital birth, offers patients a high degree of satisfaction, is associated with a low cesarean section rate, and involves low overall levels of morbidity and mortality."

SELF-SELECTION TO BIRTH CENTER CARE DOES NOT MAKE A DIFFERENCE

5. Scupholme A and Kamons AS. Are outcomes compromised when mothers are assigned to birth centers for care? *J Nurse Midwifery* **1987;32(4):211-215.** (This is the same birth center as in Abstract 10.)

This Miami birth center had the opportunity to test whether its excellent outcomes were due to self-selection by its clients. Overcrowding caused its associated hospital to assign low-risk women to the birth center, enabling researchers to compare outcomes between women who chose the center and women assigned there.

Women who were either self-selecting or assigned to the birth center were matched for age, ethnic group, parity, financial status, and level of education (*N* = 148 pairs).

When assigned women were compared with self-selected women, length of labor longer than 12 hours (47% versus 37%), use of analgesia (39% versus 43%), intrapartum transfer rate (24% versus 26%), Apgar scores, meconium in the amniotic fluid (18% versus 20%), birth weights, cesarean rates (5% versus 5%), and neonatal transfer rates (5% versus 5%) were similar. Rates were higher than the national average for intrapartum transfers (20%), probably because all women not in active labor by 18 hours after rupture of membranes were transferred for oxytocin. This was in order to forestall a pediatric policy of performing a full septic workup, including spinal tap, on every infant born 24 hours or more after membrane rupture. Expectations were that assigned women would have more complications and cases of arrested labor because they were less motivated about self-care and would carry more residual anxiety about the safety of out-of-hospital birth, but this did not happen. In fact, many patients from the assigned group liked the birth center so well that they returned for subsequent babies and referred friends and family.

MULTIPLE BIRTH CENTER STUDIES

6. Bennetts AB and Lubic R. The freestanding birth centre. *Lancet* **1982;1:378-380.**

Because most birth centers have low numbers of clients, this article collected data from 11 geographically diverse centers (N = 1938 women) that met the following criteria: (1) they were run by nurse-midwives with physician and hospital backup, (2) the philosophy was minimal intervention, and (3) only low-risk women were accepted.

The original intent was a randomized matched-pair comparison, but women who chose an out-of-hospital center refused to be randomized back into the hospital, and hospitals refused to randomize patients into birth centers. [Abstract 5, the sole randomized study in the literature, is both important and unique for this reason.] The authors "strongly desired" to study families who transferred into the hospital, but they could not get access to the requisite data. "It seems that, although there are methodological difficulties in evaluation of innovative services and programmes, the most persistent problems are primarily political. (The activities of the opposed professional groups conform to anthropological models of political activity engaged in by controlling groups the world over.)" As a result, only birth center outcomes could be reported. These were: a 15% combined intrapartum and postpartum transfer rate, a 5% instrumental delivery rate, a 5% cesarean rate, and a neonatal mortality rate of 4.6 per 1000 births.

7. Eakins PS. Freestanding birth centers in California: program and medical outcome. *J Reprod Med* **1989;34(12):960-970.**

Registrants at 16 California freestanding birth centers (FSBC) (N = 2002) (92% of the birth center deliveries in 1984-85) were compared with the national averages for birth centers. California centers differed in that three-fourths of birth center births were attended by obstetricians, and therefore procedures like EFM, instrumental delivery, and oxytocin augmentation were more likely to be performed on-site. The antepartum transfer rate for the eight centers that reported that information (1269 registrants) was 11% (10% for medical reasons) versus 14.5% nationally, and the intrapartum transfer rate for all 16 centers was 8% versus 14% nationally. There was a 0.2% maternal postpartum transfer rate and a 2% infant transfer rate. There was no maternal mortality, and neonatal mortality was 4 per 1000 births, none apparently related to birth center care. Most centers had cesarean rates ranging from 4% to 8%; the average was 4%. One center, which opened in the last few months of 1984, had an 18% cesarean rate, which dropped to 7% the next year. It attributed its high cesarean rate to "inexperience with birth center deliveries." It also had a 37% intrapartum transfer rate, which dropped to 17% the following year.

Because birth centers cost one-third to one-half less than hospital births, "the FSBC movement has the potential to challenge the dominance of hospitals in the arena of low-risk maternity care." Health insurance companies are enthusiastic about them, but malpractice insurance companies are not, despite their excellent safety records and the low incidence of suits. [This makes sense considering that malpractice insurance companies are controlled by doctors interested in protecting their economic turf.] "The current crisis in affordability and availability of professional liability insurance has become the greatest obstacle to the continued existence of FSBCs." [See what I mean?] No statewide regulations exist, but birth centers set their own guidelines. Safety factors were: prenatal screening, one-to-one nursing care during labor, family education programs, rapid transport to the hospital, on-site emergency equipment, and a peer review system for medical care providers. "The medical outcome at these centers parallels what we would expect to find for a low-risk population delivering in a hospital. Thus FSBCs . . . appear to offer personalized maternity care at an acceptable risk level."

8. Rooks JP, et al. Outcomes of care in birth centers: the National Birth Center Study. *N Engl J Med* 1989;321(26):1804-1811.

Note: Extensive and detailed data from the this study are presented in (1) Rooks JP, Weatherby NL, and Ernst EK. The National Birth Center Study. Part II—Intrapartum and immediate postpartum and neonatal care. *J Nurse Midwifery* 1992;37(5):301-330, and (2) Rooks JP, Weatherby NL, and Ernst EK. The National Birth Center Study. Part III—Intrapartum and immediate postpartum and neonatal complications and transfers, postpartum and neonatal care, outcomes, and client satisfaction. *J Nurse Midwifery* 1992;37(6):361-397.

Data were collected from 84 freestanding birth centers from mid-1985 through 1987 in order to remedy the problem that large numbers were needed to evaluate outcomes in a low-risk population. Sixty of the centers were run by nurse-midwives, 11 by obstetricians, six by other doctors such as family practitioners, three by obstetricians and nurse-midwives, three by licensed or lay midwives [some states license midwives without the prerequisite of a nursing degree], and one by a team of nurse-midwives and lay midwives. Nurse-midwives or student nurse-midwives provided care at 78.6% of the labors and 80.6% of the births at the centers.

Of the original 17,856 women who enrolled at the birth centers, 33.8% were not admitted in labor. The antepartum transfer rate for medical reasons was 14%; the rest were for other reasons such as the birth center closed, the women moved, changed their minds, or had abortions. Thus, 11,814 women were admitted in labor. The intrapartum transfer rate was 11.9%, and the postpartum transfer rate was 2.5%. The timing of transfer was unknown for 1.4%, making an overall transfer rate of 15.8%. The cesarean rate was 4.4% (9.9% nulliparas, 0.8% multiparas).

All but 5% of women drank and/or ate during labor, and 43.4% took showers and/or baths. Ninety-seven percent had friends and family present, often including children.

Only 24% of nulliparas and 6.2% of multiparas had analgesia, sedatives, or tranquilizers in labor. Only 3% had an anesthetic other than for episiotomy or tear repair. A third of the women (34.2%) had an intact perineum, 45.7% had first- or second-degree tears, 17.6% had episiotomies without additional tears, 1.6% had third-degree lacerations and 0.8% had fourth-degree lacerations.

The neonatal mortality rate was 0.8 per 1000, reduced to 0.3 per 1000 if lethal anomalies are excluded. The intrapartum death rate was 0.4 per 1000, reduced to 0.3 per 1000 if lethal anomalies are excluded. Of the stillbirths not related to anomalies, three of the four babies died in the birth center. Two involved placental abruptions [the placenta separates from the wall of the uterus prematurely and bleeds], and the other preeclampsia in labor. The fourth baby was transferred for meconium and fetal distress during first-stage labor. Two out of four of the neonatal deaths not related to anomalies were babies born in the birth center. One involved prolonged rupture of the membranes. The baby developed respiratory distress and was transferred, dying of pneumonia and hyaline membrane disease. The other was born healthy and died a week later. An autopsy did not reveal cause of death. The two who died in the hospital were transferred during labor for fetal distress.

Results were compared with five studies of low-risk hospital deliveries. The proportion of infants with low Apgar scores and the total mortality rates were comparable to the birth center, and the birth centers' cesarean rate was half that of the two hospital studies that reported cesarean rates. The authors also compared their mortality rate to birth centers excluded from the analysis because they did not conform to study standards. The mortality rate at the five excluded centers was 7.2 per 1000. [All birth centers are not alike.] "Few innovations in health service promise lower cost, greater availability, and a high degree of satisfaction with a comparable degree of safety. The results of this study suggest that modern birth centers can identify women who are at low risk for obstetrical complications and can care for them in a way that provides these benefits."

COMPARISONS BETWEEN BIRTH CENTERS AND HOSPITALS

9. Baruffi G et al. A study of pregnancy outcomes in a maternity center and a tertiary care hospital. *Am J Public Health* **1984;74(9):973-978.** (See also Abstracts 12 and 13 in Chapter 15, which use data from the same populations.)

Booth Maternity Center (BMC), located in Philadelphia, is an exception to the usual freestanding birth center in that it is a primary care hospital [a Level I hospital capable of handling the essentially normal pregnancy, birth, and newborn]. BMC has in-center physician backup and cesarean and forceps capability. It also handles larger numbers of clients than the typical birth center. On the other hand, like other birth centers, it screens out high-risk women, births are generally managed by midwives, and the approach is noninterventive.

BMC women ($N = 796$) were stratified by socioeconomic factors and grouped by pregnancy and labor risk scores. Groups were matched with women at Thomas Jefferson Memorial Hospital (TJMH) ($N = 804$), a nearby tertiary care center [Level III hospitals are equipped for high-risk pregnancy and labor and the very sickest and most premature infants]. Overall, the cesarean rate at BMC was 5.3% versus 18.2% at TJMH, and the neonatal mortality rate (uncorrected for avoidable deaths—lethal anomalies or extreme prematurity) was 3.8 per 1000 births at BMC versus 9.9 per 1000 at TJMH. [However, because TJMH accepted women who would be deemed too risky for BMC, institutional differences in cesarean and neonatal mortality rates may be misleading. Infant outcomes were broken down by risk category, which allows a better comparison basis.] The neonatal mortality rate for BMC women with low prenatal risk/low intrapartum risk was 3.0 per 1000 versus 0.0 per 1000 in the comparable group at TJMH, and the rate for low prenatal risk/high intrapartum risk BMC women was 8.0 per 1000 versus 12.8 per 1000 at TJMH [no calculations as to whether differences were statistically significant]. "While BMC departs from the classic model of the birth center, the results presented here as well as those reported previously on birth centers do not support the notion that care provided in these centers is unsafe."

10. Scupholme A, McLeod AGW, and Robertson EG. A birth center affiliated with the tertiary care center: comparison of outcome. *Obstet Gynecol* **1986;67(4):598-603.** (This is the same birth center as in Abstract 5.)

This study matched 250 low-risk women who started labor at a Miami birth center to women of similar age, parity, ethnic background, financial status, and risk status who labored at its associated tertiary care hospital. At the birth center, care was given by nurse-midwives. Women could eat, drink, and move around, and friends and family were welcome. EFM was not used nor were oxytocin, epidurals, c-sections, or forceps. Analgesia (narcotics and tranquilizers) was available, as were IVs. At the hospital there was no or minimal oral intake, and IVs were routine. Two-thirds of the women had continuous EFM, and the rest had intermittent electronic monitoring. The birth center's intrapartum transfer rate was 21.6%, mostly for no established labor within 12 hours of membrane rupture (17/54) or labor dystocia (15/54).

While the birth center women had significantly more babies weighing over 4000 g, the cesarean rate for birth center women was 6% versus 14% in the hospital group $(0.01 > p > 0.005)$. The forceps rates were similar (2% versus 3%). Oxytocin was used in 12.4% of women starting at the birth center versus 24% of the hospital group. Because interventions like oxytocin and forceps were used less often, birth center women were more likely to have second stages longer than two hours (5.3% versus 2.4%), but without detriment to maternal or infant outcomes. Analgesia usage was about the same in both groups. The postpartum hemorrhage rate was 5% at the birth center versus 2.4% in the hospital, but blood loss estimates are subjective. The neonatal transfer rate was 16%, higher than the national average. However, consultation with a doctor required transfer. Most neonatal transfers were for mild respiratory distress (12/32) or positive Coombs test [maternal antibodies to baby's blood] (19/32). The cost of birth center care was 30% less than the equivalent low-risk hospital birth.

One weakness of this study is that birth center patients are self-selecting. Superior outcomes could be due to better health behaviors in the birth center population. For example, birth center women were better educated, so education levels could not be matched between the two populations. "Outcomes for low-risk women are as good as those in the tertiary care center at less cost to the family."

11. Feldman E and Hurst M. Outcomes and procedures in low risk birth: a comparison of hospital and birth center settings. *Birth* **1987;14(1):18-24.** (This is the same birth center as in Abstract 1.)

This study compared outcomes for 77 women at 37 weeks gestation who were eligible for the Maternity Center Association's Childbearing Center in New York City with outcomes of 72 low-risk patients going to a large nearby teaching hospital. Antepartum transfers after 37 weeks (8%) and intrapartum transfers (14%) were included in the birth center data. Populations were similar in age, parity, marital status, and education through high school, and none was on Medicaid. Birth center women were more likely to have some college education. The birth center is run by nurse-midwives, and policies are like those at other birth centers. There is no use of oxytocin or EFM. Analgesia is available.

More women in the hospital group had oxytocin augmentation (59.5% versus 9.1%), amniotomy (60.9% versus 42.1%), EFM (97.0% versus 20.7%), IVs (97.2% versus 19.5%), epidurals (56.3% versus 5.2%), episiotomy (78.1% versus 47.2%), and forceps (43.7% versus 5.6%) (all P < 0.0001). [Some of the differences in oxytocin and forceps rates can be explained by the difference in epidural rates.] Narcotic analgesia rates were similar (26.8% versus 19.5%), but more hospital women had a narcotic less than two hours before birth [which could depress newborn respiration] (14.1% versus 2.6%, $p < 0.01$). There were too few cesareans to allow statistical calculation, but the hospital rate was 11.3% versus 6.5% at the birth center. [Epidurals could have played a role here too.] Labors were longer at the birth center, but thick meconium in the amniotic fluid was three times more frequent at the hospital (18.3% versus 5.2%, $p < 0.005$%). Fetal heart rate abnormalities were diagnosed more often in the hospital (23.9% versus 5.2%, $p < 0.0001$), although infant outcomes were similar. Even though outcomes were similar, transfer to neonatal intensive care was more frequent in the hospital group (5.6% versus 1.3%, NS). One fetal death occurred at term in the hospital group. Differences in population characteristics could lead to differences in the use of interventions. Compared with the hospital group, the birth center women were more educated, more likely to be having a first baby, and more likely to be white than Hispanic. However, studies show that labor interventions are positively associated with the birth center population (white, middle-class, nulliparas).

> Evidence is mounting that out-of-hospital birth centers offer an alternative as safe as hospital settings. . . . [And that] the birth center alternative provides such comparative safety with less intervention. . . . The findings raise the question of whether interventions are neutral. If there is no need for certain interventions to improve obstetrical outcome for low risk women, can their use be justified? . . . [Moreover] it is misleading to answer the question of intervention "neutrality" by assessing the risk of each procedure. The use of one intervention often creates the need for further interventions each with its associated risk.

12. Fullerton JT and Severino R. In-hospital care for low-risk childbirth: comparison with results from the National Birth Center Study. *J Nurse Midwifery* **1992;37(5):331-340.**

This study compares outcomes for women from 15 hospital-based midwifery services ($N = 2256$) with women in the National Birth Center Study (NBCS) ($N = 11,814$) [see Abstract 8]. Thus outcomes can be examined as a function of site of birth. The data set from the NBCS comprises all women who began labor at the birth centers from mid-1985 through 1987. Data were prospectively gathered from the hospital-based practices during the same time period using the same method. Logistic regression was used to control for differences in socioeconomic and medical risk factors between the two groups.

Because of missing information, the incidence of gestation longer than 42 weeks can only be estimated. Incidence was 6% for the hospital group versus 11.4% for the NBCS women, suggesting earlier intervention in the hospital group. However, this may be due to higher perinatal risk in the hospital group. NBCS women were less likely to have instrumental deliveries (2.3% versus 3.1%) or to give birth in the supine or lithotomy position (40.2% versus 21.3%). The cesarean rates were 4.4% (9.9% nulliparas, 0.8% multiparas) for NBCS women versus 9.5% (11.7% nulliparas, 3.8% multiparas) for the hospital group. After excluding nonvertex presentations and postterm births, the cesarean rate for NBCS women was 4.4% versus 7.8% for the hospital group. To eliminate the effect of complications on the use of intervention, a subset of women with no complications was compared. The NBCS midwives consistently favored less interventive and more supportive care (all P < 0.01), including analgesia (9.8% versus 20.2%), food during labor (14.9% versus 10.8%), more than four vaginal exams (44.3% versus 52.9%), external EFM (6.9% versus 50.2%), internal EFM (0.9% versus 7.7%), induction (0.4% versus 1.6%), augmentation (1.0% versus 2.2%), IVs (8.1% versus 23.5%), shower/bath during labor (40.4% versus 24.2%), amniotomy (41.2% versus 50.7%), and episiotomy (21.1% versus 33.7%). Rates of liquid intake (92.8% versus 93.3%) were similar. Among all women, the hospital group experienced higher incidences of "sustained fetal distress" (all P < 0.01) (1.8% versus 6.6%), prolapsed cord (0.03 versus 0.2%), and "great effort required to establish respirations" (0.4% versus 1.1%). Other than these, "[t]here was a remarkable similarity in the incidence of complications." Equally good maternal and infant outcomes were obtained; therefore, birth center birth had no adverse effect (on low-risk women). Women giving birth in the hospital, even women with no complications, experienced many more interventions. This not only did not improve outcomes but may have contributed to infant morbidity.

REFERENCES

AAP and ACOG. *Guidelines for perinatal care.* 1983.
——. *Guidelines for perinatal care.* 2d ed. 1988.
ACOG. *Alternative birth centers.* Dec 3-4, 1982.
APHA. Guidelines for licensing and regulating birth centers. *Am J Public Health* 1983;73(3):331-334.
Eakins PS. Freestanding birth centers: prospects and problems. *Birth* 1988;15(1):25-30.
Ernst K. Interview, Sep 20, 1991.
——. Personal communication, January 4, 1994.
Marshall VA. A comparison of two obstetric risk assessment tools. *J Nurse Midwifery* 1989;34(1):3-7.
Perez P. Personal communication, Jan 5, 1994.
Permezel JMH, Pepperell RJ, and Kloss M. Unexpected problems in patients selected for birthing unit delivery. *Aust N Z J Obstet Gynaecol* 1987;27:21-23.
Shearer MH and Eakins PS. Commentary and response: the malpractice insurance crisis and freestanding birth centers. *Birth* 1988;15(1):30-32.

17

Home Birth

Myth: *Home birth is so dangerous that it should be considered child abuse.*

Reality: *"There is no evidence to support the claim that the safest policy is for all women to give birth in hospital. . . . There is some evidence . . . that morbidity is higher amongst mothers and babies delivered and cared for in institutional facilities in general and . . . obstetric units in particular."*

Campbell and Macfarlane 1986

For years the American College of Obstetricians and Gynecologists has officially opposed home birth on grounds of safety (ACOG 1979). If the argument for universal hospitalization for childbirth is that it is safer, then it is reasonable to ask: has moving birth into the hospital decreased the risks? Before answering that, however, we must first take into account that doctors overestimate the dangers of childbirth and that their own actions cause some of the complications they see.

Labor is not nearly as dangerous as doctors make it out to be. Doctors tend to manage labor on a worst-case basis, treating every labor as though disaster could strike at any moment (Brody and Thompson 1981). With this approach, the concerns proper to high-risk conditions spill over and color thinking about all labors, regardless of risk level. For example, one in-hospital birth center that admitted only women free of complications risked out (transferred to the standard labor and delivery unit) 10 mothers during labor for nonspecific anxiety on the part of doctors (Saldana et al. 1983). The majority of adolescents also risked out due to "the anxiety of the resident or attending physician who perhaps viewed adolescence as representing a risk factor in pregnancy." Ten other mothers were transferred because of "precipitate labor," meaning they were disqualified for rapid labor and imminent birth, which makes no sense. Indeed, only 41% of the 390 women who were eligible as of the third trimester actually gave birth in the hospital's birth center. Compare this with the roughly 80% rates reported for freestanding birth centers and home births, where beliefs about the intrinsic risk of childbirth differ.

Furthermore, as Mold and Stein (1986) explain, the doctor's diffuse anxiety about labor may trigger the cascade effect, a seemingly inevitable stepwise series of events catalyzed by some characteristic of the system. For example, the worry that any fetus may suddenly develop acute distress in labor leads to using electronic fetal monitoring (EFM) in normal, healthy women. EFM restricts women to bed, which may slow labor. Amniotomy or oxytocin may then be used to speed labor up. Increased pain results, which may lead to an epidural. The epidural may further retard progress, or perhaps the oxytocin or amniotomy causes abnormal fetal heart rate tracings. The labor ends in a cesarean for failure to progress or fetal distress. According to Mold and Stein, medical cascades of this type may be triggered by the temptation to do "something—anything—decisive to diminish [the doctor's] own anxiety," efforts to feel in control by controlling the patient, and protocols that treat everybody alike and fail to individualize care. Medical staff rarely recognize that they are the source of the cascade. In illustration of this, Saldana et al. (1983) argue against home birth, pointing to the many complications that arose even in their low-risk population, all of which they believe to be due to the inherent risk of the natural process. They see nothing strange in so many healthy women with normal pregnancies having cesareans (10%), forceps deliveries (13%), or oxytocin (> 20%). Yet freestanding birth centers and home births report half or less of these rates with equally good or better outcomes.

There is nothing new in obstetricians' denying they cause complications. In this Saldana et al. merely echo the doctors of Semmelweis's time who insisted postpartum infections must be due to the constitutions of the poor mothers (in every sense of the word) they delivered, not their own failure to wash their hands plus the wounds made by forceps and episiotomies.

Returning to whether moving childbirth into the hospital made birth safer, the answer is unequivocally no. Doctors argue that the decrease in mortality and morbidity rates as birth moved into the hospital proves that the hospital is safer (Philipp 1984; Adamson and Gare 1980). Even if that statement were true, it would not mean hospital birth was responsible for the decline, but the claim is false. In the 1920s middle-class women began having babies in hospitals partly on grounds of safety. By the mid-1920s half of urban births took place there, and by 1939, half of all women and 75% of all urban women gave birth in hospitals. Despite this shift, maternal mortality did not drop below the 1915 levels of 63 maternal deaths per 10,000 births until the late 1930s, when sulfa drugs and antibiotics to treat infection were introduced and more stringent controls were placed on obstetric practices. During that same time period, urban maternal mortality rates, where hospitalization for birth was more common, were considerably higher than overall rates: 74 deaths per 10,000 births (Dye 1986). Infant deaths from birth injuries actually increased by 40% to 50% between 1915 and 1929 (Wertz and Wertz 1977).

Modern techniques and technology still have not succeeded in making hospital birth safer than home birth. Contemporary defenders of universal hospital confinement point to statistics showing higher perinatal mortality rates for out-of-hospital births (Brown 1987; Philipp 1984; Adamson and Gare 1980), but these were raw statistics and included unintended home births and births without a trained birth attendant. No study has ever shown that planned home birth with a trained attendant who took proper precautions increased the incidence of poor outcomes among low-risk women compared with low-risk women in the hospital.

In fact, hospitals may not even be the best place for women with risk factors. Tew's (1985, abstracted below) analysis of British statistics showed that perinatal mortality rates were lower for home births at every level of predicted risk except the very highest category. Tew posits that interventions used by doctors in hospitals introduced risk or that in the more relaxed, supportive home environment, with a birth attendant who believed in the normalcy of birth, problems either never arose or were resolved noninterventively.

This whole book confirms that Tew is right on the first count, and while little or no direct research has been done on the adverse effects of a stressful environment or the efficacy of supportive measures, she is almost certainly right on the second count too. Consider the effect on *any* physiological process if it were treated as labor is treated. Take digestion. In the 1950s, similar to our current belief that labor should progess at a certain rate and that deviation is pathological, many people believed that healthy individuals should move their bowels once a day, and failure to do so required treatment. As a result, the misuse of laxatives and enemas ruined normal physiological mechanisms, causing problems with constipation where there never were difficulties before.

At worst, mainstream medical belief dismisses the mother's psychological experience as irrelevant to or even in conflict with the goals of a healthy mother and a healthy baby (Adamson and Gare 1980). At best, doctors claim that women's objections to hospital birth can be met by creating a homelike environment in the hospital (Home, hospital, or birthroom? 1986; Adamson and Gare 1980). But *homelike hospital birth* is an oxymoron. Hospitals are intrinsically bureaucratic, hierarchical institutions where policies are designed to meet the hospital's needs first and women and their families a distant last. Only cosmetic changes are possible within a hospital unless its fundamental nature undergoes drastic change. Despite admitting fathers in the 1970s, candlelit dinners in the 1980s, and single-room maternity care in the 1990s, hospital staff today usually still expect women to be passive and to accommodate to the disruptions, intrusions, and inconveniences as best they may. Active management of labor is a quintessential example of this. Its principal benefit was to make staffing more predictable (see Chapter 5). By contrast, in her own home, the woman sets the rules, her needs are the focus of attention, and all nonhousehold members, including her birth attendant, are her guests and there on her sufferance.

Ultimately, the issue of the safety of home birth cannot be settled by research. While research has failed to show that home birth is dangerous, research cannot conclusively prove it to be safe. It comes down to a matter of individual choice. The real question about safety is not, "Do you want a pleasant birth at home or a safe birth in the hospital?" It is, "Do you want to give birth at home and run the minuscule risk of an emergency that might (but not necessarily would) be handled better in the hospital, or do you want to give birth in the hospital and run the considerably increased risk of infection, the certainty of additional stress, and the near certainty of having unnecessary (and potentially risky) interventions?"

SUMMARY OF SIGNIFICANT POINTS

- Raw data, such as birth certificates, give an inaccurate picture of the risks of home birth because they include a large proportion of unplanned home births and births without a trained attendant, both situations carrying extremely high risk. (Abstracts 2, 4, 7-10)

- No study of planned home births of a screened population of women with a trained attendant taking proper precautions has shown excess risk. (Abstracts 1-23)

- Because unexpected problems arise even within a screened population, those planning home birth should have appropriate backup arrangements with an obstetrician and a hospital. Home birth attendants should have the skills to monitor the labor and the baby and the skills, equipment, and medication to manage or stabilize emergencies such as a baby who does not breathe spontaneously or a mother who hemorrhages after birth. (Abstracts 3, 8, 14, 16-18, 20, 22)

- Home birth becomes dangerous only when doctors and hospitals fail to provide backup services. (Thus, their failure converts an imaginary risk into a real one.) (Abstracts 3, 14)

- Excellent outcomes with much lower intervention rates are achieved at home births. This may be because the overuse of interventions in hospital births introduces risks or the home environment promotes problem-free labors. (Abstracts 2, 5-6, 11-13, 15-19, 21-23)

- An ultrasound scan may be advisable in late pregnancy to rule out twins and breech presentation (and to confirm placental location). (Abstracts 16-17, 20-21)

- To prevent unnecessary postpartum hospital transfer, the attendant should be able to repair perineal lacerations and to perform and repair an episiotomy. (Abstract 20)

ORGANIZATION OF ABSTRACTS

Analyses of Statistics (Reviews)

The Netherlands
Great Britain

Analyses of Statistics (Studies)

The Netherlands
Great Britain
United States

Studies of Home Birth

The Netherlands
Great Britain
Australia
Canada
United States

Note: The Netherlands' unique maternity care system is often studied by researchers interested in midwifery or home birth. The Netherlands never fell prey to the economic turf wars of other developed countries that resulted in doctors' either driving out midwives or subjugating them under obstetricians. Dutch midwives have maintained full autonomy. They train directly as midwives and are not required to hold a nursing degree. They provide primary maternity care, while obstetricians are reserved for problematic pregnancies or births. Dutch insurance reimburses only for midwifery care, unless medical problems mandate referral to an obstetrician. If a woman elects an obstetrician's care, she must pay for it herself. Thus, public health policy in the Netherlands has never been shaped by the medical model—the belief that universal hospital confinement is necessary for safety and that the liberal use of interventions is both necessary and harmless. As a result, women may choose home or hospital, and home birth in the Netherlands has remained a viable option, with about one third of women having their babies at home. Insurance covers postpartum nurses' aides, a support service that also makes home birth more feasible (Eskes 1992, abstracted below; Torres and Reich 1989).

ANALYSES OF STATISTICS (Reviews)

The Netherlands

1. Eskes TK. Home deliveries in the Netherlands—perinatal mortality and morbidity. *Int J Gynaecol Obstet* **1992;38(3):161-169.**

Only Dutch studies are included in this review. In 1989, 33.4% of the 190,079 births in Holland took place at home. Midwives cared for 45.7% of women, general practitioners for 11.3%, and obstetricians for 43.0%. Midwives attended 32.9% of hospital births. In 1988 midwives referred 31.8% of their cases to obstetricians.

National perinatal mortality rates (PMR) for hospital births under obstetrical care ranged from 0.9% to 1.0% between 1983 and 1988. The PMR for midwife-attended births was 0.09% in 1988 [unclear whether this means midwives in general or just midwife-attended hospital births]. One study argued that because PMRs declined faster over time in other European countries with universal hospitalization, Holland should move toward universal hospital birth too. However, another study [Abstract 3] found regional PMRs did not correlate with percentage of hospitalization. In Enschede during 1974, the PMR under obstetrical care was 24.3 per 1000 versus 2.4 per 1000 for low-risk women having home births with midwives or general practitioners. The PMR for late referrals to the hospital was 59.1 per 1000. In Wormerveer, the overall PMR between 1969 and 1983 for a large group of midwives was 11.1 per 1000. For the 17.1% of women referred out during pregnancy it was 51.7 per 1000,and for those referred during labor it was 11.0 per 1000. For women who started labor under midwifery care, it was 2.3 per 1000, and for women giving birth under midwifery care it was 1.3 per 1000. Two studies evaluated avoidable perinatal mortality. In Nijmegen, researchers concluded that most cases of avoidable death between 1976 and 1977 were because toxemia and fetal growth retardation were not recognized early enough. In the Wormerveer study, the intended place of birth played a "minor and insignificant role" in avoidable death. As for morbidity, a large prospective study of neurologic condition in the newborn could not distinguish between care provider or place of birth. Perinatal outcome data must be used with caution. Wrong conclusions may be drawn if the population characteristics of the caregiver, fetal age, and cause of death are not considered.

Great Britain

2. Campbell R and MacFarlane A. Place of delivery: a review. *Br J Obstet Gynaecol* **1986;93(7):675-683.**

This review analyzes papers examining the association between place of birth and mortality and morbidity for British births [including Abstract 6]. They conclude that:

- The statistical association between the increase in hospital deliveries and the decline in perinatal mortality is unlikely to be a cause-and-effect relationship.

- Attempts to show that higher perinatal mortality rates in obstetric facilities prior to 1970 were because such units had more high-risk patients have failed.

- The rise in perinatal mortality rates for home births is due to the changing proportions of planned versus unplanned home birth. As more women gave birth in the hospital, a higher and higher proportion of home births were unplanned, and thus very high risk.

- Perinatal mortality rates for low-risk women planning home births are very low.
- "There is no evidence to support the claim that the safest policy is for all women to give birth in the hospital."
- There is some evidence to support the claim that the higher morbidity among mothers and babies cared for in hospitals, and particularly by obstetricians, is due to labor management.
- A majority of women who have given birth both in the hospital and at home prefer home birth, although it is likely that this group selectively contains many women who chose home birth because they had an unsatisfactory hospital experience.

ANALYSES OF STATISTICS (Studies)

The Netherlands

3. Treffers PE and Laan R. Regional perinatal mortality and regional hospitalization at delivery in the Netherlands. *Br J Obstet Gynaecol* **1986;93(7):690-693.**

The correlation between Dutch PMR and percentage of hospital births was examined for the 11 provinces, by municipalities grouped by number of inhabitants, and among the 17 cities with populations greater than 100,000. The lowest percentage of hospital births for any individual province, municipality, or city was 49.2%, the highest 95.7%. In no case did the PMR correlate with degree of hospitalization for birth. The effect of underreporting cannot be determined, but it is unlikely that many perinatal deaths at home go unreported. Notification of perinatal death is obligatory to obtain permission to bury the infant. It might be easier to avoid notification after a hospital birth because disposing of the infant without formal burial is more difficult at home. [Such births are likely to be extremely preterm infants, not cases where site of birth could affect outcome.] The conclusion that home birth does not adversely affect PMR may not apply outside the Netherlands, where there are competent midwives and midwives' assistants, and there is selection of low-risk pregnancies and good ambulance service [and, reliable obstetric backup].

Great Britain

4. Murphy JF et al. Planned and unplanned deliveries at home: implications of a changing ratio. *Br Med J* **1984;288(6428):1429-1432.**

In England and Wales perinatal mortality increased between 1975 and 1977 among babies born at home, rising higher than that of babies born in hospitals with obstetric units. This observation is cited as evidence for phasing out home birth. However, these statistics do not differentiate between planned home births and births to women who deliberately refuse hospital care, women (often teenagers) who make no plans, and women overtaken by emergency births at home, all high-risk situations. This study looks at outcomes for planned versus unplanned home birth from 1970 to 1979 among Welsh women in three major cities.

During the 1970s the overall incidence of home births fell from 2% to 0.7%. Since this represented a decrease in planned home births but the percentage of unplanned home births remained changed, a higher and higher proportion of home births were unplanned. By the end of the decade, the number of unplanned home births per year exceeded the number of those planned.

Of 315 women who began a planned home birth at home, eight (2.5%) were intrapartum transfers. Three babies died [perinatal mortality, 9.5/1000]. Among the 159 women who had unplanned or unattended home births during the same time period, 13 babies died [perinatal mortality, 81.8/1000]. [The perinatal mortality rate for hospital population was 22.9 per 1000 during the same period.]

5. Tew M. Place of birth and perinatal mortality. *J R Coll Gen Pract* 1985;35(277):390-394.

Using the raw PMRs from a 1970 British national survey, the hospital PMR was 27.8 per 1000 births versus 5.4 per 1000 for home births/general practitioner units (GPU). This was not because hospitals handled more high-risk births. When PMRs were standardized based on age, parity, hypertension/toxemia, prenatal risk prediction score, method of delivery, and birth weight, adjusted hospital PMRs for each category ranged from 22.7 per 1000 to 27.8 per 1000 while home birth/GPU rates ranged from 5.4 per 1000 to 10.5 per 1000.

The 1970 survey assigned a prenatal risk score to predict the likelihood of problems during labor. When PMRs for hospital versus home/GPU for the same level of risk (very low, low, moderate, high, very high) are compared, the hospital PMR was lower only at the very highest risk level. All differences, except in the "very high risk" category, were significant. The PMR for *high*-risk births in home/GPUs (15.5/1000) was slightly lower than that for *low*-risk births in the hospital (17.9/1000). Moreover, the PMRs in home/GPUs for very low, low, and moderate risk births were all similar, but hospital PMRs increased twofold between categories, which suggests that hospital labor management actually intensified risks.

The percentage of infants born with breathing difficulties (9.3% versus 3.3%), the death rate associated with breathing difficulties (0.94% versus 0.19%), and the transfer rate to neonatal intensive care units for infants with breathing problems who survived six hours (62.0% versus 26.2%) were all higher in the hospital (all $p < 0.001$), further evidence that hospital interventions do not avert poor outcomes.

Although no national study has been undertaken since, smaller studies confirm that increasing use of hospital confinement is not the reason for the overall drop in PMR since 1970. In fact, those years when the proportional increase in hospital births was greatest were the years when the PMR declined least and vice versa.

6. Tew M. Do obstetric intranatal interventions make birth safer? *Br J Obstet Gynaecol* 1986;93(7):659-674.

First the British annual stillbirth rates between 1969 and 1981 are analyzed. As the campaign to move birth into the hospital succeeded, the proportion of home births that were unplanned and unattended (and thus at high risk) rose, whereas the hospital birth population was increasingly diluted by low-risk women. Calculation shows that if the proportion of out-of-hospital births had remained the same in 1981 as in 1969, the stillbirth rate would have been 5.9 per 1000 instead of 6.6 per 1000. The increase in hospitalization actually retarded the decline in stillbirths.

Women transferred during labor are known to have a high PMR, which is taken as evidence that out-of-hospital birth is risky. In the 1970 national survey, the PMR for births booked at the hospital was 22.9 per 1000 versus 4.9 per 1000 for home birth/GPUs versus 58.9 per 1000 for births not booked for the hospital. Even making the unlikely assumption that all births not booked for the hospital were transfers of home/GPU births, the PMR for home/GPU becomes 19.2 per 1000, still less than the planned hospital rate of 22.9 per 1000.

[Tew then goes on to match 1970 hospital and home/GPU PNMRs by prenatal risk, as she did in Abstract 5. She concludes that obstetric management increases rather than reduces risk and the PMR would have been lower if all women had had home births.] "These findings support the often expressed theory of Michel Odent that the fetus already at increased risk is less able to withstand the stresses of obstetric intervention. . . . [In addition,] since maternal fear, stress and lack of self confidence militate against easy and successful labor, an excess of these factors could contribute to the excess of risk among hospital births."

The argument that higher PMRs are associated with intervention, but intervening forestalled an even worse PMR is not sustained. Citing induction as an example, large numbers of uncomplicated cases were subjected to interventions. Moreover, induction was used more often for the same problem inside the hospital than outside. Indiscriminate use of interventions may create, rather than abate, complications. Hospital-based technology clearly benefits low-birth-weight babies, but average-weight babies do significantly worse.

The improvement in PMR that followed improvements in maternal health status unfortunately coincided with increasing obstetric management. It was then "all too easy" to attribute the declining PMR to the benefits of obstetric management. "[Most] obstetricians . . . have become convinced that the natural process of birth is fraught with dangers which their increasingly sophisticated technological interventions are increasingly capable of minimizing. Amazingly, they have managed, without producing any valid supporting evidence, to persuade the majority of people, medical and lay, that they are right." Relatively few people now believe that "for healthy women, giving birth is a normal physiological process, which obstetric intervention cannot improve though it can harm," or that only in rare cases do obstetric interventions definitely help.

7. Campbell R et al. Home births in England and Wales, 1979: perinatal mortality according to intended place of delivery. *Br Med J* 1984;289(6447):721-724.

Data are analyzed from a survey undertaken of the 8061 babies born at home in England and Wales during 1979 for whom information could be obtained on intended place of delivery. While 67% of births occurring at home were planned, only 11% of the perinatal mortality occurred in this group. By contrast, 41% of the perinatal mortality occurred among the 15% booked for a consultant unit, and 27% of the perinatal mortality occurred among the 3% not booked at all. The differences were all significant ($p < 0.01$). The perinatal mortality rates were, respectively, 4.1 per 1000, 67.5 per 1000, 196.6 per 1000. Similarly, the highest mean birth weights were among planned home births, and the lowest were among unbooked births. The percentage of babies weighing less than 2500 g among the unbooked population was 29% compared with 18% for those booked in a consultant unit and 2.5% for births planned at home. "[This study] shows the critical importance of knowing about the intended place of delivery when trying to assess the risk of mortality associated with home delivery."

United States

8. Burnett CA et al. Home delivery and neonatal mortality in North Carolina.
JAMA **1980;244(24):2741-2745.**
This study links home births ($N = 1296$) with neonatal mortality for the years 1974-76. Home births attended by a lay midwife ($N = 768$) and those classified by questionnaire as "intended" ($N = 166$) were assumed to be planned (72%). The 51 infants weighing 2000 g or less whose births were not attended by a midwife and 199 others classified by questionnaire as "precipitate" or "failure to plan for health care" were considered unplanned home births (19%). [No mention is made of the other 9%.]

The neonatal mortality among planned home births was 6 per 1000 versus 120 per 1000 for unplanned home births. All three deaths attended by a midwife were associated with congenital anomalies. An additional three deaths occurred among planned home births that had an attendant other than a doctor or midwife. Excluding infants weighing 2000 g or less at birth, the neonatal mortality rate for hospital deliveries in North Carolina was 7 per 1000 and for midwife-attended home births it was 4 per 1000 (NS). This was despite the fact that women attended by midwives were more likely to be demographically high risk (young, black, unmarried, and less educated than the average woman in the state).

9. Hinds MW, Bergeisen GH, and Allen DT. Neonatal outcome in planned v unplanned out-of-hospital births in Kentucky. *JAMA* **1985;253(11):1578-1582.**
Observed versus expected rates were compared for neonatal mortality and low-birth-weight (LBW) at out-of-hospital Kentucky births from 1981 to 1983. The standard was Kentucky statewide rates for 1979-82. Stillbirths were not considered because out-of-hospital stillbirths are probably underreported.

There were 809 births classifiable by planning status. Compared with planned home births, unplanned home births had higher odds of LBW (OR 6.6, CL 3.9-11.2). After adjusting for maternal age and parity, LBW was half as likely to occur among planned home births as expected (OR 0.48; CL 0.29-0.73), and LBW was more likely than expected at unplanned home births (OR 2.9, CL 2.2-3.8). Neonatal mortality was greater among unplanned home births compared with planned home births (72.7 per 1000 versus 3.5 per 1000, $p = 4.4 \times 10^{-8}$), but the numbers were not big enough to establish significance for an odds ratio for observed versus expected deaths. This study does not include deaths that may have occurred after hospital transfer, but based on data from other studies, that number is likely to be too small to affect the results. The close agreement with the North Carolina study [Abstract 8] argues for the validity of the data.

10. Schramm WF, Barnes DE, and Bakewell JM. Neonatal mortality in Missouri home births. *Am J Public Health* **1987;77(8):930-935.**
Planning status was established for 3645 home births between 1978 and 1984. Planning status and attendant type were established for all 62 neonatal deaths of babies born at home, and the expected versus observed ratio was calculated after adjusting for race, age of mother, and birth weight. The standard was rates for Missouri resident physician-attended hospital births.

The LBW rate for unplanned home births (25.6%) was nearly eight times that of the planned home births (3.4%), which was half the hospital rate (6.8%). There were 17 observed deaths for planned home births compared with 8.59 expected for a relative risk of about two to one, but nearly all of the excess were planned home births with attendants who were not members of the Missouri Midwives Association (MMA) or who were categorized as "other" (family or friends). Among physicians, certified nurse-midwives, and MMA-recognized midwives, there were five neonatal deaths compared to 3.92 expected (RR 1.28, CI 0.53-3.08 (NS)). Stillbirths were not included because they are likely to be underreported among home births.

STUDIES OF HOME BIRTH

The Netherlands

11. Damstra-Wijmenga SM. Home confinement: the positive results in Holland. *J R Coll Gen Pract* 1984;34(265):425-430.
Almost all the 1692 (99.3%) inhabitants of Gröningen who gave birth in 1981 were interviewed. While the national home birth rate is 34.7%, 23.4% chose home delivery, of whom 78% (or 18.4% of the whole population) gave birth at home.

Women opting for home births were less likely to be referred to an obstetrician during both pregnancy (5.6% versus 11.7%) and labor (15.6% versus 25.4%). The same percentage of complicated labors occurred among women referred to obstetric care for medical indications (54%) as among women who elected obstetric care, although this was only 24 women. Of babies born at home, 2.8% were taken to an infant special care unit compared with 9.5% born in the hospital. There was no perinatal mortality among home-born infants. The only significant difference [*p* value not given] among indications for transfer to obstetric care during labor or the early postpartum was "lack of progress." Only 4.6% of women at home were transferred versus 11.7% of women already in the hospital. The author speculates that either midwives judged labor progress differently at home or women progressed better at home. "If these figures indicate that more complications occurred among those women who, of their own free will, opted for hospital confinement than among those who decided to have their babies at home, it might be wondered how many of these complications were induced by the medical professional during labor."

Great Britain

12. Wood LAC. Obstetric retrospect. *J R Coll Gen Pract* 1981;31:80-90.
The outcomes are reported for all 817 pregnancies of more than 28 weeks duration managed by a single British general practitioner between 1946 and 1970. As the years passed, the number of home births declined from 59% to 43% with the percentage overall being 51%. Similarly, freestanding maternity unit births declined from 35% to 19%, with the percentage overall being 29%. In total, 80% of the group gave birth outside the hospital, including 68% of the cases designated high risk.

Most of the labors (86%) were rated normal. The antenatal transfer rate jumped from 3.0% to 12.4% in the last decade of practice. The intrapartum transfer rate rose in each decade, to a maximum of 5.0% in the last decade. The overall cesarean rate was 1.6%, and the forceps rate was 9.3%. The induction rate was 7.3%, and the episiotomy rate 11.7%, with 60.1% of vaginally birthing women having an intact perineum. Perinatal mortality rates were stratified by time period and compared with the British Births Surveys' figure for the same period. Rates for the practice were substantially lower for 1946-50 (26.7/1000 versus 38/1000) and 1951-60 (18.8/1000 versus 33/1000), and they were similar during the last decade (25.6/1000 versus 23/1000). "I would not claim that these results are at all exceptional; many general practitioners working in similar conditions have done better. Nor would I decry the value of the new techniques in the small proportion of abnormal pregnancies and labours that do occur, but I would question the current assumptions about the superiority of these methods in all cases."

13. Shearer JM. Five year prospective survey of risk of booking for a home birth in Essex. *Br Med J* 1985;291(6507):1478-1480.
This prospective study compared 202 healthy multiparas 20 to 35 years of age who chose home birth with a population of 185 similar women who chose hospital birth. Subjects were recruited from 26 general practices between 1978 and 1983. Women giving birth at home were attended by midwives. [The article does not say who attended hospital deliveries, more likely a doctor.] Of women planning home birth, 8% were transferred antenatally and 3% intrapartum.

"Significantly" fewer women at home were induced (8% versus 19% [no p value]). Women giving birth at home were less likely to have episiotomies (13% versus 28%, $p < 0.001$) and more likely to have an intact perineum (44% versus 29%, $p < 0.01$). Five-minute Apgars were similar. All three cesareans (1%) occurred among the home birth group—one for a brow presentation and two for antepartum hemorrhage. There was no perinatal mortality. "Although the numbers are too small to draw firm conclusions, the results suggest that there is no appreciable increased risk to the mothers or their babies in booking for a home birth. They certainly do not support any 'self evident' risk that has been suggested in the reports mentioned above." [If hospital births were mostly attended by doctors, these differences may reflect differences between midwife and physician management.]

14. Ford C, Iliffe S, and Franklin O. Outcome of planned home births in an inner city practice. *BMJ* 1991;303(6816):1517-1519.
In this London practice, antenatal care for women desiring home births was shared between midwives and general practitioners. At the birth, the doctor visited early in labor and then returned during second stage. Among 277 women planning home births between 1977 and 1989, six had miscarriages, 26 (9.4%) risked out during pregnancy, 26 of the 245 remaining (10.6%) were transferred during labor (22 delay in labor, 4 fetal distress), and 4 of the 219 giving birth at home (1.8%) were postpartum transfers (two postpartum hemorrhage, one retained placenta, one suturing of extensive tear). Compared with multiparas, nulliparas were equally likely to risk out during pregnancy (9% versus 10%) but more likely to risk out during labor (30% versus 1%, $p = 0.00002$). No adverse neonatal outcomes were related to home birth. Nulliparas should be discouraged from home birth because of their high intrapartum transfer rate. "However, as nulliparous women have a legal right to opt for home birth, . . . refusal to support them simply shifts the problem to colleagues . . . obliged by their contracts to visit their patients in an emergency." In cases of obstetric risk, the care of someone knowledgeable and enthusiastic "seems more appropriate than the late arrival of an apprehensive and resentful doctor summoned by unsupported midwives."

Australia

15. Howe KA. Home births in south-west Australia. *Med J Aust* **1988;149(6):296-302.**

The outcomes of 165 home births between 1983 and 1986 from the practices of all six midwives located in southwest Australia are reviewed. Sixteen percent were transferred to the hospital for birth complications. The cesarean rate was 1.2%, the assisted vaginal delivery rate was 4.8%, the induction rate was 0%, and the augmentation rate was 3%. One baby died of congenital anomalies, and another had good Apgar scores but then developed respiratory difficulties. The baby was transported to the hospital and made a spontaneous recovery.

It is interesting to speculate on the reasons for such consistently favourable results in studies on home birth. One hypothesis is that the common obstetric interventions at best do not improve outcome and at worst are hazardous; this implies that their use should be reduced drastically. Alternatively, the intervention rates may be appropriate for the hospital population but are not necessary for women who are giving birth at home; this implies that one or more factors are operating at home to facilitate the progress of normal labor. Suggested factors are: the surroundings at home are more relaxed . . . ; the relationship between the home-birth midwife and the patient is much stronger and therefore perhaps more "therapeutic" . . . ; and the home-birth mothers are more strongly motivated than are their hospital counterparts, and this motivation is a strong positive factor in terms of outcome.

16. Crotty M et al. Planned homebirths in South Australia 1976-1987. *Med J Aust* **1990;153:664-671.**

This review included all planned home births registered with a group of five general practitioners and 11 midwives. Outcomes were compared with South Australia hospital births in 1983. Of 799 women booked, 174 mothers or babies were transferred (21.8%). Most women (83%) gave birth at home. Of the hospital births, 37.5% were antepartum, and 62.5% were intrapartum transfers. Women planning home deliveries were more likely to be low risk than the comparison group with regard to age, life-style, and socioeconomic group. However, 6.9% used marijuana and 0.3% used narcotics, and some had risk factors including prior cesarean delivery, stillbirth, LBW baby, second-trimester miscarriage, recurrent miscarriage, or prior sudden infant death syndrome.

Interventions were less likely among those planning home birth ($p < 0.001$) including sonograms (25.3% versus 84.4%), induction (4.8% versus 21.1%), instrumental delivery (4.1% versus 15.2%), cesarean (5.5% versus 18.8%), epidural (8.4% versus 26.1%), and episiotomy (8.3% versus 60.3%). Labor longer than 24 hours was more common (4.0% versus 2.6%, $p < 0.05$), as was postpartum hemorrhage (9.4% versus 3.7%, $p < 0.001$). Oxytocic agents were given in third stage only 17.3% of the time. This suggests that routine postpartum injection of oxtocin could reduce the incidence of hemorrhage. Three breech babies were born at home—one the second baby in an undiagnosed set of twins. Two undiagnosed sets of twins were born at home, and a third set was transferred prior to delivery. The perinatal mortality rate was 16.2 per

1000. Stratifying by birth weight and correcting for lethal anomalies, the expected rate was calculated to be 2.17 deaths. Eleven deaths actually occurred. However, only four of these were born at home: a known hydrocephalic baby, a baby transferred to hospital when fetal heart tones were lost in labor (autopsy, diagnosis: tear of umbilical artery), a change from vertex to face presentation in second stage (no autopsy, diagnosis: intrapartum asphyxia), and a baby born in poor condition following an uncomplicated labor (autopsy, diagnosis: asphyxia, unknown cause). Several potential problems with home birth care were identified: booking high-risk pregnancies, the low use of sonograms, possible delay in transfer, low use of oxytocics in third stage, and lack of autopsies when cause of death is not obvious.

17. Woodcock HC et al. Planned homebirths in western Australia 1981-1987: a descriptive study. *Med J Aust* 1990;153:672-678.

Data for this analysis of planned home births ($N = 995$) came from statutory home birth notification forms linked to midwifery records, perinatal and infant death certificates, and a congenital malformation registry. Because women planning home birth were mostly white, the comparison group was singleton western Australia Caucasian births in the same years. Parity distribution and marital status were similar to the comparison group. Women planning home birth tended to be older and taller. The home birth population included women with previous preterm birth, stillbirth, neonatal or subsequent death, and scarred uterus.

Of the 778 births at home with records, 96.5% were attended by a midwife, and 2.1% occurred before arrival of the midwife. A doctor was also present at 17.1%. Overall, 24.6% of mothers or babies were transferred, of whom 21.8% were antenatal and 59.4% were intrapartum (including seven breeches) transfers. Intervention was less likely among those planning home birth including induction (2.5% versus about 26%), elective cesarean (0.6% versus 7.1%), and emergency cesarean (3.6% versus 6.7%). All but four births at home were spontaneous vaginal cephalic deliveries (99.5%). The four were three forceps deliveries and one undiagnosed breech born while waiting for an ambulance. The postpartum hemorrhage rate for the planned home birth population was 8.5%, but data were missing on 48.2% of the transfers (no comparison data). For those who gave birth at home, it was 8.4%. This high rate may be due to failure to inject oxytocics after birth. The perinatal mortality rate was 10.1 per 1000 versus 9.7 per 1000 among the comparison group. No perinatal death appeared related to the place of birth. No emergency transfer was associated with preventable mortality. Because virtually all planned home births were identified, it is unlikely that serious adverse outcomes were missed.

Canada

18. Tyson H. Outcomes of 1001 Midwife-attended home births in Toronto, 1983-1988. *Birth* 1991;18(1):14-19.

All 26 midwives in practice between 1983 and 1988 were contacted, and the outcomes for all women who were not risked out prior to labor for were examined. Of the 1001 births, 83.5% took place at home with no postpartum complications. Including transfers, 93% were spontaneous vaginal births. The forceps rate was 3.4%, and the cesarean rate was 3.5%. Among all vaginal births, 17.9% had episiotomies, of which most were performed by physicians at hospital births. Only 0.5% had third-degree lacerations and 55.2% had an intact perineum. The midwives did the suturing at home except for six women (0.7%) who were transferred postpartum for suturing of difficult lacerations. Two infants died [neonatal mortality 2/1000]. One baby's mother was transferred for vaginal bleeding early in labor and underwent nine hours of care before having an emergency cesarean for fetal distress; the other baby was born at home with unsuspected asphyxia, was transferred, and died three days later.

United States

19. Mehl LE et al. Outcomes of elective home births: a series of 1,146 cases. *J Reprod Med* 1977;19(5):281-290.
This study reported outcomes for 1970-75 for three physician groups and two lay midwife groups in the San Francisco area. No analgesia, forceps, or IV oxytocin were used at home. Meconium in the absence of fetal heart rate irregularities was not an indication for transfer. Nor were twins and breech babies automatically excluded. Comparison data, where available, were for California in 1973.

The antepartum transfer rate for medical reasons was 4.1%. Eleven percent were transferred intrapartum and 0.9% postpartum. The cesarean rate was 2.4% compared with a California primary cesarean rate of about 5%. The forceps rate was 1.5%. The episiotomy rate was 7.8%, and 12.9% of women had lacerations requiring repair. There was no association between length of labor and Apgar scores [long labor did not harm the baby, as is popularly believed], and none of the 14 cases of prolonged ruptured membranes led to infection. [Inducing women with ruptured membranes and no contractions is not necessary to prevent infection. See Chapter 10.] The preterm birth rate was 3% versus 5.3% for California white women 20 to 29 years old. Only 1.3% of babies weighed less than 2501 g (including two sets of twins) versus 6.4% for California. The perinatal mortality rate was 9.5 per 1000 versus 20.3 per 1000 for California. "Evidence from this study population strongly suggests that home delivery is a safe alternative for medically screened, healthy women."

20. Sullivan DA and Beeman R. Four years' experience with home birth by licensed midwives in Arizona. *Am J Public Health* 1983;73(6):641-645.
The study examines outcomes for 1449 women accepted for care by 26 midwives between 1978 and 1981. The midwives were not allowed to administer medications [they could not administer drugs to control postpartum bleeding] or perform any operative procedure [they could neither perform episiotomies nor repair lacerations].

The total transfer rate prior to birth was 14%, which includes 25 women transferred for "other indications (including non-medical)." Of the 1243 women who gave birth at home, 175 (14%) had a laceration that required transfer to hospital for suturing, of which all but eight were no worse than an episiotomy. Overall, 18% were transferred after birth for medical attention, but only 3% were admitted to the hospital. Of the newborns, 5% were transferred for medical care, but only 2% were admitted to the hospital. There were two neonatal and three fetal deaths [perinatal mortality 3.5/1000]. Two were due to congenital anomalies, one was a breech birth conducted unsupervised at home by a "granny" midwife [a midwife with no formal training], one was an antepartum death where the midwife falsely reported a heartbeat so her client could give birth at home, and one was unknown cause (a fetal heartbeat was heard late in second stage, but the baby could not be resuscitated). The midwives had no access to hospital records, so aside from knowing there were no maternal or newborn deaths among those transferred, there is no information on interventions or outcomes for the 206 women transferred before birth. "Arizona's experience illustrates that home births can be a safe alternative for low-risk pregnancies if they are attended by an adequately trained practitioner, even if that practitioner is not a physician."

21. Koehler MS, Solomon DA, and Murphy M. Outcomes of a rural Sonoma County home birth practice: 1976-1982. *Birth* 1984;11(3):165-169.

Outcomes are reported for the 521 women who were clients of an obstetrician-lay midwife home birth practice. The antepartum transfer rate was 13%, not all of which were for pregnancy complications. For example, seven women had an elective repeat cesarean. The intrapartum transfer rate was 7%. Excluding elective repeat cesareans, the cesarean rate was 5%, "considerably lower than the community average." The episiotomy rate was 11%. All four preterm births were planned hospital births.

The perinatal mortality rate was 5.7 per 1000. Of the three perinatal deaths, one was a fetal death at 34 weeks gestation, one was a stillborn where the membranes ruptured spontaneously in early labor in a double-footling breech and the umbilical cord prolapsed [came down ahead of the baby], and one was a baby with no spontaneous respiration. The baby was resuscitated and transported to the hospital but subsequently died. Judith Lumley, in an editorial comment on this paper says, "Most obstetric reviewers would regard the delivery of a footling breech at home . . . as a major avoidable factor in the death of the infant."

22. Anderson R and Greener D. A descriptive analysis of home births attended by CNMs in two nurse-midwifery services. *J Nurse Midwifery* 1991;36(2):95-103.

Outcomes are reported for two Texas home birth midwifery practices during 1987. Of the 108 women (21.3% nulliparas) planning a home birth in the third trimester, 98 gave birth at home. Five (4.6%) were transferred to a hospital (one antepartum fetal demise of unknown cause, one gestational diabetes, one "patient's choice," two failure to progress (FTP) in active labor), one gave birth in a freestanding birth center, and place of birth was unknown in four. All obstetric interventions took place within the hospital. Rates were 2% oxytocin, 1% analgesia, 1% epidural, 4.6% EFM, 1% episiotomy, and 2.9% cesarean (two for FTP, one for fetal distress). Only seven women gave birth supine or in the lithotomy position, of whom three were in the hospital. The most common midwifery interventions were: 32.7% bath/shower, 18.3% amniotomy at more than 6 cm dilation, and 12.5% nonoxytocic labor induction (castor oil, cervical stimulation, enema, nipple stimulation, herbs). Complications included 4.8% rupture of membranes longer than 24 hours, 1% heavy meconium, 2.9% fetal distress, 5.7% second stage longer than 2 hours (all gave birth at home), 3.8% shoulder dystocia, 1% postpartum blood loss more than 500 cc, and 1% third-degree laceration (not the episiotomy). Three babies (3%) weighed less than 2500 g. Three babies were born at home before 37 weeks gestation because the mothers did not want to go to the hospital and the midwife estimated fetal weight to be over 2500 g. However, two weighed less than 2500 g. No infant had a 5-minute Apgar below 8. The only neonatal morbidity was 3.8% jaundice and 3.8% cephalohematoma.

23. Duran AM. The safety of home birth: the Farm study. *Am J Public Health* 1992;82(3):450-453.

This study compares outcomes between 1707 lay midwife-attended births from 1971 to 1989 at the Farm (a commune located in rural Tennessee) with a sample of doctor-attended hospital births from the 1980 US National Natality/National Fetal Mortality

Survey (NNS/NFMS) (*N* = 14,033). At the Farm, women labor without analgesia. Friends and family attend. Women are encouraged to remain active and to eat and drink. No time limits are put on labor, and occasionally labors last two to three days. Women with preexisting diabetes, hypertension, Rh-negative blood, obesity, anemia, and, prior to 1985, previous cesarean section were excluded. Excluded from the NNS/NFMS sample were women attended by nonphysicians, women with no prenatal care, and women with risk factors that would preclude birth at the Farm. The power to detect odds ratios of 1.5 or more for the birth route and labor complications was greater than 99%, for low 5-minute Apgars it was 75% (99% for OR > 2), and for perinatal mortality it was 62% (98% for OR > 2).

Transfer rates were 1.6% antepartum, 7.4% intrapartum, and 4.5% postpartum for a total rate of 13.5%. No significant differences were found for either crude or adjusted odds ratios for perinatal death, bleeding, birth injury, respiratory distress syndrome, or 5-minute Apgar below 7. However, the Farm cesarean rate was 1.5% versus 16.5% for the NNS/NFMS sample (OR 0.09, CI 0.08-0.10). [The Farm data extend to 1989 but are compared with 1980 data. The national cesarean rate rose to about 24% by the mid-1980s, so the gap is really much wider.] "The results of this study suggest that for relatively low-risk pregnancies, home birth with attendance by lay midwives is not necessarily less safe than . . . hospital-physician delivery. Support by the medical and legal communities for those electing, and those attending, home births should not be withheld on the grounds that this option is inherently unsafe."

REFERENCES

ACOG. Statement on Home Delivery. 1979.

Adamson GD and Gare DJ. Home or hospital births? *JAMA* 1980;243(17):1732-1736.

Brody H and Thompson JR. The maximin strategy in modern obstetrics. *J Fam Practice* 1981;12(6):977-986. (abstracted in Chapter 15)

Brown RA. Midwifery and home birth: an alternative view. *Can Med Assoc J* 1987;137(10):875-877.

Dye NS. The medicalization of birth. In *The American way of birth.* Eakins P, ed. Philadelphia: Temple University Press, 1986.

Home, hospital or birthroom? *Lancet* 1986;2(8505):494-496.

Mold JW and Stein HF. The cascade effect in the clinical care of patients. *New Engl J Med* 1986;314(8):512-514.

Philipp E. Planned and unplanned deliveries at home. *Br Med J* 1984;288:1996-1997

Saldana LR et al. Home birth: negative implications derived from a hospital-based birthing suite. *South Med J* 1983;76(2):170-173.

Tew M. We have the technology. *Nursing Times* 1985;81(47):22-24.

Tew M and Damstra-Wijmenga SMI. Safest birth attendants: recent Dutch evidence. *Midwifery* 1991;7:55-63.

Torres A and Reich MR. The shift from home to institutional childbirth: a comparative study of the United Kingdom and the Netherlands. *Int J Health Serv* 1989;19(3):405-414.

Wertz RW and Wertz DC. *Lying-in: A history of childbirth in America.* New York: Schocken Books, 1977.

18

The Nature of Evidence (Reprise): Why the Gap Between Belief and Reality?

Myth: *Obstetrics is a science whose practices are grounded in medical research.*

Reality: *"[W]e find a pervasive assumption, shared by medical practitioners and their clients alike, that [obstetric] practices are . . . scientifically grounded. Even though a given medical practitioner, at any one time, may not just then have the data at hand which support his conviction, he knows that they exist. . . . [O]n examination, the evidence on which his conviction is based is sometimes non-existent, and if it does exist, is frequently far from clear-cut."*

Jordan 1993

Obstetrics claims to be a science, deriving from rational, objective assessment of the facts. Yet as we have seen, it is riddled with paradoxes and inconsistencies that few among its adherents notice. It claims to be based on medical research, yet this book shows that where evidence exists (and often it does not!), it all too frequently lies solidly on one side while practice lies on the other. Obstetrics claims to have the best interests of women and babies at heart, yet as this book makes clear, it routinely subjects them—and always has—to unproven or dangerous therapies, treatments, and drugs. The justifications it openly offers for some of its practices—defensive medicine, inadequate staff, patient choice—benefit doctors and nurses at the expense of their patients and defend practices admitted to be harmful. It professes that its primary responsibility is to women, yet it routinely expects—even compels—women to submit to all sorts of painful and risky treatments, including major surgery, on behalf of someone else: the fetus. Seen in one light, obstetrics, far from serving the needs of childbearing women, could be described as a kind of sanctioned violence against them. Manifestly, obstetrics is not what it claims to be. Why, then, is there an enormous gap between what obstetrics claims to be and what it actually is? And if it is not a science, is there an alternate theory that better explains how and why obstetrics operates as it does?

Robbie Davis-Floyd (1992), a medical anthropologist, expanding on the work of Brigitte Jordan (1983) and others before her, offers just such a theory. Obstetrics, she says, is a set of internally consistent rituals designed to reinforce certain core values held by the culture as a whole.

OBSTETRICS AS RITUAL

All cultures, Davis-Floyd explains, develop sets of rituals as a means of managing the awe and fear birth and death inevitably produce in the human mind. Rituals provide a meaning, a path, a way to feel that such events are knowable, even controllable. Similarly, other transition periods, when people pass from one state to another—puberty, adulthood, marriage, motherhood—also inspire rituals. These rituals serve to reinforce cultural values for all participants, to provide a bridge between the old and the new state of being, and to instill the competence and confidence initiates need as they attain a new status or role.

There is nothing wrong with cultural constructs of this type. Every society creates them. Davis-Floyd's point, with which I (and others) agree, is that because of the beliefs on which they are based, the values inculcated, and the practices expressive of those values, Western birth rituals often work to the detriment of women and babies. They are both physically and psychologically harmful.

The physical risks are obvious. To cite two glaring examples, nearly one in four American women gives birth by major abdominal surgery, and virtually all women are given at least one drug during labor that has potential adverse fetal effects (Woodward et al. 1982).

The psychological hazards are less obvious. Rites that mark life transitions normally empower the initiate; this one accomplishes exactly the opposite. Studies find that satisfaction with the birth experience relates to taking an active role in the process and using little or no pain medication (Humenick 1981; Humenick and Bugen 1981; Green 1993; DiMatteo, Kahn, and Berry 1993). Obstetrics expects the mother passively to accept the attentions of medical staff and discourages natural childbirth. Starting off motherhood handicapped by feelings of discontent and disempowerment is likely to have profound although, in our culture, generally unacknowledged effects. Postpartum depression, extending even into the second year after the birth, correlates with the number and invasiveness of medical interventions and the woman's feelings that her needs and wishes had been ignored (Lumley 1992). Thousands of women, more deeply traumatized by their experience, express the same emotions, even use the same words, as those who have been sexually assaulted or abused (Kitzinger 1990).

What, then, are the beliefs that Davis-Floyd argues are infused through what she calls an American (and I would broaden to a Western) rite of passage? The first is very old. It is that women are not merely different from men; they are physically and mentally inferior. Women are defective simply because they are not men. Other dualities that play a role in the obstetric approach to childbirth—man versus nature, mind versus heart, action versus inaction—are similarly rank-ordered on the grounds that the inferior polarity is characteristic of women.

The second belief arose when a great revolution in thinking gave birth to science and medicine as we understand it. Until the seventeenth century, the natural world, including the human body, was an awe-inspiring mystery of God, not to be tampered with. The birth of a child was a miracle, too, but respect carried over to neither the natural process nor women. Childbirth, like menstruation, was a polluting process, and men had nothing to do with it except to accuse midwives and herb women of practicing witchcraft. With the new thinking, the natural world and the human body became conceptualized as mechanisms that could be explored, picked apart, understood, and improved. As Davis-Floyd put it:

> [I]f a society chooses to see itself and the universe it inhabits as mechanistic, then it will need to see as equally mechanistic the human bodies that comprise it. The problem here, of course, is that bodies are not machines. . . . And so it became both the cultural mission and the vested interest of Western medicine to prove the ultimate truth and viability of this model by making the body *appear to be* as mechanistic as possible. . . . Along with the responsibility for maintaining the consistency of our dominant belief system, doctors hold another social duty that had previously been the responsibility of the priest—namely, that of inculcating individual members of society with the basic tenets of this belief system.

This mechanistic model was superimposed over the old one. Therefore, if the human body became a type of machine, then by extension a woman's body became a defective, untrustworthy machine. It was inclined to break down and functioned poorly even when working properly. During pregnancy the added stresses made the female "machine" especially prone to failure. This opened the way for obstetrics, the manly art of interfering, as opposed to midwifery, the womanly art of supporting.

One of the more potent myths of obstetrics is that women and babies died in huge numbers until obstetricians saved them from the ravages of the natural process and the ignorance of midwives. Quite the contrary is true. The endless parade of procedures and drugs that obstetricians have inflicted on women and babies since that time, including the much-lauded forceps, have maimed and killed more women and babies than ever have been saved by their use (Wertz and Wertz 1977; Ashford 1986).

Recently the belief that man could dominate and improve on nature has elevated technology into a god. This has led to the final hubris: no longer need the creation of new life be left to the inadequate bodies of women subject to the whims of the natural process. Scientific knowledge wielded by experts will take over. Thus, babies become the product of society—in short, the sole creation of men.

Davis-Floyd (1994) explains that this transformation is accomplished by what Peter Reynolds calls in his book, *Stealing Fire: The Mythology of the Technocracy*, the "one-two punch." First, technology renders a natural process dysfunctional, as when building a dam prevents salmon from swimming upstream. Then technology rebuilds the process as a cultural construct: Men remove the salmon, have them spawn artificially, grow the eggs in trays, and release the baby salmon downstream. "The cultural management of American birth," writes Davis-Floyd, "is a perfect example of the One-Two Punch."

Davis-Floyd (1992) describes a typical hospital birth, showing how at each step of the way, no valid scientific rationale exists, but the procedure works effectively as ritual. Each element of the typical hospital birth helps to convince the woman and her caretakers that childbirth is a risky business and that women are not really giving birth; medical staff are delivering the baby.

DAVIS-FLOYD'S THEORY FITS

As a general principle, the more numerous and varied the phenomena a theory explains, the more validity it gains. The belief that obstetrics is a science fits the facts of obstetric practice poorly. However, Davis-Floyd's anthropological theory—that obstetrics is a collection of rituals designed to reinforce core cultural values—does an excellent job of making sense of much that is otherwise inexplicable.

The anthropological model explains why, except for a tiny minority, obstetricians have ignored the fact that medical research shows that intervening is usually unnecessary and frequently causes harm. Belief systems bring order and sense to the chaos of real events by filtering reality to make it conform to or support the tenets of the belief system. In that service, those who have internalized the beliefs will explain away phenomena that do not fit, will not notice inconsistencies, or simply will not "see" something "inconvenient" that is there.

It also explains why normally assertive women meekly acquiesce to, even defend, a system that treats them as fetal containers, bullies them, patronizes them, ignores their wishes, strips them of the rights normally accorded competent adults, and puts them and their babies at risk to boot. In fact, provided medical staff are reasonably pleasant about it, most women do not even notice that this is what is happening. Women have been indoctrinated with the same belief system their obstetricians have. Although this is true of women generally, it becomes clearest when we look at women professionals, the women most highly assimilated into a male-dominated world. Studying 32 such women, Davis-Floyd (1994) found that most of them had incorporated the male values of efficiency and control. They espoused rigid, oppositional separations of mind and body and mother and child and believed in the superiority of technology over nature. They felt profound distrust of the chaotic, powerful processes of pregnancy and childbirth—which meant rejecting the very essence of their female natures—and they embraced highly interventive and technological pregnancy and birth management as heartily as the most authoritarian, sexist, and misogynistic obstetrician could do. A few of them even went to the extreme of demanding—and getting—elective cesareans.

Davis-Floyd's theory explains how childbearing came under the purview of doctors. Childbearing, after all, is a *normal* physiologic function. Why should pregnant and laboring women routinely need a *surgeon*'s supervision, let alone a doctor's, or, for that matter give birth in a hospital? As Pamela Eakins (1986) writes, "In American culture, disease is viewed as any deviation . . . from what is believed to be the normal or average condition." Pregnancy and childbirth are not "normal" conditions because they are not shared by males, the pattern for normal. Ergo pregnancy and childbirth are pathological and thus, by definition, a medical matter.

It also explains why pregnant women, who are healthy, competent adults, are supposed to cede their autonomy to medical staff. We expect sick or injured people to submit themselves to those who have the knowledge and skills to make them well (Annas 1989). Pregnant women are supposed to behave submissively partly because they are women and that is their "proper" role, but partly because by defining childbearing as inherently pathological, we have converted normal childbearing women into "patients."

The anthropological perspective explains why women do not really have choices, although they are told they do. Richards (1982) writes, "Arguing for choice [in childbirth] can be too much like getting a shop to stock two kinds of frozen fish fingers when the issue may be to find somewhere that sells fresh fish." Belief systems only admit options that do not contradict their beliefs. So a hospital with a 27% cesarean rate, routine IVs, routine electronic fetal monitoring, and no midwives on staff can advertise without seeing the contradiction, "We deliver more babies because we deliver more choices."

It also explains the reaction to women who want "fresh fish" or to the medical professionals who provide it. Richards again: "Characteristic of many conversations between doctor and mother is the use of that peculiar royal 'we' by the doctor. 'We would not want to do anything that might jeopardize the baby.'" Of course, everyone wants a healthy baby, "but, especially if the mother does not sound too keen to submit to whatever is being proposed, there is also an implicit message that it is only the doctor who has the true interests of the mother, or, more especially, the child, at heart." Jordan (1983), an anthropologist, observes in her analysis of birth in different cultures, "The sense of superiority and moral requiredness that is built into every functioning system keeps its practitioners specifically uninformed about alternate ways of doing birth, since any tampering with the 'correct' way is likely to be regarded as unethical, exploitative, dangerous, bad medicine, and the like."

It explains, too, compulsory cesarean section. In no other case besides pregnancy do doctors attempt legally to force one person to undergo a medical procedure of any kind, let alone major surgery, to benefit a third party. By so doing, obstetricians classify the woman's rights on the same level as an animal's, and, since you cannot harvest organs for transplant without permission, lower than those of a corpse. Yet as late as 1993 doctors took a woman to court for just this reason (they lost the case and the baby was born healthy three weeks later) (San Jose Mercury News 1993), and as late as 1989 Elkins et al. argued that the threat of fetal death or disability gave doctors the right to override the mother's autonomy. (Elkins et al. stipulated that the physician must assess "the reasonableness and rationality" of the patient's refusal, but, of course, refusing a cesarean after being told the fetus was endangered would constitute an unreasonable and irrational act by definition.) Such an aberration makes sense in a belief system operating on the metaphor that the woman is an inherently defective mechanism and that the obsetrician's role is to ensure she produces a quality product.

Obstetrics as a belief system explains why, instead of rationally debating the merits of alternatives, the alternatives themselves are attacked as if they were religious heresies. In a sense, they are. Depending on the triviality or gravity of the case, dissenters will be subjected to the same types of social sanctions: ridicule, shaming, shunning, or persecution, for these are the defense mechanisms that keep belief systems in place.

Elizabeth Janeway (1971), a sociologist, tells us that social systems assign roles in reciprocal pairs. The principal player expects the proper response from the other players. If one of them misses a cue, confusion and distress result. If the lapse is relatively minor, the usual reaction is to laugh it off. (Thus, a woman who does not want an epidural may be portrayed as misguided, or perhaps selfish, for subjecting her baby to the stresses of her pain.) If the departure is more serious, shaming may be the tactic. (Thus, a woman who refuses electronic monitoring may be told she is taking an irresponsible chance with her baby.) If the role breaker is perceived to be outside the belief system, then he or she threatens the very order of the universe, and persecution is likely to result. (Thus, an obstetrician who champions home birth may be shunned by colleagues, and a midwife who is not a certified nurse-midwife may be prosecuted in many states.)

Continuing with the theatrical metaphor, the other actors may smother role breakers' attempts to rewrite the "play" by co-opting them (Declercq 1983). The reformers may be given jobs with no real power, or the institution may adopt the rhetoric but not the substance of reform, as in "homelike" hospital birth, or those aspects that do not pose a threat to the belief system may be incorporated and treated as if it were the whole proposed change, as happened when fathers were admitted to labor and delivery wards.

The evolution of Lamaze education is a case in point. Although they did not know or intend this, the early Lamaze teachers were subversives. The idea that women should be accompanied by their husbands and that they could cope with labor without analgesia seems innocuous enough, but it challenged the dominant model that birth was analogous to an operation (an analogy that has now become fact for 1 million women each year in the U.S. alone), and it introduced another male who might dispute the doctor's authority. Resistance was fierce: "Husbands in the delivery room? Infection will run rampant! They'll faint; they'll get in the way!" "Natural childbirth? What kind of weirdo masochist are you?" But the public clamor for change was too much to resist outright, so Lamaze was co-opted. Today most Lamaze classes are taught by nurses and are either under the direct supervision of hospitals or doctors or the teacher depends on their referrals. As a result, unmedicated births are few and far between. As for fathers, as Coleman Romalis (1981) describes, they too were co-opted. They were brought into the service of controlling the mother by a message that played on their protective instincts and their desires to identify with authority: "You and I together," intimates the doctor, "will take care of the 'little woman.'" "But it is like a fly assisting a spider; even while cooperating . . . with the doctor . . . the father himself is rendered silent and captive."

This process is happening again. Unless midwifery can establish itself as independent from obstetric control, which it shows few signs of doing, midwives are headed down the same track (see Chapter 15).

The anthropological model explains the discrepancies between stated values and real values. According to Jordan (1993), such discrepancies are rarely deliberate. The subjective nature of a belief system introduces a systematic bias, opening unconscious gaps between what is done and what people think is being done. In the same year that only 20% of women with a prior cesarean had a vaginal birth after a cesarean (VBAC), 92% of obstetricians surveyed said they "encouraged" VBAC (see Chapters 3 and 4). Or consider episiotomy; try to name another surgical procedure, short of a life-or-death crisis, that is performed without obtaining consent.

It explains, too, why simply providing authoritative information supportive of reducing the use of technology or intervention usually has little or no effect on practice, a phenomenon noted with surprise and sometimes with frustration (see Chapter 3; also Pierre et al. 1991; Kanouse and Jacoby 1988; Greer 1988). Similarly, it explains why birth alternatives that would have no effect on medical care but would merely better meet the needs of laboring women encounter fierce resistance and demand elaborate strategies to implement them successfully (Mackey 1991). Conversely, it also explains why changes that increase the use of technology or replace one intervention with another are readily accepted without or in spite of the evidence. Thus, EFM became the standard of practice without research validation, and its use continues to increase despite over a decade of research showing no benefits and considerable harm compared with auscultation (see Chapter 7). So, too, obstetricians hail active management of labor as the replacement for cesarean for labor dystocia (see Chapter 5). The belief system dictates what is accepted. Anything congruent with it requires no proof. Anything counter to it will not be accepted whether proof is offered or not. Writes Jordan (1983), "The [status of] any given controversy is decided not on the basis of the kind of evidence that is produced by bio-medical research (though that evidence will be put in the service of the enterprise) but rather its status will depend on how well it fits with the socio-political realities and the ideological belief system of its time and place."

Davis-Floyd's theory explains the inversions and perversions of language. Doctors do not deliver babies; women give birth, except in the case of that oxymoron, "cesarean birth." "Birth injuries" are often doctor inflicted, not caused by the birth itself. "Birth asphyxia" frequently results from preexisting problems, nor is it, in most cases, a real or dangerous lack of oxygen. "Failure to progress" usually means "failure to wait." And "respiratory embarrassment" is a euphemism for the paralysis of breathing muscles sometimes caused by an epidural. In each case, failure is the fault of the mother or the natural process, success is attributed to the doctor, and doctor-caused harm is denied or buried. This is just what one would expect from a belief system in which the doctor is always right.

Do not underestimate the power of subliminal linguistic messages. When obstetricians talk about "managing labor" instead of caring for laboring women, they are revealing a hidden truth: "You're in labor?" says the obstetrician in one cartoon. "I'm in management!" When they ask, "Which do you want: a safe birth or a pleasant experience?" they frame the issue in such a way that the woman cannot answer, "I want both." The same hospital that had the 27% cesarean rate gives laboring women anticipating vaginal birth a generic form entitled, "Consent for Operation, Anesthesia, and Medical Services," which says, "This operation is known as _____," and further adds that signing means the woman understands "the risks associated with it, the potential for harm, and alternative treatment." This is no accident. That form is one step in a process that teaches women that birth is not conceptually different from an operation while simultaneously reminding staff of that point. Insurance lingo refers to "pregnancy disability," lumping pregnant women together with people who have health problems. Pregnancy is obviously an "ability," even a super-ability compared with what men can do, but how better to reinforce that we have no category for a condition that applies exclusively to females and that whatever is not shared by males is abnormal? "Informed consent" itself, although not specific to obstetrics, implies that once you are informed, you will consent. Look how the meaning would shift if it were called "informed decision making."

Hilda Bastion (1992) in an editorial on how obstetric language dehumanizes and controls women writes:

> I am constantly amazed at the list of things women are told they have "failed" at: they can "fail" to dilate, to progress, to home birth, to breastfeed—and their babies can "fail" to thrive. Bits and pieces of them can "fail" as well: contractions can be "inadequate" as can their pelvis. Their cervix can be "incompetent" (or merely "unfavorable"). . . . [A]n examination of [the] somewhat aggressive language may reveal ways of thinking about care which are inappropriate in themselves. "Allowing" a woman a "trial" of labour, for example. . . . Why is it necessary to tell one particular group of women that they are "on trial" and regard them in this way? Indeed, it is hard to imagine any circumstance in which it is appropriate to put a woman or her uterus "on trial" (after a second stage "arrest" perhaps!)

She believes this terminology to be merely insensitive, not intentional, but it is a deliberate and vivid expression of underlying attitudes toward women and childbirth.

Obstetrics as a belief system explains why not intervening has the burden of proving itself rather than the other way around. In the Alice in Wonderland world of obstetrics, you have to show that letting mothers walk around and choose positions of comfort is better than confining them to their backs in bed. You have to prove that giving women their healthy babies after birth is superior to whisking them off to the nursery. The belief system makes intervention the norm, its "rightness" a given.

It explains magical thinking. When a doctor can relate without seeing the illogic that his partner did a cesarean on a woman for no other reason than that her previous child had died of multiple congenital anomalies and they wanted to guarantee her a normal baby, then you know nothing rational is at work (Summey 1986). While his position may seem extreme, it could arise only where cesarean surgery is commonly believed to be superior to vaginal birth.

It also explains why adverse signs are considered problems only if they arise naturally but not if the obstetrician caused them. When discussing postdates pregnancy, doctors warn that insufficient amniotic fluid may lead to fetal distress because of umbilical cord compression, but no one worries about this when intentionally rupturing membranes (amniotomy). Loss of normal fetal heart rate variability, which may signal adverse changes in fetal neurologic status, perturbs doctors only when it appears spontaneously but not as a result of narcotic pain medication. Poor labor progress is cause for alarm except when the mother has had an epidural. Nor do doctors find the fairly common drop in maternal blood pressure or slowing of the fetal heart rate that may follow an epidural of much concern. They know what they will do to fix it and what they will do if that does not work or if their treatment causes another problem—up to and including a cesarean section. Like the rooster thinking the sun rises because he crows, rituals create the illusion of control. Obstetrician-induced complications feel safe, manageable, an acceptable risk. Doctors can predict them; they know what caused them and what they will do next.

Davis-Floyd's model explains the slavish reliance on tests and technology and the rejection of other sources of knowledge, especially information provided by the mother herself. That would be expected in a belief system that all but worshiped technology and devalued women. In an extreme example of how obstetricians disregard women, Sheila Kitzinger (1987) quotes a dialogue between a doctor and woman recorded by Ann Oakley:

DOCTOR (reading case notes): Ah, I see you've got a boy and a girl.

PATIENT: No, two girls.

DOCTOR: Really? Are you sure? I thought it said . . . (checks in case notes) Oh, no, you are quite right, two girls.

It explains what drives malpractice suits. The practice of obstetrics essentially has the doctor say to the woman, "If you do not do what I tell you, I can't guarantee you a healthy baby." If she holds up her end of the bargain and the baby is damaged or dies, then clearly the doctor must have fallen down on the job. Obstetricians complain bitterly that their patients demand perfect babies, but they have only themselves to blame. They created that expectation with this unwritten contract. A lawsuit may be justified, of course, but the propensity to sue over every damaged baby looks in one light like nemesis for the hubris of taking credit for the birth of a healthy child.

It explains the fierce rejection of the idea that how the mother feels can influence the labor. Labor has been limited to a mechanical process; feelings do not affect machines. The one exception is the assertion that the stress hormones released by the pain of labor can harm the baby (see Chapter 13). This fits with the belief that the natural process is inherently damaging and provides a compelling rationale for epidural anesthesia, the high-tech solution. Meanwhile, it ignores that the unpleasant environment, numerous restrictions, and impersonal care of hospitals cause considerable stress.

Every live baby and mother (and it is amazing how tough women are) provides reinforcement that the system works to those imbued with its beliefs. Every injury or death, Davis-Floyd (1992) says, "will lead [obstetricians] to intensified performance of the rituals designed to prevent such failure, rather than to their rejection," doing in their zeal, the evidence suggests, more damage than they ever prevent. So as we saw with prenatal testing, the high false-positive rate serves to convince obstetricians that inducing or performing a cesarean rescued the baby, not that the baby was fine all along (see Chapter 9). And as we found with gestational diabetes, the failure to improve outcomes leads only to calls for more stringent measures (see Chapter 8). Obstetricians all too frequently are like the man who was waving his arms in figure eights. When asked what he was doing, he replied, "Keeping elephants away." "But there are no elephants for miles," exclaimed his questioner. The man smiled craftily. "Works, doesn't it?"

WHY THIS BOOK?

One possible explanation is that the whole obstetric edifice arose from a giant case of womb envy. As keepers of the unknowable creative mystery of pregnancy and birth, women have powers in which no man can ever share. What do men do in the face of that incontrovertible fact? They do what people often do when they see that someone can do something special, something so wonderful and awe inspiring that it makes them feel envious and inadequate. They stick out their chests and say it does not matter; they are better anyway. They say they are really running the show; disaster would ensue without them. They usurp powers and honors that do not belong to them by right. "Thank you, Doctor," says the properly indoctrinated woman, "for delivering [or saving] my baby." What does it matter if you cannot do the wonderful thing if you can make everyone think you can?

The obstetric belief system has enabled men to achieve this goal, and fundamental change cannot occur without an equally fundamental change in consciousness. Without this, women will endlessly trade their mess of pottage for yet another bowl of pottage and never recover their birth rights. Manual dilation of the cervix will give way to oxytocin, will give way to cesarean section, will give way to active management of labor (Ashford 1986), will give way to who knows what next.

This book has been part of my attempt to change that consciousness among both medical professionals and childbearing women. For those already in my camp, I trust it validated their perspective. For those not sure what they thought, I hope it persuaded them, either by revealing what lies behind the kindly mask or because the research evidence convinced them. And for those inspired to become agents for change, either on their own behalf or that of others, the knowledge presented here of what truly motivates obstetric practice and its practitioners may enable them to craft more effective arguments—efficiency or cost-effectiveness rather than comfort, for example—and design better strategies for implementing change. Readers may also use the information it contains to convince others who are open-minded enough to believe in following where the research evidence leads. At the very least, this last chapter may prevent readers from being co-opted and prepare them for hostile responses even from those they thought were on their side.

A belief system works somewhat like blinders in that one can only see what is straight ahead and somewhat like colored glasses in that everything is tinted and some things are invisible, but the wearer does not notice. I make no claim to be free of this subjectivity. My claim to legitimacy lies on other grounds: the queerest inversion of all is that we have the quintessential female process being defined and controlled by males according to a singularly male perspective. This in itself would not be so bad, but it is doing untold physical and psychological damage to women, the worst of which is that women have internalized its mysogynistic beliefs. My critique of obstetric care (and those of others) derives from a commonly held feminine perspective that would reclaim childbearing as an empowering act, one in which women would be cherished, nourished, supported, celebrated, and respected. "Honor labor," says the familiar bumper sticker. Yes, let's.

REFERENCES

Annas GJ. *The rights of patients*. Carbondale, IL: Southern Illinois University Press, 1989.

Ashford JI. A history of accouchement forcé: 1550-1985. *Birth* 1986;13(4):241-249.

Bastion H. Confined, managed and delivered: the language of obstetrics. *Br J Obstet Gynaecol* 1992;99:92-93.

Davis-Floyd RE. The technocratic body: American childbirth as cultural expression. *Soc Sci Med* 1994;38(8):1125-1140.

———. *Birth as an American rite of passage*. Berkeley: University of California Press, 1992.

Declercq ER. The politics of co-optation: strategies for childbirth educators. *Birth* 1983;10(3):167-172.

DiMatteo MR, Kahn KL, and Berry SH. Narratives of birth and the postpartum: an analysis of the focus group responses of new mothers. *Birth* 1993;20(4):204-211.

Eakins PS. Introduction: The American way of birth. In *The American way of birth*. Eakins PS, ed. Philadelphia: Temple University Press, 1986.

Elkins E et al. Court-ordered cesarean section: an analysis of ethical concerns in compelling cases. *Am J Obstet Gynecol* 1989;161(1):150-154.

Green JM. Expectations and experiences of pain in labor: findings from a large prospective study. *Birth* 1993;20(2):65-72.

Greer AL. The state of the art versus the state of the science. *Int J Tech Assess Health Care* 1988;4:5-26.

Humenick SS. Mastery: The key to childbirth satisfaction? A review. *Birth* 1981;8(2):79-83.

Humenick SS and Bugen LA. Mastery: The key to childbirth satisfaction? A study. *Birth* 1981;8(2):84-89.

Janeway E. *Man's world, woman's place: A study in social mythology*. New York: Morrow, 1971.

Jordan B (revised and expanded by Davis-Floyd R). *Birth in four cultures*. 4th ed. Prospect Heights, IL: Waveland Press, 1993.

———. *Birth in four cultures*. 3d ed. Montreal: Eden Press, 1983.

Kanouse DE and Jacoby I. When does information change practitioners' behavior? *Int J Tech Assess Health Care* 1988;4:27-33.

Kitzinger S. A workshop with Sheila Kitzinger. Presented at Innovations in Perinatal Care: Assessing Benefits and Risks, ninth conference presented by *Birth*, San Francisco, Nov 1990.

———. *Your baby, your way*. New York: Pantheon Books, 1987.

Lumley J. Events and experiences in childbirth: Is there an association with postpartum depression? Paper presented at Innovations in Perinatal Care: Assessing Benefits and Risks, tenth conference presented by *Birth*, Boston, October 31-November 1 1992.

Mackey MC. Strategies for change: nursing implementation of the birthing room. *J Perinatol* 1991;11(3):262-267.

Pierre KD et al. Obstetrical attitudes and practices before and after the Canadian Consensus Conference Statement on Cesarean Birth. *Soc Sci Med* 1991;32(11):1283-1289.

Richards MPM. The trouble with "choice" in childbirth. *Birth* 1982;9(4):253-260.

Romalis C. Taking care of the little woman. In *Childbirth: Alternatives to medical care*. Romalis S, ed. Austin: University of Texas Press, 1981.

San Jose Mercury News. Dec 13, 15, 17, 30, 1993.

Summey PS. Cesarean birth. In *The American way of birth*. Eakins PS, ed. Philadelphia: Temple University Press, 1986.

Wertz RW and Wertz DC. *Lying-in: A history of childbirth in America*. New York: Schocken Books, 1977.

Woodward L et al. Exposure to drugs with possible adverse effects during pregnancy and birth. *Birth* 1982;9(3):165-172.

Glossary

< : less than

> : more than

≥ : greater than or equal to

≤ : less than or equal to

± : plus or minus

Abruptio placentae: *see* placental abruption

Acidosis: an accumulation of lactic acid in the blood when lack of oxygen causes anaerobic metabolism

Active management of labor: a protocol developed in an Irish hospital, it is designed to keep the first-time laboring woman from exceeding the average rate of progress, i.e., 1 cm per hour during the dilation phase and two hours to push out the baby

Active phase labor: *see* labor, phases of

Ambulate: to walk

Amnionitis: inflammation resulting from infection of the amniotic sac, which is one of the fetal membranes. *See also* chorioamnionitis

Amniotomy: artificial rupture of membranes

Analgesia: pain relief

Anesthesia: loss of sensation

Anoxia: lack or almost complete lack of oxygen, sometimes also used to describe a moderate decrease in oxygen, which is more properly called "hypoxia"

Antepartum: before labor

Anterior position: *see* cephalic presentation

Antiemetic: preventing or arresting vomiting

Apgar score: a means of assessing the health status of the newborn by scoring for color, heart rate, muscle tone, reactivity, and respiration efforts. Scoring is routinely done one and five minutes after birth. Scores range from 0 to 10, and a score of 7 or less at five minutes indicates the need for additional medical care

AROM or ARM: artificial rupture of membranes

Asphyxia: impaired or absent respiratory exchange of oxygen or carbon dioxide

Aspiration: inhalation of vomitus into the lungs, a potential complication of general anesthesia

Asynclitism: the fetal head is at an angle—tipped toward one shoulder or with the chin not tucked down on the chest

Atony: lack of muscle tone, muscle weakness

Augmentation of labor: stimulation of a labor that began spontaneously, usually by IV oxytocin

Auscultation: listening to body sounds (in obstetrics commonly the fetal heartbeat) with a stethoscope or hand-held ultrasound device

Bishop score: an evaluation of readiness for labor based on cervical dilation, efface-ment, consistency, position with respect to the vagina (the cervix moves from posterior to anterior), and station of the presenting fetal part

Bolus (IV): a large amount of (IV) fluid given rapidly, as before an epidural or preoperatively

Brachial paralysis *or* brachial plexus injury: injury to a network of nerves serving the arm, shoulder, and chest

Bradycardia: abnormally slow heart rate

Braxton-Hicks contractions: mild, nonlabor uterine contractions

Breech presentation: the fetus is head up instead of the normal head down

> **frank breech**: buttocks down in pike position, flexed at the hips with legs straight
>
> **complete breech**: buttocks down, flexed at both hips and knees; may convert to an incomplete breech during labor
>
> **incomplete breech**: usually a footling breech, with one or both feet or knees presenting to the birth canal

Caput succedaneum: a pressure-caused, fluid-filled swelling under the scalp of the fetal head

Cardiotocogram: electronic fetal monitor tracing

Cardiotocography: electronic fetal monitoring

Case control study: *see* retrospective study

Case report: reports of a single case or cases of an unusual event

Cephalic presentation: the baby presents head down; its position is described by the location of the back of the baby's skull (occiput) with respect to the mother

> **anterior position**: the baby faces the mother's back, the favorable position for dilation and birth, i.e., left occiput anterior (LOA) (most common) or right occiput anterior (ROA)

> **posterior position**: the baby faces the mother's belly, i.e., left occiput posterior (LOP) or right occiput posterior (ROP)

> **transverse position**: the baby faces between anterior and posterior, i.e., occiput transverse (OP)

Cephalopelvic disproportion: the baby's head is too big to pass through the mother's pelvis

Chorioamnionitis: inflammation resulting from infection of the fetal membranes. *See also* amnionitis

CI: confidence interval

CL: confidence limits

Clavicular fracture: broken collarbone

Clinical trial: researchers take two or more similar groups, submit them to different treatments (or no treatment, i.e., "controls"), and compare outcomes.

Confidence limits *or* interval: the range of possible values for an odds ratio or relative risk within 95% confidence limits, meaning there is only a 5% chance that the true value falls outside the range. If the range does not intersect 1, the ratio is significant.

Contraction stress test: a fetal surveillance test that looks at the fetal heart rate response to contractions; contractions may be elicited by nipple stimulation or an oxtocin drip

Cord prolapse: *see* umbilical cord prolapse

Crystalloids: nonprotein IV solutes including glucose, salt, or those found in Ringer's lactate

CST: contraction stress test

Cystocele: a herniation of the posterior bladder through the anterior vaginal wall

Dehiscence: the opening of a wound, specifically in obstetrics the opening of a uterine cesarean scar; sometimes distinguished from "uterine rupture" by being symptomless. When used in this sense, "dehiscence" is synonymous with "window."

Delivery, types

> **assisted**: forceps or vacuum extraction

> **cesarean**: major abdominal surgery

> **instrumental**: usually forceps or vacuum extraction; occasionally includes cesarean section as well

operative: forceps, vacuum extraction, or cesarean section; sometimes the phrase "operative vaginal delivery" excludes cesarean section

spontaneous: the mother gives birth without assistance.

Dilation, cervical: the cervix opens

Dorsal: of or relating to the back

Double-blind: neither the researcher nor the subject knows whether the subject had an intervention or was in the control group

Dubowitz score: a means of assigning gestational age by certain physical characteristics and responses of the newborn

Dyspareunia: coital pain

Dystocia: difficult childbirth, often used to mean "slow labor progress"

Dystocia, shoulder: the head is born, but the shoulders are impacted

ECV: external cephalic version

Edema: an accumulation of an excessive amount of watery fluid in the tissues

Effacement, cervical: the cervix shortens and becomes soft and thin in preparation for and during labor

EFM: electronic fetal monitoring

Electronic fetal monitoring: monitoring the fetal heart rate with a machine that either picks up signals through an external ultrasound device or an internal monitor lead attached to the baby's scalp. Contractions can be monitored by an external pressure sensor or an internal pressure catheter. Data are displayed on a screen and on a paper tracing.

Emesis: vomiting

Epidural space: a space lying outside the first of the two membranes (the dural membrane) that sheathe the spinal cord. When epidural anesthesia is administered, medication is delivered into this space.

Episiotomy: a perineal incision to enlarge the vaginal opening for childbirth

mediolateral: the cut goes down and off to one side

midline (also called median): the cut goes straight down toward the rectum

Estriol assay: a measurement of estrogen metabolite levels in maternal urine; a fall was believed to indicate problems, but the test is inaccurate and has been discredited

Expectant management: watching and waiting, usually for the onset of spontaneous labor

External cephalic version: turning a breech baby to vertex by manipulating it through the abdominal wall

Extradural: the same as "epidural"

False-negative rate: the percentage of people diagnosed by a test as healthy who, in fact, have the disease

False-positive rate: the percentage of people diagnosed by a test as diseased who, in fact, are healthy

Fetal mortality rate: the number of fetal deaths divided by the sum of live births plus fetal deaths during the same period

FHR: fetal heart rate

First-degree laceration: *see* laceration, perineal

First-stage labor: from the onset of progressive contractions to full dilation of the cervix (10 cm)

Fourth-degree laceration: *see* laceration, perineal

FTP: failure to progress

Hartmann's solution: the British version of Ringer's lactate, an electrolyte replacement IV fluid

Hematoma: a blood-filled swelling

Hospital   (level of maternity care services)

> **primary care (Level I)**: a hospital with the capability of caring for the essentially normal mother and infant
>
> **secondary care (Level II)**: a hospital with the capability of caring for mothers and infants with some complications and the ability to stabilize very sick mothers or babies or premature infants for transport to a tertiary care center
>
> **tertiary care (Level III)**: a hospital with the staffing and equipment to handle high-risk expectant mothers and infants

Hyperbilirubinemia: high bilirubin count, neonatal jaundice

Hyperglycemia: high blood sugar level

Hyperstimulus: overstimulation, particularly of uterine contractions

Hypertension: high blood pressure

Hypertonic: overly contracted (as in "hypertonic uterus")

Hypoglycemia: low blood sugar level

Hyponatremia: low blood sodium level

Hypotension: low blood pressure

Hypoxia: insufficient oxygen

Hypoxic-ischemic encephalopathy: abnormal neurologic symptoms believed to be caused by the consequent damage of insufficient oxygenated blood reaching the brain

Instrumental delivery: *see* delivery, types

Intrapartum: during labor

Intubation: putting a tube down the throat to create an airway and, in the case of general anesthesia, to deliver more controlled doses of anesthetic

IUGR: intrauterine growth retardation

Ketosis: the body's metabolic response to starvation or to diabetes, a disease that prevents the body from metabolizing sufficient amounts of glucose. Fats are metabolized instead, producing ketones.

Ketonuria: the presence of excessive amounts of ketones in the urine

Labor, phases of

> **latent phase**: early labor; labor from the onset of dilation to 3 to 5 cm dilation, at which time the intensity of labor and the rapidity of dilation increase

> **active phase**: labor from the point at which the tempo of labor increases, generally beginning at 3 to 5 cm dilation

> **transitional phase**: the last two or three centimeters of dilation are sometimes distinguished from the rest of the dilation phase of labor by this term

Laceration, perineal

> **first degree**: into the skin

> **second degree**: into the underlying muscle (the equivalent of an episiotomy)

> **third degree**: the definition varies. It may include any laceration involving the anal sphincter and/or rectum, or it may be limited to tears into but not through the sphincter. Sometimes it includes tears through the sphincter but not into the rectal mucosa.

> **fourth degree**: Where third degree is limited to tears into the sphincter, fourth degree is used to mean tears through the sphincter or into the rectal mucosa.

Lactacidosis: acidosis due to lactic acid formation

Latent phase labor: *see* labor, phases of

Lithotomy position: positioning for delivery on the back with legs in stirrups

LOA: left occiput anterior

LOP: left occiput posterior

LMP: last menstrual period

Macrosomia: overly large babies commonly defined as birth weight of 4000 g or more (8 lb 13 oz)

Meconium: the baby's first bowel movement, which accumulates during pregnancy. It is black and sticky. Sometimes the baby passes meconium into the amniotic fluid, a possible sign of fetal distress. If the baby inhales (aspirates) the meconium into its lungs upon taking its first breath, the irritation and the particles may cause a type of pneumonia.

Meta-analysis: a study that uses sophisticated statistical techniques to pool data from several small studies

Methodology: the details of how a study was conducted

Morbidity: injury, disease, or complications, often following a medical procedure

Multigravida: a woman who has had more than one pregnancy

Multipara: a woman who has given birth to more than one child

Neonatal mortality rate: the number of deaths occurring during the first 28 days after birth (sometimes the first 7 days) divided by the number of live births in the same population over the same time, usually expressed per thousand live births

Nonstress test: a fetal surveillance test that looks at the fetal heart rate response to Braxton-Hicks contractions or fetal movements

Normoglycemic: normal blood sugar level

Normotensive: normal blood pressure

NPO: an abbreviation of the Latin term *non per os*, which means "nothing by mouth"

NST: nonstress test

Nuchal: having to do with the back of the neck, i.e., a nuchal arm is trapped behind the baby's head

Nulligravida: a woman who has never been pregnant

Nullipara: a woman who has never given birth, sometimes used interchangeably with *primipara* or *primigravida*

Observational study: usually a statistical report

Occiput anterior: *see* cephalic presentation

Occiput posterior: *see* cephalic presentation

Odds ratio: the odds of having the risk factor if the condition is present divided by the odds of having the risk factor if the condition is absent

Oligohydramnios: deficient amount of amniotic fluid

Oligouria: deficient urine output

OP: occiput posterior

Operative delivery: *see* delivery, types

OR: odds ratio

OT: occiput transverse

Para: short for *parity*

Paresthesia: abnormal sensation

Parity: the condition of having given birth to one or more children

Pelvimetry: measurement of the diameters of the pelvis

Perinatal mortality rate: usually defined as the number of deaths occurring between 28 weeks gestation and 7 days after birth divided by the number of stillborn infants of at least 28 weeks gestation plus all liveborn infants in the same population regardless of gestational age; usually expressed per 1000

Perineum: the block of tissue between the bottom of the vagina and the anus

Phototherapy: using ultraviolet light to treat neonatal jaundice

Pitocin: synthetic oxytocin, the hormone that stimulates contractions

Placebo effect: from the Latin "I shall please," the improvement seen after taking an inert substance

Placenta accreta: abnormal attachment of the placenta to the muscular wall of the uterus

Placenta increta or percreta: the placenta grows into or even completely through the uterine wall

Placenta previa: the placenta implants low, partially or completely overlaying the cervix. This causes hemorrhage when the cervix begins to dilate.

Placental abruption: The placenta separates from the wall of the uterus prematurely. The separation may be partial or complete.

Polycythemia: too many red blood cells

Postdates: generally defined as birth after 42 weeks gestation, sometimes earlier

Postmature: past the optimal time for birth and thus believed to be prone to certain complications believed due to a failing placenta

Postterm: generally defined as birth after 42 weeks gestation, sometimes earlier; often improperly used as synonymous with *postmature*

Posterior presentation: *see* cephalic presentation

Postpartum: after birth

Postprandial: after eating

Power: the ability to detect a true difference in the sample data

Predictive value: the percentage of subjects who will correctly be identified as having (*positive predictive value*) or not having (*negative predictive value*) a disease, given its prevalence among that particular population

Preeclampsia: a pregnancy complication characterized by water retention, protein in the urine, and high blood pressure

Premature rupture of membranes: spontaneous rupture of the fetal membranes before the onset of labor

Presentation: the part of the baby presenting to the birth canal. This is almost always the head but may be the buttocks, feet, knees, face, brow, or shoulder. *See also* cephalic presentation; breech presentation

Preterm: birth prior to 37 weeks gestation

Primary cesarean: a first cesarean, as opposed to a repeat cesarean

Primary cesarean rate: the total number of cesareans divided by the total number of women giving birth who had not previously had a cesarean

Primary care center (Level I hospital): *see* hospital

Primigravida: a woman having her first pregnancy, often used interchangeably with *nullipara* and *primipara*

Primipara: a woman who has given birth for the first time, often used interchangeably with *primigravida* and *nullipara*

PROM: premature rupture of membranes

Prospective study: Prospective studies assemble a population with certain characteristics in common and then follow them to see if they are more likely to have some particular outcome compared with controls who are similar in other respects, but do not share the target characteristics.

Pruritis: itching

Pudendal block: the vagina is numbed by passing a long needle through the wall of the vagina and injecting local anesthestic around the pudendal nerve

P value: the probability that the observed difference is due to chance. Usually values below 0.05, or 5%, are considered significant, meaning that the results are unlikely to be due to chance.

Pyrexia: elevated body temperature, fever

Randomized controlled trial: a clinical trial in which subjects are randomly assigned to study group(s) or control group

RCT: randomized controlled trial

Recall bias: the propensity for memory to play tricks

Rectocele: herniation of the anterior rectal wall through the posterior vaginal wall

Recumbent: lying down

Relative risk: the probability of developing the outcome if the risk factor is present divided by the probability of developing the problem if it is absent

Retrospective study: a study that collects a population with a particular outcome or problem and then delves into the past for characteristics or events they have in common that are not shared by members of a control group not having that outcome or problem

RhoGAM: an immune globulin that prevents Rh negative mothers from forming antibodies to the blood of an Rh-positive fetus

Ringer's lactate: an electrolyte replacement IV fluid

Ripening, cervical: the cervix becomes soft, effaced, and begins to dilate

ROA: right occiput anterior

ROP: right occiput posterior

RR: relative risk

Rupture: in obstetrics, the opening of the uterine scar; sometimes used to mean all varieties, including symptomless windows, sometimes used to mean only scar openings accompanied by symptoms (such as bleeding or fetal distress) that pose a risk to mother or baby.

SD: standard deviation

Secondary care center (Level II hospital): *see* hospital

Second-degree laceration: *see* laceration, perineal

Second stage: the stage of labor that begins with full cervical dilation and ends with the birth of the baby

Sensitivity (of a test): the percentage of the population tested that will be accurately identified as diseased

Shoulder dystocia: *see* dystocia, shoulder

Significant difference: The observed difference is considered a true difference, not the result of chance. The usual cutoff probability value (p value) is $p < 0.05$.

Specificity (of a test): the percentage of the population that will be correctly diagnosed as disease free

Spontaneous delivery: *see* delivery types

Stages of labor: *see* first stage; second stage; third stage

Standard deviation: a measure of variability or dispersion within the group. Assuming normal distribution (a bell-shaped or Gaussian curve), about 95% of all values will be found within two standard deviations on either side of average.

Station: the location of the presenting fetal part with respect to the ischial spines of the mother's pelvis. Location at the spines is 0 station. Minus station is centimeters above the spines (as in -1, -2), and plus station is centimeters below the spines (as in +1, +2).

Stress incontinence: an involuntary loss of urine in response to laughing, sneezing, or coughing

Subarachnoid space: the space below both of the membranes covering the spinal cord

Supine: lying on the back

Supine hypotension: When a pregnant woman lies supine, the weight of the uterus and baby compress the great blood vessels serving her lower body and the uterus. This can cause adverse changes in the fetal heart rate.

Tachycardia: abnormally fast heart rate

Tachypnea: abnormally rapid breathing

Term: a full-length pregnancy, usually defined as between 37 weeks and 42 weeks gestation. Earlier than 37 weeks is usually considered preterm, and later than 42 weeks is usually considered postdates or postterm. *Premature* and *postmature* are sometimes incorrectly used as synonymous with *preterm* and *postterm*.

Tertiary care center (Level III hospital): *see* hospital

Third-degree laceration: *see* laceration, perineal

Third stage: the stage of labor that begins with the birth of the baby and ends with the birth of the placenta

Tocodynamometry: measurement of the force of uterine contractions

Tocolytic: a uterine relaxant drug

TOL: trial of labor

Transition: *see* labor, phases of

Type I error: the statistical error of finding a significant difference when no true difference exists

Type II error: the statistical error of not finding a significant difference when a true difference exists

Umbilical cord prolapse: The umbilical cord comes down ahead of the baby. This obstetrical emergency is more common when the baby is not head down or membranes rupture before the head is well applied to the cervix.

Uterine dehiscence: *see* dehiscence

Uterine rupture: *see* rupture

VBAC: vaginal birth after cesarean

Vertex presentation: baby presents head down

Index

About the Author

HENCI GOER is an ASPO-certified childbirth educator and doula (professional provider of labor support). A medical writer for the past ten years, she has written numerous pamphlets and magazine articles for her fellow professionals and for expectant couples, and in 1993, the National Association of Childbearing Centers presented her with its annual Media Award. Currently, she serves on *Childbirth Instructor Magazine*'s Advisory Board and abstracts medical journal articles for an electronic health database.

ISBN 0-89789-242-9

EAN

HARDCOVER BAR CODE